Imaging Atlas of
Human Anatomy

FOURTH EDITION

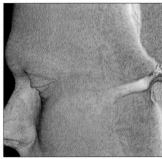

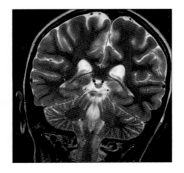

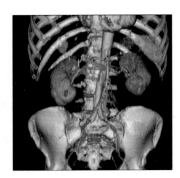

Jamie Weir MBBS, DMRD, FRCP(Ed), FRANZCR(Hon), FRCR
Emeritus Professor of Radiology
University of Aberdeen
Aberdeen, UK

Peter H Abrahams MBBS, FRCS(Ed), FRCR, DO(Hon)
Professor of Clinical Anatomy, Warwick Medical School, UK
Professor of Clinical Anatomy, St George's University, Grenada, West Indies
Extraordinary Professor, Department of Anatomy, University of Pretoria, South Africa
Fellow, Girton College, Cambridge, UK
Examiner, MRCS, Royal College of Surgeons, UK
Family Practitioner, Brent, London, UK

Jonathan D Spratt MBBChir, MA(Cantab), FRCS(Eng), FRCS(Glasg), FRCR
Chief Radiologist, County Durham and Darlington NHS Foundation Trust
Examiner in Anatomy, Royal College of Radiologists, UK
Examiner, MRCS, Royal College of Surgeons, UK
Fellow in Anatomical Radiology, Northumbria University, UK
Visiting Professor of Anatomy, St George's School of Medicine, Grenada and St Vincent

Lonie R Salkowski MD
Associate Professor of Radiology and Anatomy
University of Wisconsin School of Medicine and Public Health
Madison, Wisconsin, USA
Clinical Professor, College of Health Sciences
University of Wisconsin-Milwaukee
Milwaukee, Wisconsin, USA

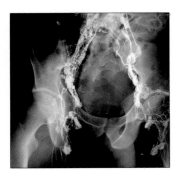

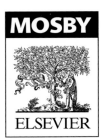

MOSBY

ELSEVIER

MOSBY

ELSEVIER

An imprint of Elsevier Limited

First edition 1992
Second edition 1997
Third edition 2003

The right of Jamie Weir, Peter H Abrahams, Jonathan D Spratt and
Lonie R Salkowski to be identified as authors of this work has been asserted by
them in accordance with the Copyright, Designs and Patents Act 1988.

ISBN: 978-0-7234-3457-3
  Reprinted 2010
International Edition ISBN: 978-0-8089-2388-6

British Library Cataloguing in Publication Data

Imaging atlas of human anatomy. -- 4th ed.
  1. Human anatomy--Atlases. 2. Diagnostic imaging.
  I. Weir, Jamie.
  611'.00222-dc22

  ISBN-13: 9780723434573

Library of Congress Cataloging in Publication Data

A catalog record for this book is available from the Library of Congress

Notice

Medical knowledge is constantly changing. Standard safety precautions must be
followed, but as new research and clinical experience broaden our knowledge,
changes in treatment and drug therapy may become necessary or appropriate.
Readers are advised to check the most current product information provided by
the manufacturer of each drug to be administered to verify the recommended
dose, the method and duration of administration, and contraindications. It is
the responsibility of the practitioner, relying on experience and knowledge of the
patient, to determine dosages and the best treatment for each individual patient.
Neither the Publisher nor the authors assume any liability for any injury and/or
damage to persons or property arising from this publication.

The Publisher

ELSEVIER your source for books,
journals and multimedia
in the health sciences

www.elsevierhealth.com

Working together to grow
libraries in developing countries

www.elsevier.com | www.bookaid.org | www.sabre.org

ELSEVIER   BOOK AID
International   Sabre Foundation

The
Publisher's
policy is to use
**paper manufactured
from sustainable forests**

Typeset by IMH(Cartrif), Loanhead, Scotland
Printed in China
Last digit is the print number: 9 8 7 6 5 4 3 2

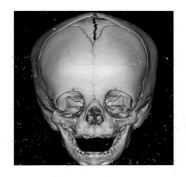

IMAGING ATLAS OF
HUMAN
ANATOMY

FOURTH EDITION

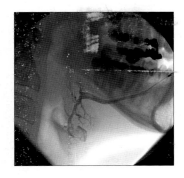

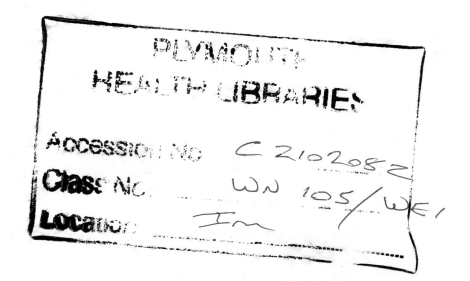

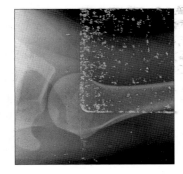

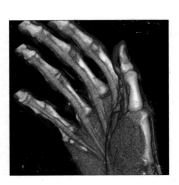

Commissioning Editor: Madelene Hyde
Development Editor: Sharon Nash
Project Manager: Frances Affleck
Design: Kirsteen Wright
Marketing Managers: Jason Oberacker (US) and Ian Jordan (UK)

Contents

Preface to the fourth edition

There is increasing importance placed on the interpretation of radiological anatomy in a world that has seen considerable changes in medical student training programmes over the last decade, combined with the reduction in cadaver dissection.

We have updated and revised this atlas, by the addition of new images and techniques, to reflect these trends. The 'Author' team has also changed. We wish to record our sincere thanks to Drs Hourihan, Belli, Moore and Owen for their previous contributions and introduce you to our two new co-authors, Dr Jonathan Spratt from Durham, UK and Dr Lonie Salkowski from Madison, WI, USA. Both are radiological anatomists of high repute and most of the new material emanates from their work.

The format for this fourth edition remains the same but the layout of the chapters on the abdomen and pelvis has been revised to reflect current radiological and anatomical practice; the new chapters being cross-sectional imaging of the abdomen and pelvis and non cross-sectional imaging of the abdomen and pelvis.

A new section on nuclear medicine, by Dr Salkowski, has also been added.

We are adding for the first time, a website of pathology to complement this radiological atlas. It consists of a series of 34 PowerPoint tutorials related to the eight anatomical chapters and based on nine 'concepts'. These 'concepts' have been designed to help you understand the relationship between normal anatomy and altered, abnormal anatomy that is the discipline of pathology. This material has been produced with the help of Dr Jennifer Allison who started this project as a medical student. A selection of these tutorials is available free with the atlas (please see inside front cover for access details) and the remainder will be available for a small charge from the same site.

The nine concepts are as follows:

1. 'things pushed'
2. 'things pulled'
3. 'things added'
4. 'things missing'
5. 'things larger than normal'
6. 'things smaller than normal'
7. 'things that have an abnormal structure, either locally or diffusely'
8. 'things that have an abnormal shape, either locally or generally'
9. 'things you cannot see despite knowing they are present pathologically, i.e. you are either using the wrong imaging technique or you will never see any abnormality because the disease is only microscopic and has not induced any visible anatomical (or physiological) change'.

Further explanations together with numerous examples to demonstrate these 'concepts' are on the website. We believe the ongoing reliance placed by clinicians on the imaging of pathological processes will be facilitated by this novel and exciting approach and the addition of pathology combined with this extensively revised radiological anatomy text will enhance the understanding of imaging to the benefit of both you, the reader, and your patient. As this book and accompanying website are for you, the student, we encourage and welcome corrections or suggestions and ideas for future editions.

Jamie Weir, Peter H Abrahams, Jonathan Spratt and Lonie Salkowski
January 2010

Preface to the first edition

Imaging methods used to display normal human anatomy have improved dramatically over the last few decades. The ability to demonstrate the soft tissues by using the modern technologies of magnetic resonance imaging, X-ray computed tomography, and ultrasound has greatly facilitated our understanding of the link between anatomy as shown in the dissecting room and that necessary for clinical practice. This atlas has been produced because of the new technology and the fundamental changes that are occurring in the teaching of anatomy. It enables the preclinical medical student to relate to basic anatomy while, at the same time, providing a comprehensive study guide for the clinical interpretation of imaging, applicable for all undergraduate and postgraduate levels.

Several distinguished authors, experts in their fields of imaging, have contributed to this book, which has benefited from editorial integration to ensure balance and cohesion. The atlas is designed to complement and supplement the *McMinn's Clinical Atlas of Human Anatomy* 6th edition.

Duplication of images occurs only where it is necessary to demonstrate anatomical points of interest or difficulty. Similarly, examples of different imaging modalities of the same anatomical region are only included if they contribute to a better understanding of the region shown. Radiographs that show important landmarks in limb ossification centre development, together with examples of some common congenital anomalies, are also documented. In certain sections, notably MR and CT, the legends may cover more than one page, so that a specific structure can be followed in continuity through various levels and planes.

Human anatomy does not alter, but our methods of demonstrating it have changed significantly. Modern imaging allows certain structures and their relationships to be seen for the first time, and this has aided us in their interpretation. Knowledge and understanding of radiological anatomy are fundamental to all those involved in patient care, from the nurse and the paramedic to medical students and clinicians.

Jamie Weir and Peter H Abrahams
February 1992

Acknowledgements

Thank you to all of our previous contributors of images to the previous editions of this atlas and to Dr Alison Murray who has kindly granted permission for use of images used in the online pathology tutorials. New material and labelling have been added by Dr Richard Wellings, University Hospital, Coventry and Warwickshire and Dr Andrew Hine, N.W. London Hospitals and we are very grateful for their help. The two images in the introduction, the body MRA and the MR tractography, were kindly supplied by Toshiba Medical Systems.

Dedication

To our students – past, present and future

Introduction

Guide to ossification tables

Ossification tables, such as the one shown on the right, appear throughout this book.

The key to these tables is as follows:

(c) = cartilage
(m) = membrane
miu = months of intrauterine life
wiu = weeks of intrauterine life
mths = months
yrs = years

And the rule to remember is: girls before boys.

Magnetic resonance imaging

Magnetic resonance imaging (MRI) produces images by magnetising the patient in the bore of a powerful magnet and broadcasting short pulses of radiofrequency (RF) energy at 46 MHz to resonate mobile protons (hydrogen nuclei) in fat, protein and water. The protons produce RF echoes when their resonant energy is released and their density and location can be exactly correlated by complex mathematical algorithms into an image matrix.

The spinning proton of the hydrogen nucleus acts like a tiny bar magnet, aligning either with or against the magnetic field producing a small net magnetic vector. RF energy is used to generate a second magnetic field, perpendicular to the static magnetic field, which rotate or 'flip' the protons away from the static magnetic field. Once the RF pulse is switched off, the protons flip back to their original position of equilibrium ('relaxation'), emitting the RF energy they had acquired into the antenna around the patient, which is then digitised, amplified and, finally, spatially encoded by the array processor.

MRI systems are graded according to the strength of the magnetic field they produce. Routine high-field systems are those capable of producing a magnetic field strength of 1.5–3 T (Tesla) using a superconducting electromagnet immersed in liquid helium. Open magnets for claustrophobic patients and limb scanners use permanent magnets between 0.2 and 0.75 T. For comparison, earth's magnetic field varies from 30 to 60 uT. MRI does not present any recognised biological hazard. Patients who have any form of pacemaker or implanted electro-inductive device must not be examined. Other prohibited items include ferromagnetic intracranial aneurysm slips, certain types of cardiac valve replacement and intra-ocular metallic foreign bodies. Many extra cranial vascular clips and orthopaedic prostheses are now 'MRI friendly', but these may cause local artefacts. Loose metal items must be excluded from the examination room – pillows containing metallic coiled springs have been known to near suffocate patients!

Although beyond the remit of the current edition of this book, new methods of analysing normal and pathologic brain anatomy are now

CLAVICLE (m)	Appears	Fused
Lateral end	5 wiu	20+ yrs
Medial end	15 yrs	20+ yrs
SCAPULA (c)		
Body	8 wiu	15 yrs
Coracoid	<1 yr	20 yrs
Coracoid base	Puberty	15–20 yrs
Acromion	Puberty	15–20 yrs

at the forefront of research, namely MRS, fMRI and mMRI, the latter taking on a new direction since the description of the human genome.

Magnetic resonance spectroscopic imaging (MRS) assesses function within the living brain. MRS takes advantage of the fact that protons

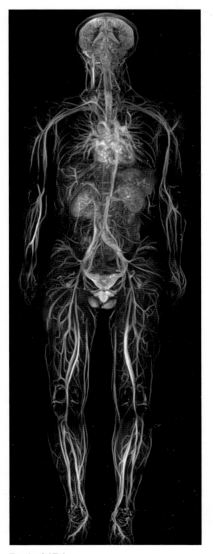

Body MRA.

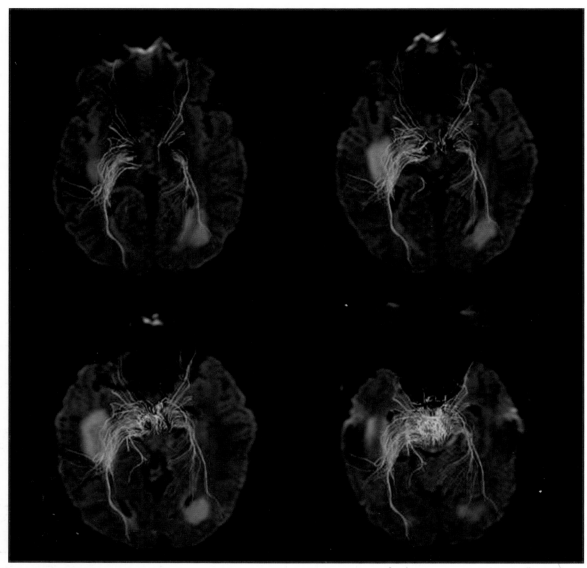

MR tractography.

residing in differing chemical environments possess slightly different resonant properties (chemical shift). For a given volume of brain the distribution of these proton resonances can be displayed as a spectrum. Discernible peaks can be seen for certain neurotransmitters: *N*-acetylaspartate varies in multiple sclerosis, stroke and schizophrenia while choline and lactate levels have been used to evaluate certain brain tumours.

Functional MRI (fMRI) depends on the fact that haemoglobin is diamagnetic when oxygenated but paramagnetic when deoxygenated. These different signals can be weighted to the smaller vessels, and hence closer to the active neurons, by using larger magnetic fields. In molecular imaging (mMRI) biomarkers interact chemically with their surroundings and alter the image according to molecular changes occurring within the area of interest, potentially enabling early detection and treatment of disease and basic pharmaceutical development, also allowing for quantitative testing.

High-field-strength magnets of course give significant improvement in spatial resolution and contrast. MR images have been acquired

at 8 T of the microvasculature of the live human brain allowing close comparison to histology, having significant implications in the treatment of reperfusion injury and in the physiology of solid tumours and angiogenesis. There is every reason to believe that continued efforts to push the envelope of high-field-strength applications will open new vistas in what appears to be a never-ending array of potential clinical applications.

Ultrasound

In contrast with the other images in this book, ultrasound images do not depend on the use of electromagnetic wave forms. It is the properties of high-frequency sound waves (longitudinal waves) and their interaction with biological tissues that go to form these 'echograms'.

A sound wave of appropriate frequency (diagnostic range 3.5–20 MHz) is produced by piezo-electric principles, namely that certain crystals can change their shape and produce a voltage potential, and vice versa. As the beam passes through tissues, two important effects determine image production: attenuation and reflection. Attenuation is caused by the loss of energy due to absorption, reflection, refraction out of the capture of the receiver with resulting reduction in signal intensity. Reflection of sound waves within the range of the receiver produces the image, the texture of which is dependent upon tiny differences in acoustic impedance between different tissues. Blood flow and velocity can be measured (using the Doppler principle) in duplex mode.

Techniques such as harmonic imaging and the use of ultrasound contrast agents (stabilised microbubbles) have enabled non-invasive determination of myocardial perfusion to be recently discovered. These contrast agents clearly improve the detection of metastases in the liver and spleen. Ultrasound is the most common medical imaging technique for producing elastograms in which stiffness or strain images of soft tissue are used to detect or classify tumours. Cancer is 5–28 times stiffer than the background of normal soft tissue. When a mechanical compression or vibration is applied, the tumour deforms less than the surrounding tissue. Elastography can be used for example to measure the stiffness of the liver in vivo or in the detection of breast or thyroid tumours. A correlation between liver elasticity and the cirrhosis score has been shown.

Only a handful of key ultrasound images have been included in the book to illustrate a particular point or area, as the real-time nature of ultrasound precludes further coverage. Interpretation of the anatomy from static ultrasound images is more difficult than that from other imaging modalities because the technique is highly operator-dependent and provides information on tissue structure and form different from that of other imaging techniques.

Nuclear medicine

Historically the field of nuclear medicine began in 1946 when radioactive iodine was administered as an 'atomic cocktail' to treat thyroid cancer. Since that time, nuclear medicine has advanced and was recognized by the American Medical Association as a medical specialty in 1971.

Diagnostic radiology creates an image by passing radiation through the body from an external source. Nuclear medicine, unlike diagnostic radiology, creates an image by measuring the radiation emitted from tracers taken internally. Thus the image is created from the radiation emitted from the patient. Overall the radiation dosages are comparable and vary depending on the examination.

Nuclear medicine also differs from most other imaging modalities in that the tests demonstrate the physiological function of a specific area of the body. In some instances this physiological information can be fused with more anatomical imaging of CT or MRI thus combining the strengths of anatomy and function for diagnosis.

Rather than a contrast media for imaging, nuclear medicine uses radiopharmaceuticals, which are pharmaceuticals that have been labelled with a radionuclide. These radiopharmaceuticals are administered to patients by intravenous injection, ingestion, or inhalation. The method of administration depends on the type of examination and the organ or organ process to be imaged. By definition, all these radiopharmaceuticals emit radiation. This emitted radiation is detected and imaged with specialised equipment such as gamma cameras, positron emission tomography (PET), and single photon emission computed tomography (SPECT). Radiation in certain tests can be measured from parts of the body by the use of probes, or samples can be taken from patients and measured in counters.

The premise of nuclear medicine imaging involves functional biology, thereby not only can studies be done to image a disease process but they can also be used to treat diseases. Radiopharmaceuticals that are used for imaging emit a gamma ray (γ) and those used for treatment emit a beta (β) particle. Gamma rays are of higher energy to pass through the body and be detected by a detection camera, whereas beta particles travel only short distances and emit their radiation dose to the target organ. For example, technetium-99m or iodine-123 may be used to detect thyroid disease, but certain thyroid diseases or thyroid cancer may be treated solely or in part by treatment with iodine-131. The difference in the agent used depends on the type and energy levels of the radiation particle that the radioisotope emits.

Radionuclides, or the radioactive particle, used in nuclear medicine are often chemically bound to a complex called a tracer so that when administered it acts in a characteristic way in the body. The way the body handles this tracer can differ in disease or pathologic processes and thus demonstrate images different from normal in disease states. For example, the tracer used in bone imaging is methylene-diphosphonate (MDP). MDP is bound to technetium-99m for bone imaging. MDP attaches to hydroxyapatite in the bone. If there is a physiological change in the bone from a fracture, metastatic bone disease or arthritic change, there will be an increase in bone activity and thus more accumulation of the tracer in this region compared with the normal bone. This will result in a focal 'hot spot' of the radiopharmaceutical on a bone scan.

Technetium-99m is the major workhorse radioisotope of nuclear medicine. It can be eluted from a molybdenum/technetium generator stored within a nuclear medicine department allowing for easy access. It has a short half-life (6-hours), which allows for ease of medical imaging and disposal. Its pharmacological properties allow it to be easily bound to various tracers and it emits gamma rays that are of suitable energy for medical imaging.

In addition to technetium-99m, the most common intravenous radionuclides used in nuclear medicine are iodine-123 and 131, thallium-201, gallium-67, 18-fluorodeoxyglucose (FDG) and indium-111 labeled leukocytes. The most common gaseous/aerosol radionuclides used are xenon-133, krypton-81m, technetium-99m (Technegas) and technetium-99m DTPA.

The images obtained from nuclear medicine imaging can be in the form of one or many images. Image sets can be represented as time sequence imaging (e.g. cine) such as dynamic imaging or cardiac gated sequences, or by spatial sequence imaging where the gamma camera is moved relative to the patient such as in SPECT imaging. Spatial sequence imaging allows the images to be presented as a slice-stack of images much like CT or MRI images are displayed. Spatial sequence imaging can also be fused with concomitant CT or MR imaging to provide combined physiologic and anatomical imaging. Time and spatial sequence imaging offer a unique perspective and information of physiological processes in the body.

A PET (positron emission tomography) scan is a specialised type of nuclear medicine imaging that measures important body functions, such as blood flow, oxygen use, and sugar (glucose) metabolism to evaluate how well organs and tissues are functioning. PET imaging involves short-lived radioactive tracer isotopes that are chemically incorporated into biologically active molecules. The most common molecule used is fluorodeoxyglucose (FDG), which is a sugar. After injection into the body, these active molecules become concentrated into the tissues of interest. After this waiting time, which is about an hour for FDG, imaging can proceed. Imaging of FDG occurs as the isotope decays. The isotope undergoes positron emission decay. As the positron is emitted, it travels only a few millimeters and annihilates with an electron and in so doing produce a pair of gamma photons moving in opposite directions. The PET scan detectors process only those photon pairs that are detected simultaneously (coincident detection). This data is then processed to create an image of tissue activity with respect to that particular isotope. These images can then be fused with CT or MR images.

A limitation of PET imaging is the short half-life of the isotopes. Thus close access to a cyclotron for generation of the isotopes plays an important role in the feasible location of PET imaging. Typical isotopes used in medical imaging and their half-lives are: carbon-11 (~20 min), nitrogen-13 (~10 min), oxygen-13 (~2 min) and fluorine-18 (~110 min).

Angiography/Interventional radiology

Angiographic imaging began in 1927 by Egas Moniz, a physician and neurologist, with the introduction of contrast X-ray cerebral angiography. In 1949 he was awarded the Nobel Prize for his work. The field of angiography however was revolutionised with the advent of the Seldinger technique in 1953, in which no sharp needles remained inside the vascular lumen during imaging.

Although the field of angiography began with X-ray and fluoroscopic imaging of blood vessels and organs of the body by injecting radio-opaque contrast agents in to the blood, it has evolved to so much more. Many of the procedures performed by angiography can be diagnostic, as newer techniques arose, it has allowed for the advent of minimally invasive procedures performed with image guidance and thus the name change of the discipline to Interventional radiology (or vascular and interventional radiology).

Angiograms are typically performed by gaining access to the blood vessels, whether this is through the femoral artery, femoral vein or jugular vein depends on the area of interest to be imaged. Angiograms can be obtained of the brain as cerebral angiograms, of the heart as coronary angiograms, of the lungs as pulmonary angiograms, and so on. Imaging of the arterial and venous circulation of the arms and legs can demonstrate peripheral vascular disease. Once vascular access is made, then catheters are directed to the specific location to be imaged in the body by the use of guide wires. Contrast agents are injected through these catheters to visualise the vessels or the organ with X-ray imaging.

In addition to diagnostic imaging, treatment and/or interventions can often be performed through similar catheter based examinations. Such procedures might involve angioplasties where a balloon mechanism is placed across an area of narrowing, or stenosis, in a vessel or lumen. With controlled inflation of the balloon, the area of narrowing can be widened. Often to keep these areas from narrowing again, stents can be placed within the lumen of the vessel or even in the trachea or oesophagus.

Imaging in diagnostic or interventional procedures can be still images or motion (cine) images. The technique often used is called digital subtraction angiography (DSA). In this type of imaging, images are taken at 2–30 frames per second to allow imaging of the flow of blood through vessels. A preliminary image of the area is taken before the contrast is injected. This 'mask' image is then electronically subtracted from all the images leaving behind only the vessels filled with contrast. This technique requires the patient to remain motionless for optimal subtraction.

Angiograms can be performed of the heart to visualise the size and contractility of the chambers and anatomy of the coronary vessels. The thorax can also be studied to evaluate the pulmonary arteries and veins for vascular malformations, blood clots and possible origins of hemoptysis. The neck is often imaged to visualise the vessels that supply the brain as they arise from the aortic arch to the cerebral vessels, in the investigation of atherosclerotic disease, vascular malformations and tumoral blood supplies. Renal artery imaging can elucidate the cause of hypertension in selected patients, as can imaging of the mesenteric vessels discover the origin of gastrointestinal bleeding or mesenteric angina.

In addition to angiograms and venograms, the field of interventional radiology also performs such procedures as coil-embolisation of aneurysms and vascular malformations, balloon angioplasty and stent placement, chemoembolisation directly into tumours, drainage catheter insertions, embolisations (e.g. uterine artery embolisation for treatment of uterine fibroids), thrombolysis to dissolve blood clots, tissue biopsy (percutaneous or transvascular), radiofrequency ablation and cryoablation of tumours, line insertions for specialised vascular access, inferior vena cava filter placements, vertebroplasty, nephrostomy placement, gastrostomy tube placement for feeding, dialysis access, TIPS (transjugular intrahepatic porto-systemic shunt) placement, biliary interventions, and, most recently, endovenous laser ablation of varicose veins.

Computed tomography

The limitation of all plain radiographic techniques is the two dimensional representation of three dimensional structures: the linear attenuation co-efficient of all the tissues in the path of the X-ray beam form the image.

Computed tomography (CT) obtains a series of different angular X-ray projections that are processed by a computer to give a section of specified thickness. The CT image comprises a regular matrix of picture elements (pixels). All of the tissues contained within the pixel attenuate the X-ray projections and result in a mean attenuation value for the pixel. This value is compared with the attenuation value of water and is displayed on a scale (the Hounsfield Scale). Water is said to have an attenuation of 0 Hounsfield units (HU); air typically has an HU number of −1000; fat is approximately −100 HU; soft tissues are in the range +20 to +70 HU; and bone is usually greater than +400 HU.

Modern multislice helical CT scanners can obtain images in sub-second times and imaging of the whole body from the top of the head to the thighs can take as little as a single breath hold of only a few seconds. The fast scan times allow dynamic imaging of arteries and veins at different times after the injection of intravenous contrast agents. The continuous acquisition of data from a helical CT scanner allows reconstruction of an image in any plane, commonly sagittal and coronal, as displayed in many of the forthcoming chapters. This orthogonal imaging greatly improves the understanding of the three dimensional aspects of radiological anatomy and now forms part of the standard practice of assessing disease.

Digital images are stored in an archive and form part of an electronic storage record that is becoming commonplace throughout the world, namely a PACS (Picture Archiving and Communication System). PACS allows interrogation of images via an electronic network so that those images (and reports) may be visualised at a distance, for example, on the wards or at another hospital. The Electronic Patient Record (EPR), where all patient information is stored, is developing rapidly and gaining acceptance allowing a marked improvement in data handling.

No specific preparation is required for CT examinations of the brain, spine or musculoskeletal system. Studies of the chest, abdomen and pelvis usually require intravenous contrast medium that contains iodine, so enhancing the arteries and veins and defining their relationships to a greater extent. Opacification of the bowel in CT studies of the abdomen and pelvis can be accomplished by oral ingestion of a water-soluble contrast medium from 24 hours prior to the examination to show the colon, combined with further oral intake 0–60 minutes prior to the scan, for outlining the stomach and small bowel. Occasionally, direct insertion of rectal contrast to show the distal large bowel may be required.

Generally all studies are performed with the patient supine and images are obtained in the transverse or axial plain. Modern CT scanners allow up to 25 degrees of gantry angulation, which is particularly valuable in spinal imaging. Occasionally, direct coronal images are obtained in the investigation of cranial and maxillofacial abnormalities; in these cases the patient lies prone with the neck extended and the gantry appropriately angled, but this technique has largely been superseded by the orthogonal imaging described above.

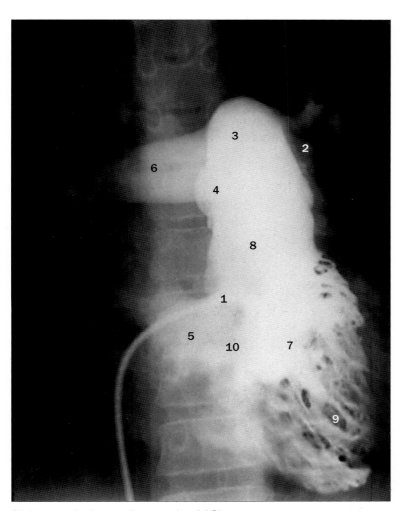

Right ventricular angiogram (p. 112).

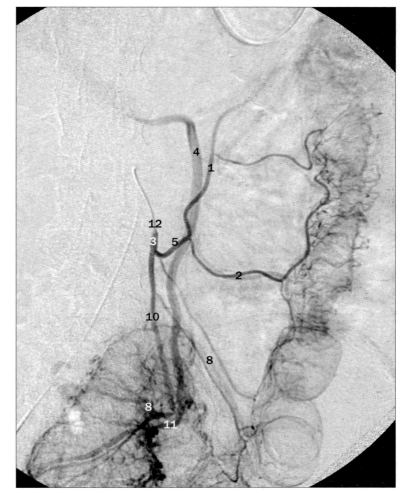

Inferior mesenteric arteriogram (p. 186).

1 Head, neck and brain

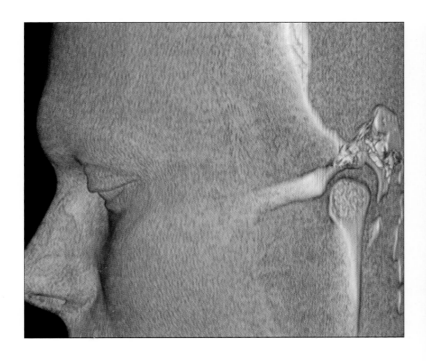

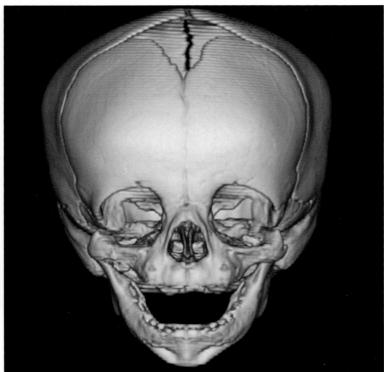

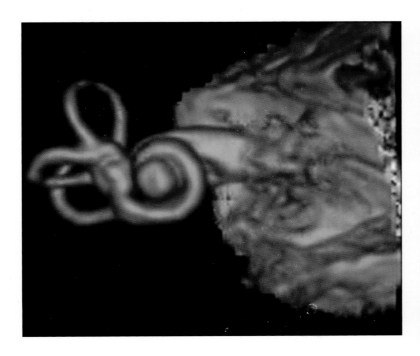

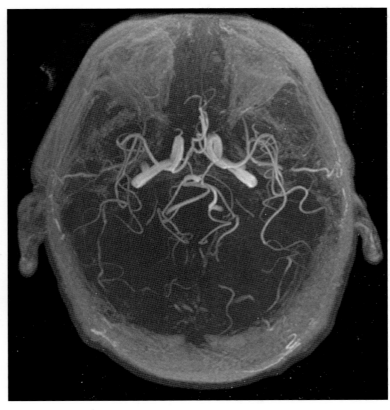

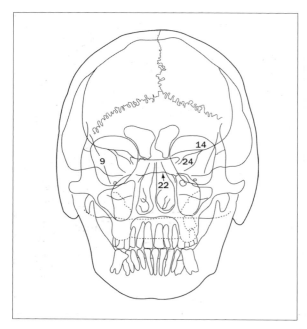

(a) Skull, occipitofrontal projection.
(b) Skull, demonstrating the foramina rotunda, occipitofrontal projection.

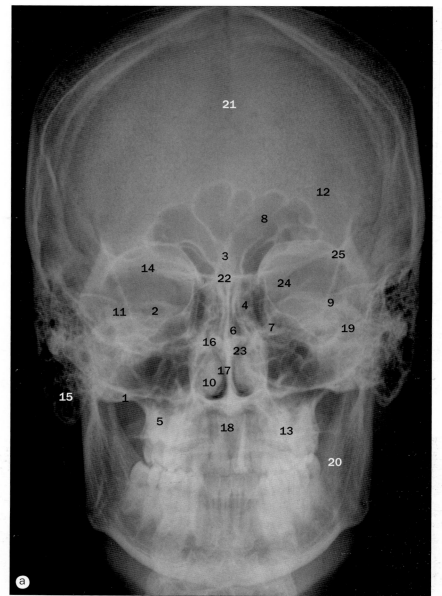

1 Basi-occiput
2 Body of sphenoid
3 Crista galli
4 Ethmoidal air cells
5 Floor of maxillary sinus (antrum)
6 Floor of pituitary fossa
7 Foramen rotundum
8 Frontal sinus
9 Greater wing of sphenoid
10 Inferior turbinate
11 Internal acoustic meatus
12 Lambdoid suture
13 Lateral mass of atlas (first cervical vertebra)
14 Lesser wing of sphenoid
15 Mastoid process
16 Middle turbinate
17 Nasal septum
18 Odontoid process (dens) of axis
    (second cervical vertebra)
19 Petrous part of temporal bone
20 Ramus of mandible
21 Sagittal suture
22 Planum sphenoidale
23 Sphenoid air sinus
24 Superior orbital fissure
25 Temporal surface of greater wing of sphenoid

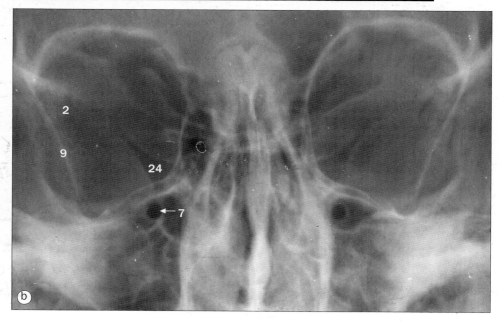

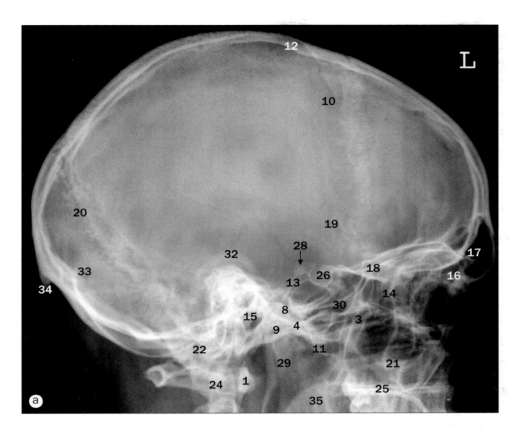

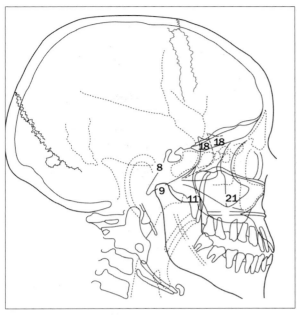

(a) Skull, lateral projection.

Pituitary fossa (sella turcica), (b) of a 7-year-old child, (c) of a 23-year-old woman, lateral projections.

1 Anterior arch of atlas (first cervical vertebra)
2 Anterior clinoid process
3 Arch of zygoma
4 Articular tubercle for temporomandibular joint
5 Basilar part of occipital bone
6 Basisphenoid/basi-occiput synchondrosis
7 Carotid sulcus
8 Clivus
9 Condyle of mandible
10 Coronal suture
11 Coronoid process of mandible

12 Diploë
13 Dorsum sellae
14 Ethmoidal air cells
15 External acoustic meatus
16 Frontal process of zygoma
17 Frontal sinus
18 Greater wing of sphenoid
19 Grooves for middle meningeal vessels
20 Lambdoid suture
21 Malar process of maxilla
22 Mastoid air cells
23 Middle clinoid process

24 Odontoid process (dens) of axis (second cervical vertebra)
25 Palatine process of maxilla
26 Pituitary fossa (sella turcica)
27 Planum sphenoidale
28 Posterior clinoid process
29 Ramus of mandible
30 Sphenoidal sinus
31 Tuberculum sellae
32 Pinna of ear
33 Inion
34 External occipital protruberance
35 Soft palate

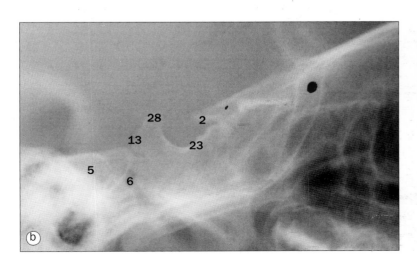

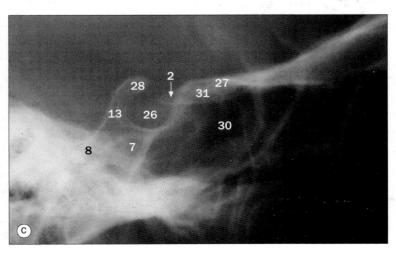

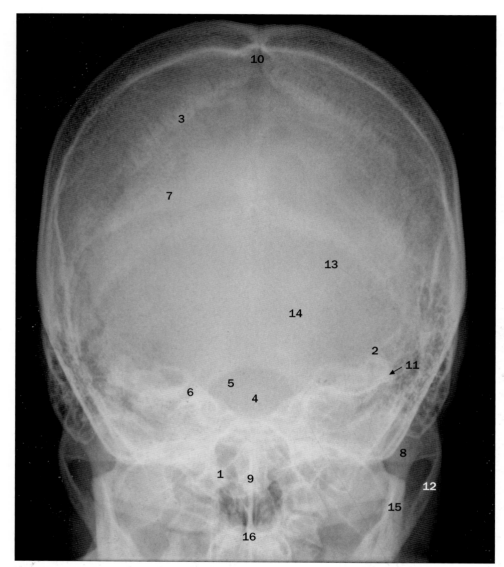

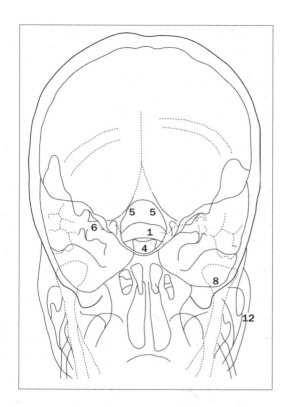

Skull, 30° fronto-occipital (Townes') projection.

1 Arch of atlas (first cervical vertebra)
2 Arcuate eminence of temporal bone
3 Coronal suture
4 Dorsum sellae
5 Foramen magnum
6 Internal acoustic meatus
7 Lambdoid suture
8 Mandibular condyle
9 Odontoid process (dens) of axis (second cervical vertebra)
10 Sagittal suture
11 Superior semicircular canal
12 Zygomatic arch
13 Groove for transverse sinus
14 Squamous occipital bone
15 Mandible
16 Nasal septum

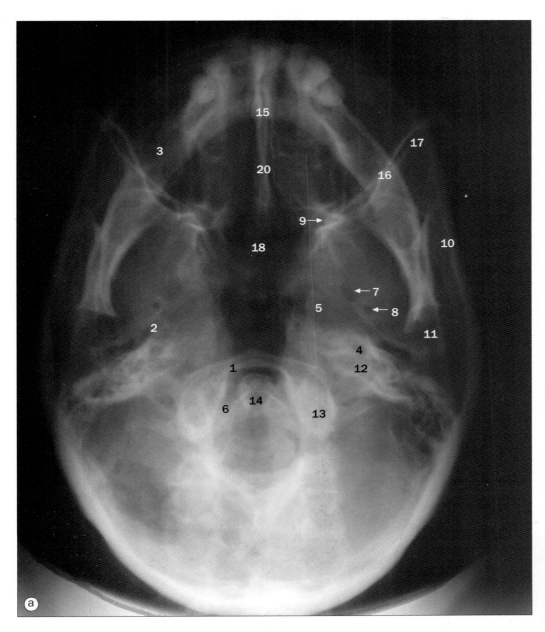

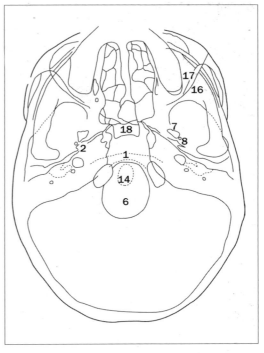

(a) Skull, submentovertical projection.
(b) Skull, with additional angulation for zygomatic arches, submentovertical projection.

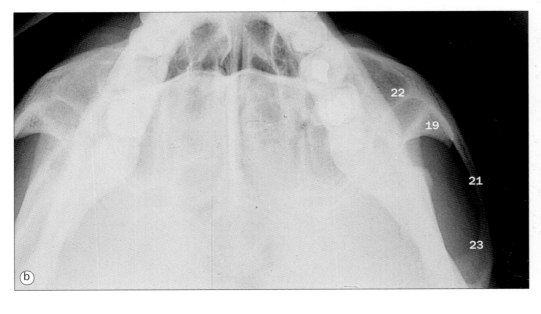

 1 Anterior arch of atlas (first cervical vertebra)
 2 Auditory (Eustachian) tube
 3 Body of mandible
 4 Carotid canal
 5 Foramen lacerum
 6 Foramen magnum
 7 Foramen ovale
 8 Foramen spinosum
 9 Greater palatine foramen
10 Greater wing of sphenoid
11 Head of mandible
12 Jugular foramen
13 Occipital condyle
14 Odontoid process (dens) of axis (second cervical vertebra)
15 Perpendicular plate of ethmoid
16 Posterior margin of orbit
17 Posterior wall of maxillary sinus (antrum)
18 Sphenoidal sinus
19 Temporal process of zygomatic bone
20 Vomer
21 Zygomatic arch
22 Zygomatic bone
23 Zygomatic process of temporal bone

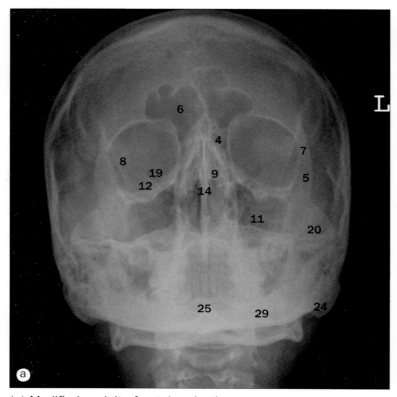

(a) Modified occipito frontal projection.

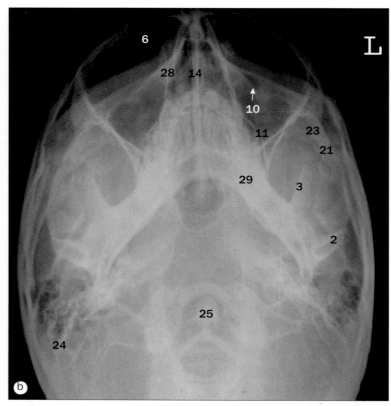

(b) Occipito mental projection.

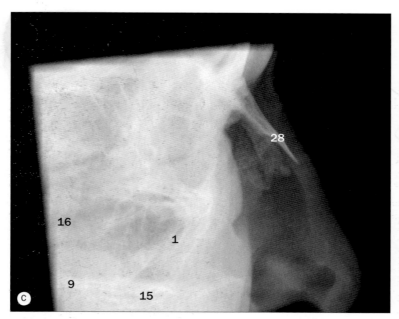

(c) Lateral nasal bones projection.

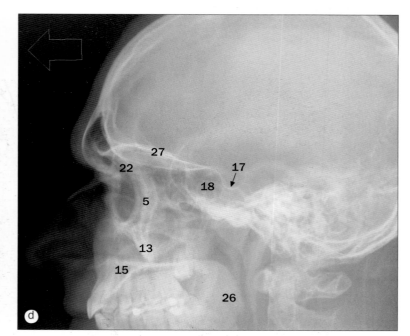

(d) Lateral sinus projection.

1 Anterior wall of maxillary sinus (antrum)	11 Left maxillary sinus (antrum)	21 Zygomatic arch
2 Condyle of mandible	12 Lesser wing of sphenoid	22 Zygomatic process of frontal bone
3 Coronoid process of mandible	13 Malar process of maxilla	23 Zygomatic process of temporal bone
4 Ethmoidal sinuses	14 Nasal septum	24 Mastoid process
5 Frontal process of zygomatic bone	15 Palatine process of maxilla	25 Odontoid peg
6 Frontal sinuses	16 Posterior wall of maxillary sinus (antrum)	26 Soft palate
7 Frontozygomatic suture	17 Sella turcica	27 Floor of anterior cranial fossa
8 Greater wing of sphenoid	18 Sphenoidal sinus	28 Nasal bones
9 Horizontal plate of palatine bone	19 Superior orbital fissure	29 Mandible
10 Infra-orbital foramen	20 Temporal process of zygomatic bone	

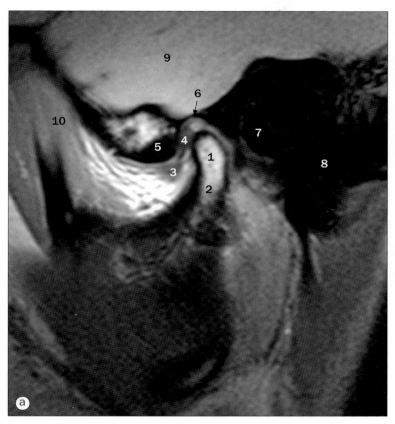

(a) Temporomandibular joint MR: closed.

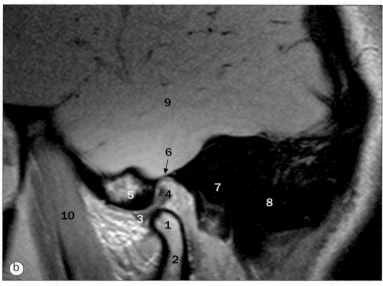

(b) Temporomandibular joint MR: open.

MR of the temporomandibular joint with the subject looking to the left.

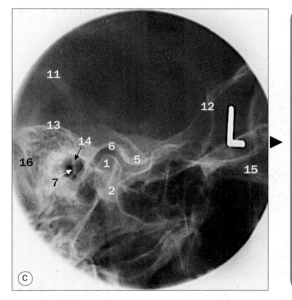

(c) Radiograph of temporomandibular joint: closed.

1 Condylar head
2 Condylar neck
3 Anterior band of disc
4 Posterior band of disc
5 Articular eminence
6 Mandibular fossa
7 External auditory canal
8 Mastoid process of temporal bone
9 Temporal lobe of brain
10 Temporalis muscle
11 Pinna of ear
12 Greater wing of sphenoid
13 Tegmen tympani
14 Malleus
15 Zygomatic process of temporal bone
16 Sinus plate

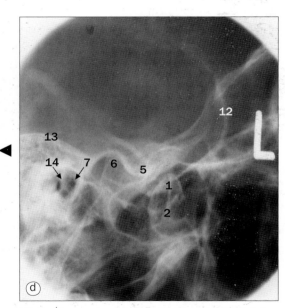

(d) Radiograph of temporomandibular joint: open.

Radiographs of the temporomandibular joint with the subject looking to the right.

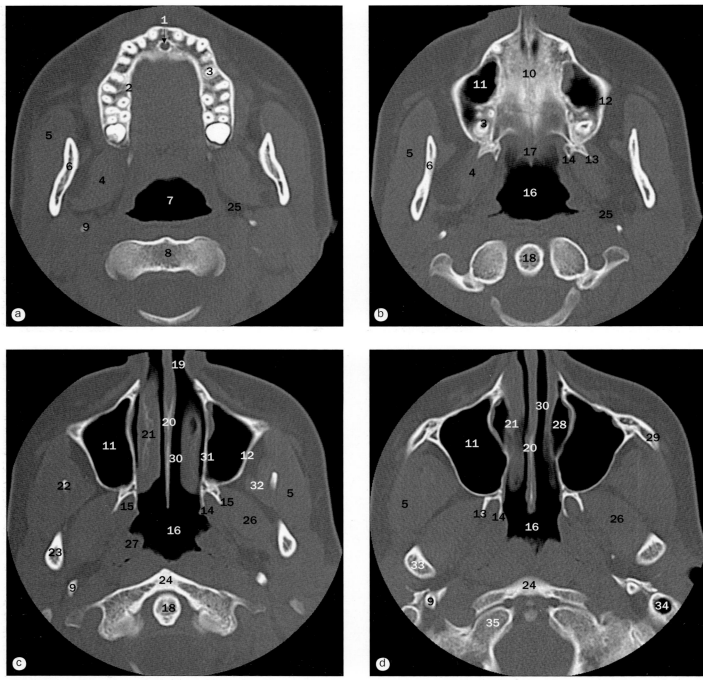

Facial bones and paranasal sinuses, axial CT images demonstrated at the following levels: **(a)** alveolar process of the maxilla, **(b)** hard palate, **(c)** nares, **(d)** maxillary sinus, **(e)** middle turbinate, **(f)** zygomatic arch, **(g)** sphenoid sinus, **(h)** ethmoid sinus.

1 Incisive canal	**14** Medial pterygoid plate	**26** Lateral pyterygoid muscle
2 Alveolar rim	**15** Pterygoid fossa	**27** Torus tubarius
3 Alveolar recess	**16** Nasopharynx	**28** Inferior meatus (at location of
4 Medial pterygoid muscle	**17** Vomer	nasolacrimal opening)
5 Masseter muscle	**18** Odontoid process (dens)	**29** Zygoma
6 Ramus of mandible	**19** Nares	**30** Nasal cavity
7 Oropharynx	**20** Nasal septum	**31** Medial wall of maxillary sinus (antrum)
8 Body of C2	**21** Inferior turbinate	**32** Temporalis muscle
9 Styloid process	**22** Coronoid process of mandible	**33** Condylar head of mandible
10 Hard palate	**23** Condylar neck of mandible	**34** Mastoid air cells
11 Maxillary sinus (antrum)	**24** Anterior arch of atlas (first cervical	**35** Occipital condyle
12 Lateral wall of maxillary sinus (antrum)	vertebra)	**36** Middle turbinate
13 Lateral pterygoid plate	**25** Parapharyngeal space	**37** Middle meatus

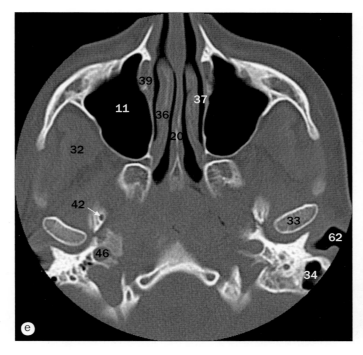

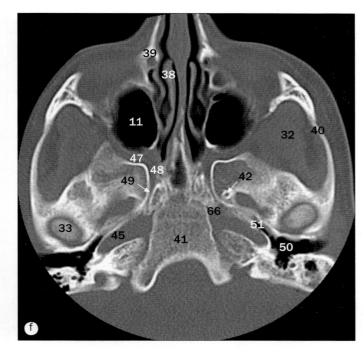

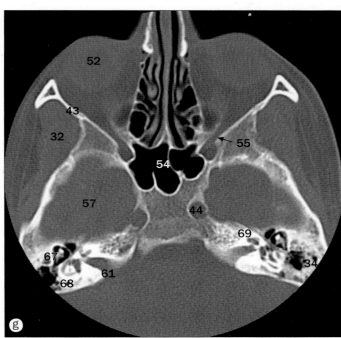

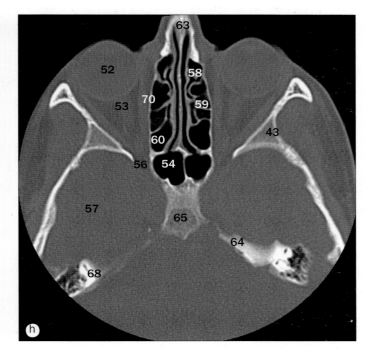

38 Superior turbinate	48 Foramen rotundum	60 Posterior ethmoidal air cells
39 Nasolacrimal duct	49 Vidian canal	61 Internal auditory canal
40 Zygomatic arch	50 Middle ear cavity	62 External auditory canal
41 Clivus	51 Eustachian tube	63 Nasal bone
42 Foramen spinosum	52 Globe of eye	64 Petrous apex
43 Greater wing of sphenoid	53 Optic nerve	65 Floor of sella
44 Cavernous internal carotid artery	54 Sphenoid sinus (antrum)	66 Foramen lacerum
45 Horizontal petrous internal carotid artery canal	55 Inferior orbital fissure	67 Ossicles of middle ear (incus and malleus)
46 Vertical petrous internal carotid artery canal	56 Superior orbital fissure	68 Semicircular canals of inner ear
47 Pterygopalatine fossa	57 Temporal lobe	69 Cochlea of inner ear
	58 Anterior ethmoidal air cells	70 Lamina papyracea
	59 Middle ethmoidal air cells	

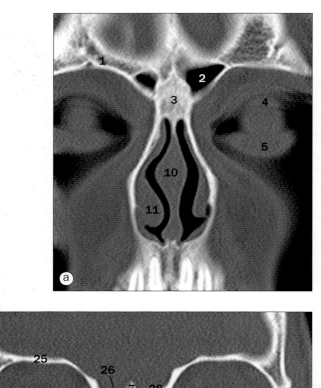
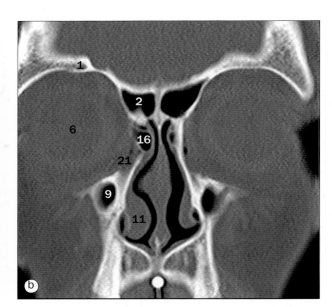
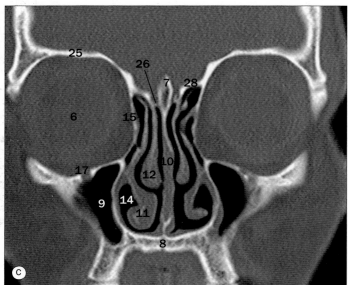
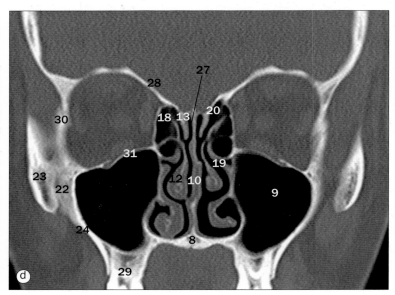

Paranasal sinuses, coronal CT images demonstrated at the following levels: (**a**) frontal sinuses, (**b**) nasolacrimal duct, (**c**) cribriform plate, (**d**) anterior ethmoids, (**e**) middle ethmoids, (**f**) pterygopalatine fossa, (**g**) sphenoid sinus, (**h**) nasopharynx.

1 Frontal bone	**11** Inferior turbinate (concha)
2 Frontal sinus (antrum)	**12** Middle turbinate (concha)
3 Nasal bone	**13** Superior turbinate (concha)
4 Upper eyelid	**14** Inferior meatus
5 Lower eyelid	**15** Lamina papyracea
6 Globe of eye	**16** Air in nasolacrimal sac
7 Crista galli	**17** Inferior orbital canal
8 Hard palate	**18** Anterior ethmoid air cells
9 Maxillary sinus (antrum)	**19** Middle meatus
10 Nasal septum	**20** Superior meatus

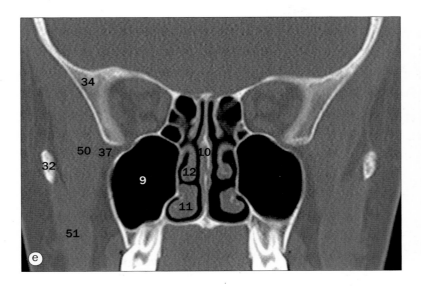
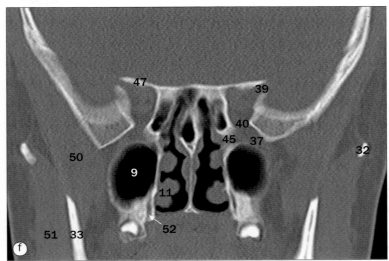
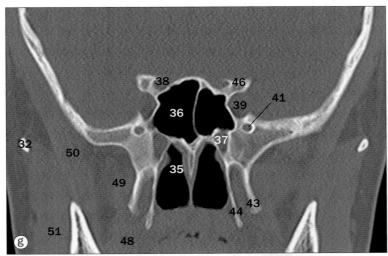
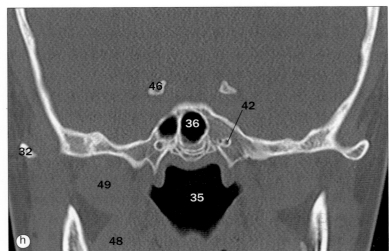

Paranasal sinuses, coronal CT images demonstrated at the following levels: (a) frontal sinuses, (b) nasolacrimal duct, (c) cribriform plate, (d) anterior ethmoids, (e) middle ethmoids, (f) pterygopalatine fossa, (g) sphenoid sinus, (h) nasopharynx.

21 Nasolacrimal duct	32 Zygomatic arch	43 Lateral pterygoid plate
22 Maxilla	33 Ramus of mandible	44 Medial pterygoid plate
23 Zygoma	34 Greater wing of sphenoid	45 Sphenopalatine foramen
24 Lateral wall of maxillary sinus	35 Nasopharynx	46 Anterior clinoid process
25 Orbital roof, frontal bone	36 Sphenoid sinus (antrum)	47 Lesser wing of sphenoid
26 Cribriform plate, ethmoid bone	37 Pterygopalatine fossa	48 Medial pterygoid muscle
27 Perpendicular plate, ethmoid bone	38 Optic canal	49 Lateral pterygoid muscle
28 Fovea ethmoidalis, frontal bone	39 Superior orbital fissure	50 Temporalis muscle
29 Upper alveolar ridge of maxilla	40 Inferior orbital fissure	51 Masseter muscle
30 Lateral orbital wall, zygomatic bone	41 Foramen rotundum	52 Greater palatine foramen
31 Orbital floor, maxillary bone	42 Vidian canal	

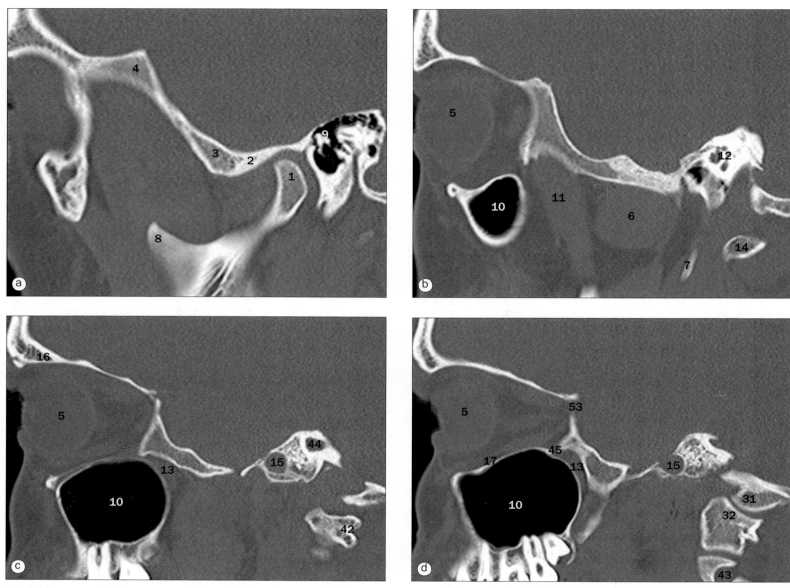

(a)–(h) Paranasal sinuses, sagittal CT images, from lateral to midline.

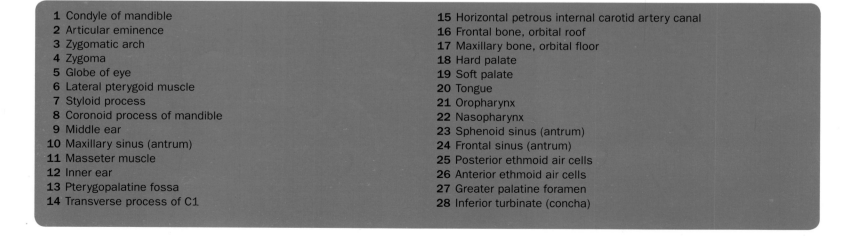

1 Condyle of mandible
2 Articular eminence
3 Zygomatic arch
4 Zygoma
5 Globe of eye
6 Lateral pterygoid muscle
7 Styloid process
8 Coronoid process of mandible
9 Middle ear
10 Maxillary sinus (antrum)
11 Masseter muscle
12 Inner ear
13 Pterygopalatine fossa
14 Transverse process of C1

15 Horizontal petrous internal carotid artery canal
16 Frontal bone, orbital roof
17 Maxillary bone, orbital floor
18 Hard palate
19 Soft palate
20 Tongue
21 Oropharynx
22 Nasopharynx
23 Sphenoid sinus (antrum)
24 Frontal sinus (antrum)
25 Posterior ethmoid air cells
26 Anterior ethmoid air cells
27 Greater palatine foramen
28 Inferior turbinate (concha)

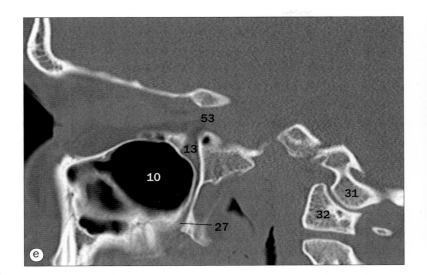

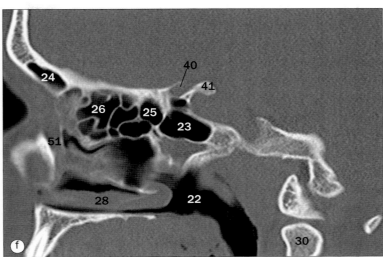

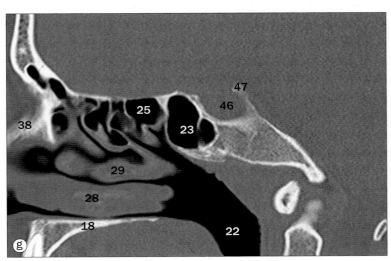

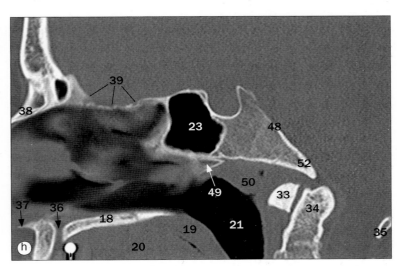

(a)–(h) Paranasal sinuses, sagittal CT images, from lateral to midline.

29 Middle turbinate (concha)
30 Base of C2
31 Occipital condyle
32 Lateral mass of C1
33 Anterior arch of C1
34 Dens (odontoid process)
35 Posterior arch of C1
36 Incisive foramen (contains nasopalatine nerve – V2 sensory branch)
37 Anterior nasal spine of maxillae
38 Nasal bone
39 Cribriform plate
40 Optic canal

41 Anterior clinoid
42 Tubercles of transverse process of C1
43 Transverse foramen of C2
44 Internal auditory canal
45 Inferior orbital fissure
46 Hypophyseal fossa
47 Dorsum sellae
48 Clivus
49 Vomer
50 Pharyngeal tonsil
51 Nasolacrimal duct
52 Basion
53 Superior orbital fissure

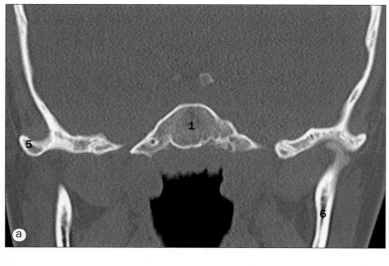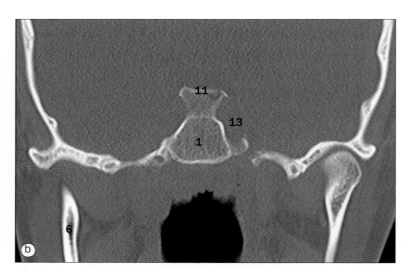

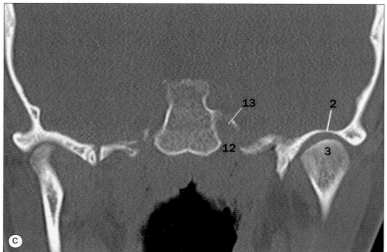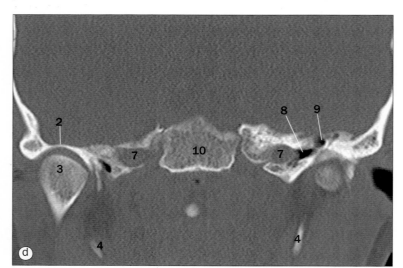

(a)–(h) Coronal CT images, from anterior to posterior.

1 Sphenoid body	**9** Epitympanum
2 Condylar fossa of temporomandibular joint	**10** Basi-occiput (lower clivus)
3 Mandibular condyle head	**11** Dorsum sellae
4 Styloid process	**12** Foramen lacerum
5 Zygomatic arch	**13** Location of vertical portion of internal carotid artery
6 Mandibular ramus	**14** Anterior arch of C1
7 Horizontal petrous internal carotid artery	**15** Dens (odontoid process)
8 Hypotympanum	**16** Body of C2

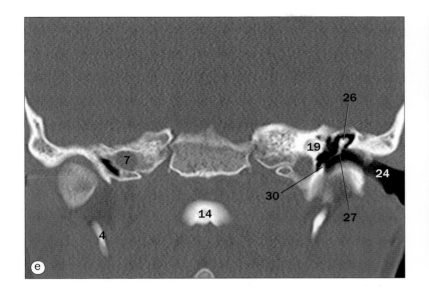

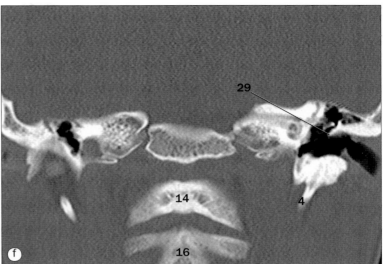

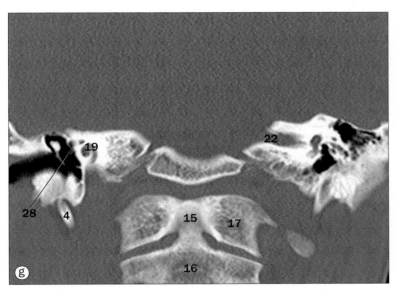

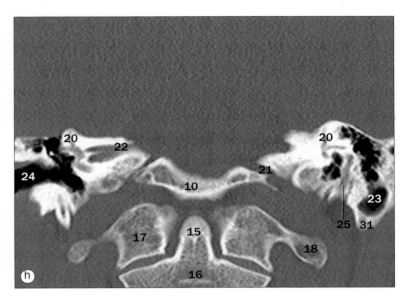

(a)–(h) Coronal CT images, from anterior to posterior.

17 Transverse process of C1	**25** Stylomastoid foramen (location of mastoid segment of CN7)
18 Lateral mass of C1	**26** Incus
19 Cochlea	**27** Malleus
20 Semicircular canal	**28** Tendon of tensor tympani muscle
21 Jugular foramen	**29** Scutum
22 Internal acoustic canal	**30** Tympanic annulus
23 Mastoid air cells	**31** Mastoid tip
24 External auditory canal	

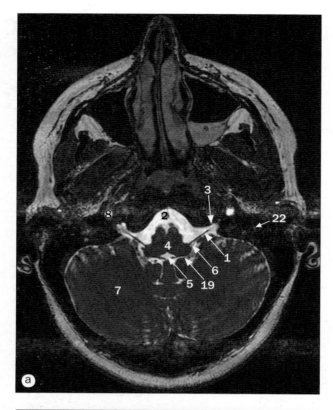

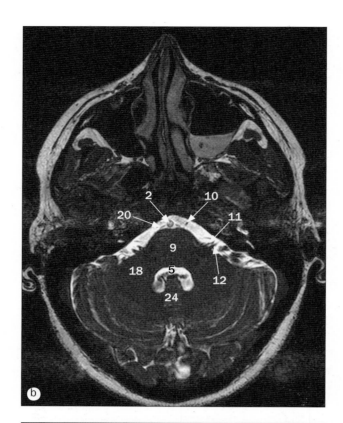

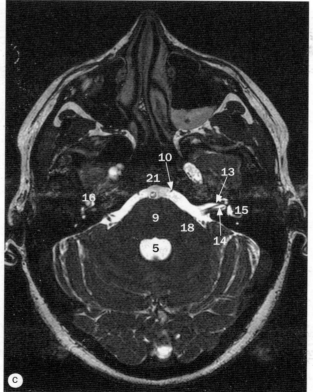

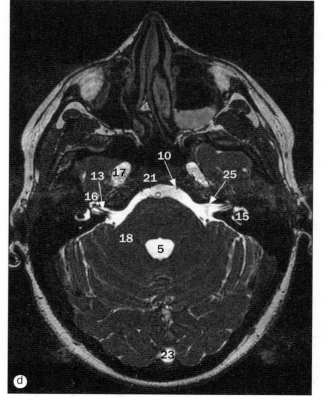

(a)–(h) Axial MR images, from inferior to superior.

1 Glossopharyngeal nerve (CN9)	**5** Fourth ventricle	**9** Pons
2 Basilar artery	**6** Vagus nerve (CN10)	**10** Abducens nerve (CN6)
3 Jugular foramen	**7** Cerebellar hemisphere	**11** Facial nerve (CN7)
4 Medulla	**8** Internal carotid artery	**12** Vestibulocochlear nerve (CN8)

The legends for pages 16–19 are common for all 4 pages.

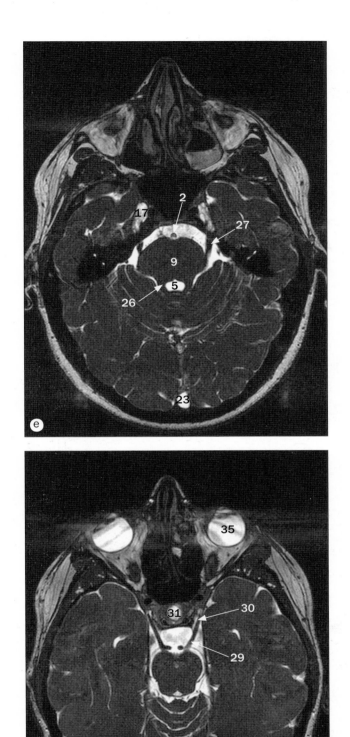
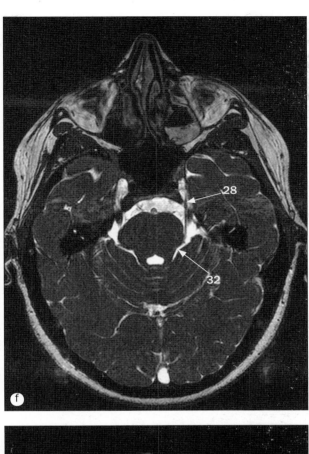
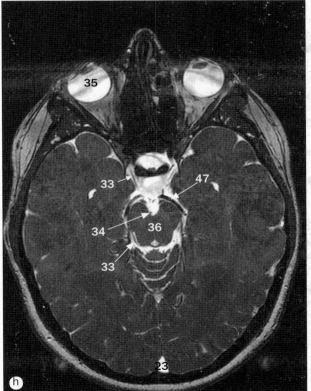

(a)–(h) Axial MR images, from inferior to superior.

13 Cochlear nerve	**17** Meckel's cave	**21** Clivus
14 Vestibular nerve	**18** Middle cerebellar peduncle	**22** Facial nerve in stylomastoid foramen
15 Semicircular canals	**19** Foramen of Luschka	**23** Superior sagittal sinus
16 Cochlea	**20** Anterior inferior cerebellar artery	**24** Vermis

The legends for pages 16–19 are common for all 4 pages.

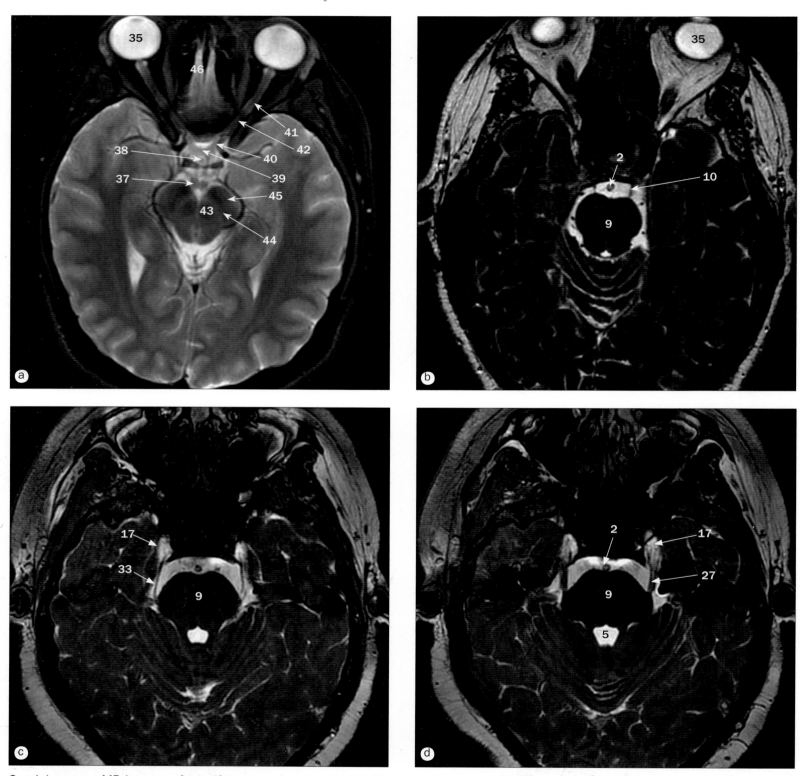

Cranial nerves, MR images of (a) olfactory and optic nerves, (b) oculomotor nerve, (c) trochlear nerve, (d) trigeminal nerve, (e) and (f) abducens, facial and auditory nerves, (g) glossopharyngeal nerve, (h) hypoglossal nerve.

25 Internal auditory canal	31 Pituitary
26 Superior cerebellar peduncle	32 Ambient cistern
27 Preganglionic segment of CN5 (trigeminal)	33 Trochlear nerve (CN4)
28 CN5 enters Meckel's cave	34 Interpeduncular cistern
29 Oculomotor nerve (CN3)	35 Globe of eye
30 CN3 in oculomotor cistern	36 Midbrain

The legends for pages 16–19 are common for all 4 pages.

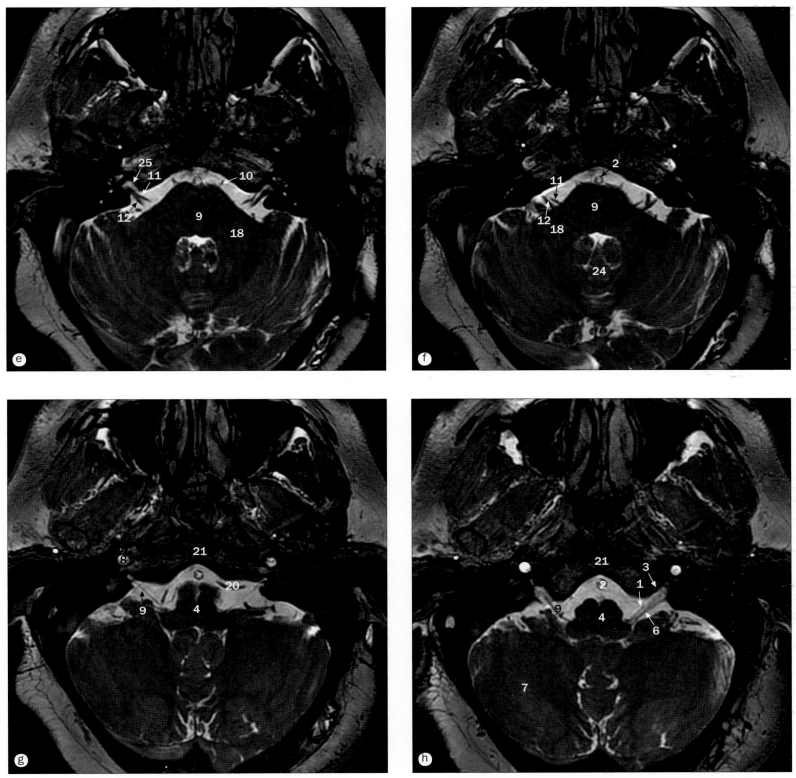

Cranial nerves, MR images of **(a)** olfactory and optic nerves, **(b)** oculomotor nerve, **(c)** trochlear nerve, **(d)** trigeminal nerve, **(e)** and **(f)** abducens, facial and auditory nerves, **(g)** glossopharyngeal nerve, **(h)** hypoglossal nerve.

37 Mammillary body		**43** Red nucleus of midbrain
38 Infundibulum		**44** Substantia nigra
39 Optic chiasm		**45** Cerebral peduncle
40 Optic nerve, intracranial portion		**46** Olfactory tract and bulb (CN1)
41 Optic nerve, intra-ocular segment		**47** Posterior cerebral artery
42 Optic nerve, intracanalicular segment		

The legends for pages 16–19 are common for all 4 pages.

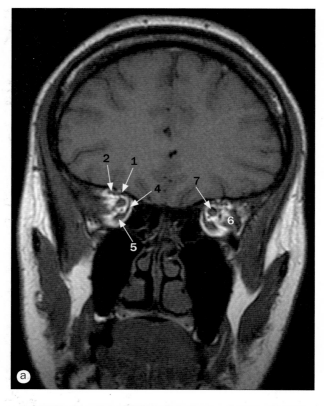

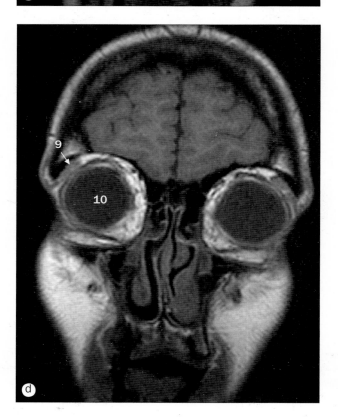

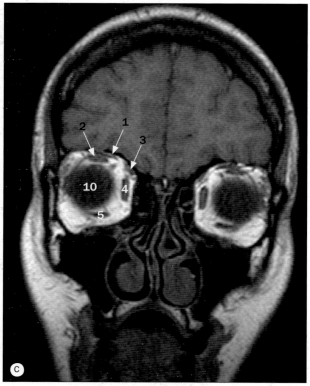

(a)–(d) Coronal MR images, from posterior to anterior.

1 Levator palpebrae superioris muscle	**6** Lateral rectus muscle
2 Superior rectus muscle	**7** Optic nerve/sheath complex
3 Superior oblique muscle	**8** Superior ophthalmic vein
4 Medial rectus muscle	**9** Lacrimal gland
5 Inferior rectus muscle	**10** Globe of eye

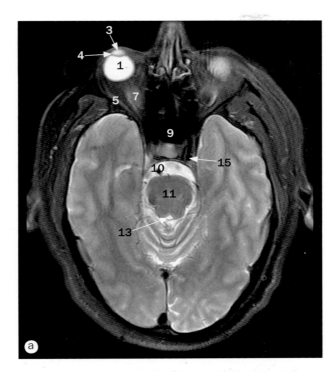

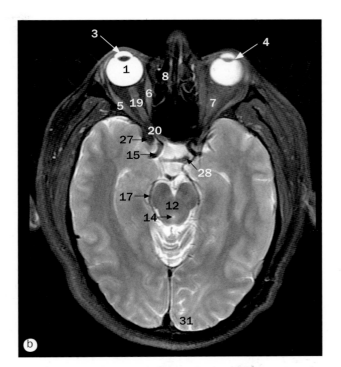

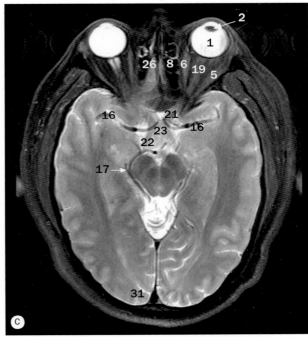

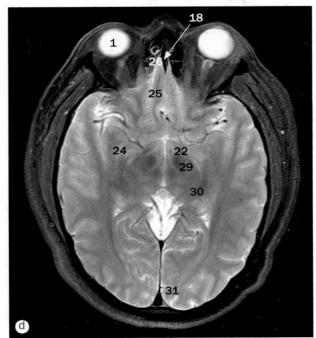

(a)–(d) Orbit, axial MR images, from inferior to superior.

1 Vitreous chamber of globe	12 Midbrain	23 Optic chiasm
2 Lens	13 Superior recess fourth ventricle	24 Anterior commissure
3 Anterior chamber of globe	14 Cerebral aqueduct	25 Gyrus rectus
4 Ciliary body	15 Internal carotid artery	26 Olfactory nerve (CN1)
5 Lateral rectus muscle	16 Middle cerebral artery	27 Anterior clinoid process
6 Medial rectus muscle	17 Posterior cerebral artery	28 Dorsum sellae
7 Superior rectus muscle	18 Crista galli	29 Cerebral peduncle
8 Ethmoid air cells	19 Optic nerve (intra-orbital segment)	30 Medial and lateral geniculate bodies
9 Sphenoid sinus (antrum)	20 Optic nerve (intracanalicular segment)	31 Visual (calcarine) cortex
10 Basilar artery	21 Optic nerve (intracranial segment)	
11 Pons	22 Optic tract	

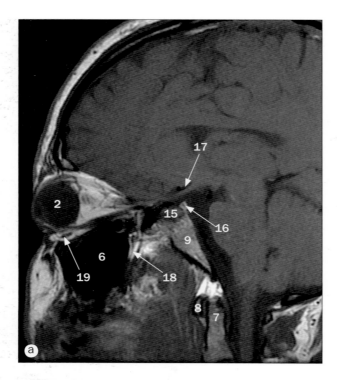

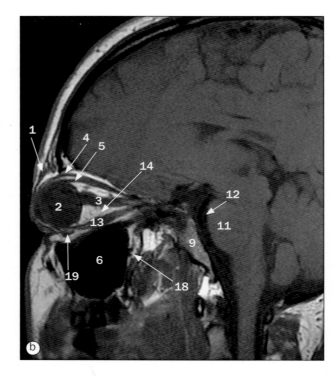

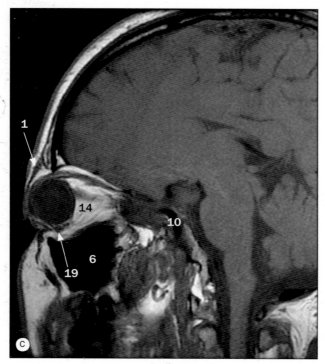

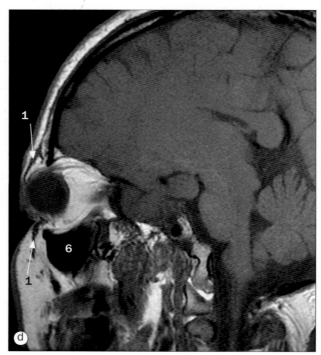

(a)–(d) Orbit, sagittal MR images, from medial to lateral.

 1 Orbicularis oculi muscle
 2 Globe
 3 Optic nerve, intraocular segment
 4 Levator palpebrae superioris
 5 Superior rectus muscle
 6 Maxillary sinus (antrum)
 7 Dens (odontoid process)
 8 Anterior arch of C1
 9 Clivus
10 Internal carotid artery

11 Pons
12 Basilar artery
13 Inferior rectus muscle
14 Retrobulbar fat
15 Sella turcica/pituitary
16 Dorsum sellae
17 Optic nerve, intracranial segment
18 Pterygopalatine fossa
19 Inferior oblique muscle

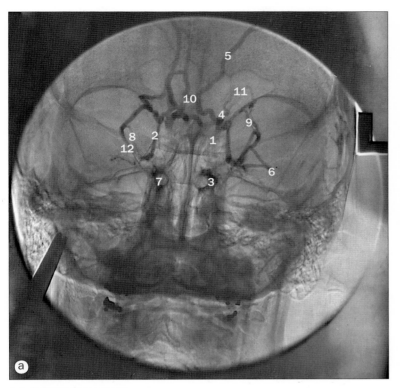

(a) Orbital venogram. ▲

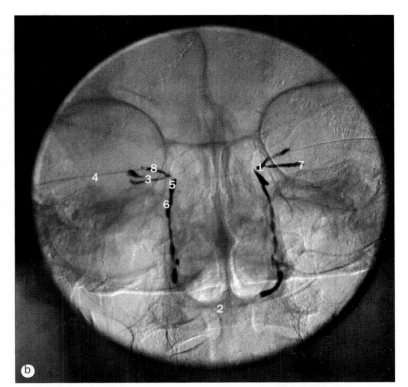

(b) Macrodacryocystogram. ▲

1 Angular veins
2 Anterior collateral vein
3 Cavernous sinus
4 First part of superior ophthalmic vein
5 Frontal veins
6 Inferior ophthalmic vein
7 Internal carotid artery
8 Medial collateral vein
9 Second part of superior ophthalmic vein
10 Superficial connecting vein
11 Supraorbital vein
12 Third part of superior ophthalmic vein

1 Common canaliculus		5 Lacrimal sac
2 Hard palate		6 Nasolacrimal duct
3 Inferior canaliculus		7 Site of lacrimal punctum
4 Lacrimal catheters		8 Superior canaliculus

1 Anterior chamber	10 Optic nerve
2 Aqueous humour	11 Retina and choroid
3 Cornea	12 Retro-orbital fat
4 Ethmoidal sinuses	13 Sclera
5 Eyelid	14 Suspensory ligament of the lens
6 Lateral rectus muscle	15 Temporalis muscle
7 Lens	16 Vitreous
8 Medial rectus muscle	
9 Ophthalmic artery	

▶

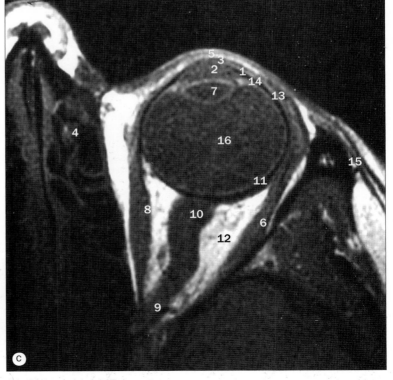

(c) Globe, axial MR image.

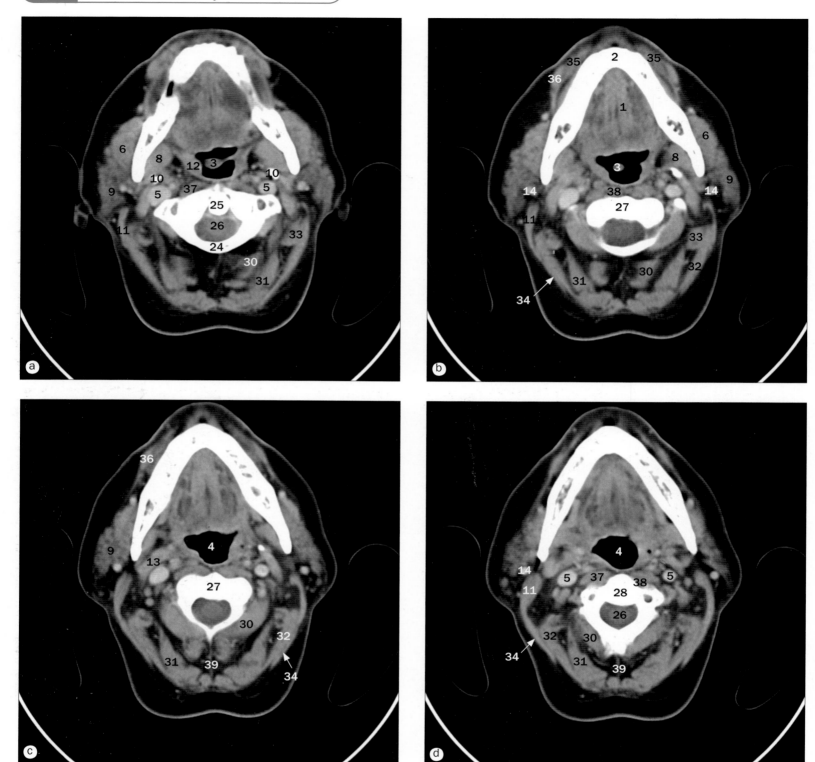

(a)–(h) Nasopharynx and oropharynx, axial CT images.

1 Genioglossus muscle	**8** Medial pterygoid muscle	**15** External jugular vein
2 Body of mandible	**9** Parotid gland	**16** Anterior belly of digastric muscle
3 Uvula	**10** Styloid process	**17** Epiglottis
4 Oropharynx	**11** Sternocleidomastoid muscle	**18** Vallecula
5 Internal jugular vein	**12** Palatine tonsil	**19** Hypopharynx
6 Masseter muscle	**13** Posterior belly of digastric muscle	**20** Mylohyoid muscle
7 Submandibular gland	**14** Retromandibular vein	**21** Platysma muscle

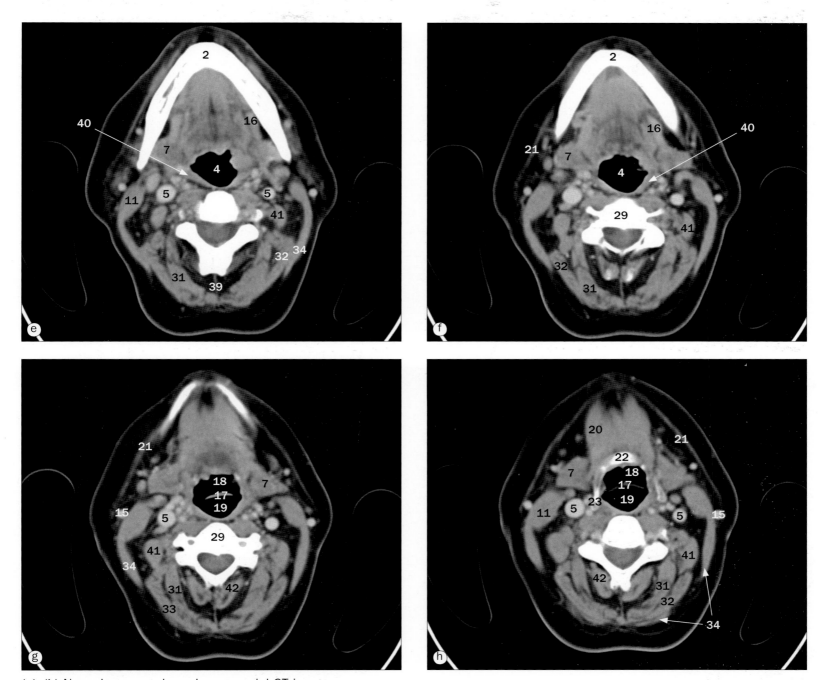

(a)–(h) Nasopharynx and oropharynx, axial CT images.

22 Hyoid body	**30** Obliquus capitis inferior muscle	**38** Longus colli muscle
23 Greater horn of hyoid	**31** Semispinalis capitis muscle	**39** Nuchal ligament
24 Posterior arch of C1	**32** Splenius capitis muscle	**40** Superior constrictor muscle of pharynx
25 Dens (odontoid process)	**33** Longissimus capitis muscle	**41** Levator scapulae muscle
26 Spinal cord	**34** Trapezius muscle	**42** Spinalis capitis muscle and multifidus
27 Body of C2	**35** Orbicularis oris muscle	muscle
28 Body of C3	**36** Levator anguli oris muscle	
29 Body of C4	**37** Longus capitis muscle	

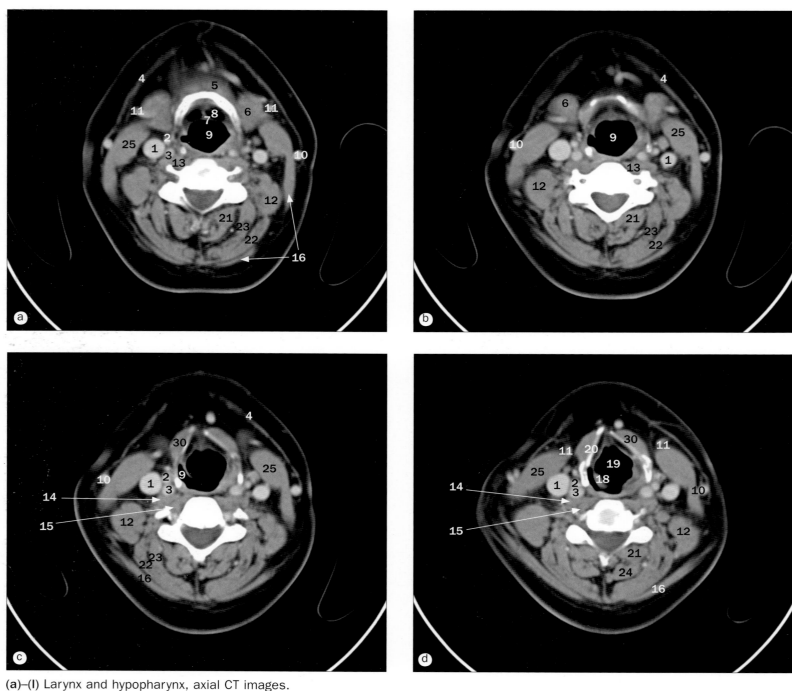

(a)–(l) Larynx and hypopharynx, axial CT images.

1 Internal jugular vein	8 Vallecula
2 External carotid artery	9 Hypopharynx
3 Internal carotid artery	10 External jugular vein
4 Platysma muscle	11 Anterior jugular vein
5 Geniohyoid muscle	12 Levator scapulae muscle
6 Submandibular gland	13 Longus capitus and colli muscles
7 Epiglottis	14 Longus capitus muscle

The legends for pages 26–28 are common for all 3 pages.

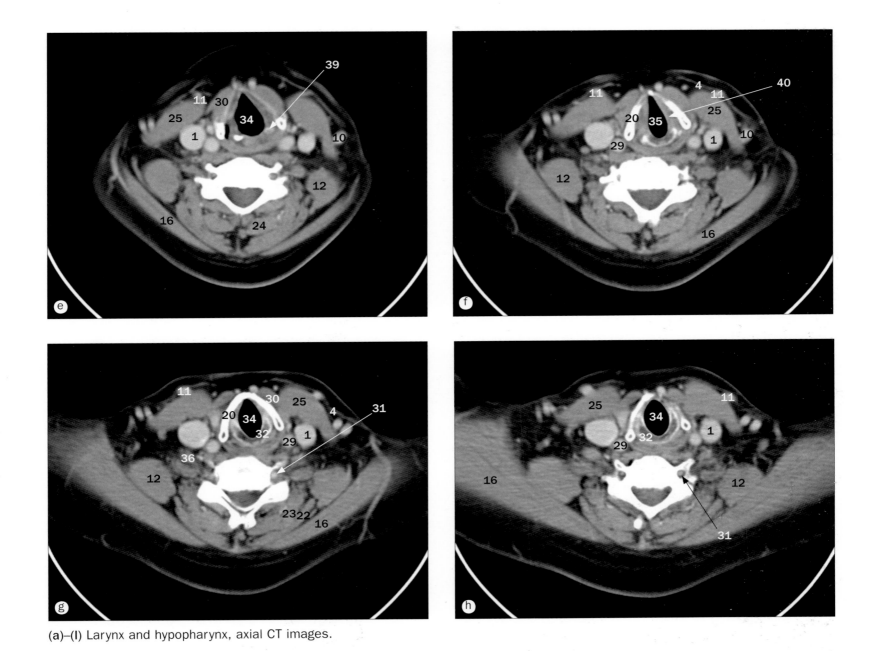

(a)–(l) Larynx and hypopharynx, axial CT images.

15 Longus colli muscle	**22** Splenius capitis muscle
16 Trapezius muscle	**23** Semispinalis capitis muscle
17 Clavicle	**24** Semispinalis cervicis muscle
18 Aryepiglottic fold	**25** Sternocleidomastoid muscle
19 Laryngeal vestibule	**26** Sternohyoid muscle
20 Thyroid cartilage lamina	**27** Thyroid gland
21 Spinalis cervicis muscle	**28** Oesophagus

The legends for pages 26–28 are common for all 3 pages.

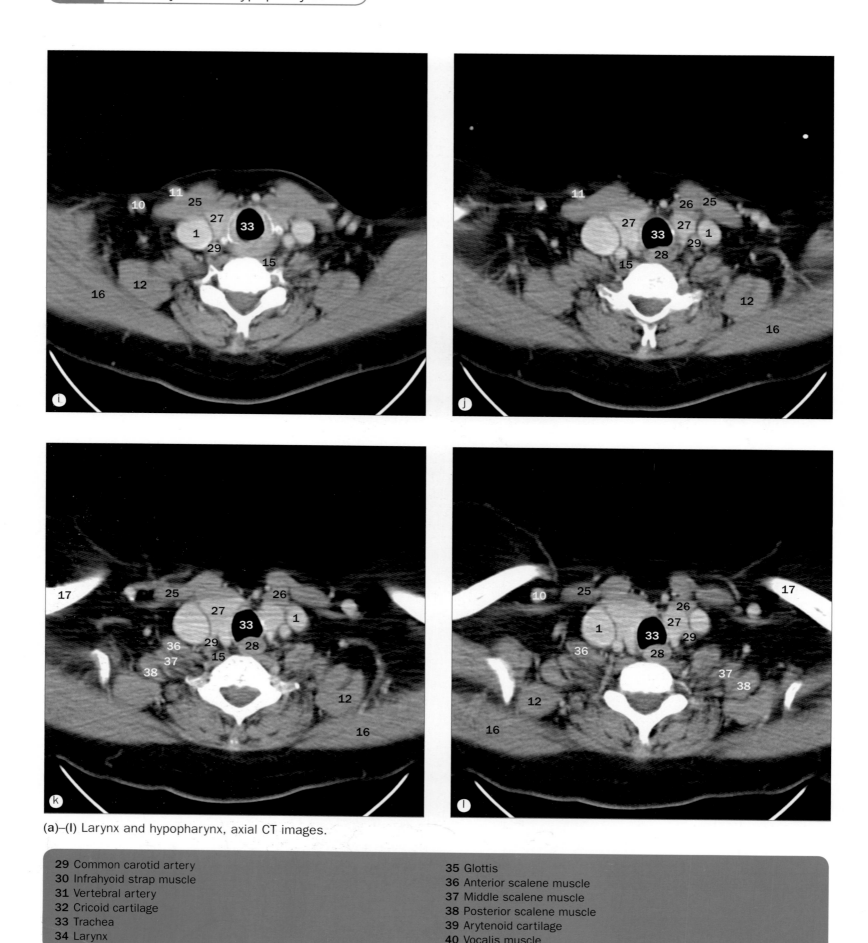

(a)–(l) Larynx and hypopharynx, axial CT images.

29 Common carotid artery	**35** Glottis
30 Infrahyoid strap muscle	**36** Anterior scalene muscle
31 Vertebral artery	**37** Middle scalene muscle
32 Cricoid cartilage	**38** Posterior scalene muscle
33 Trachea	**39** Arytenoid cartilage
34 Larynx	**40** Vocalis muscle

The legends for pages 26–28 are common for all 3 pages.

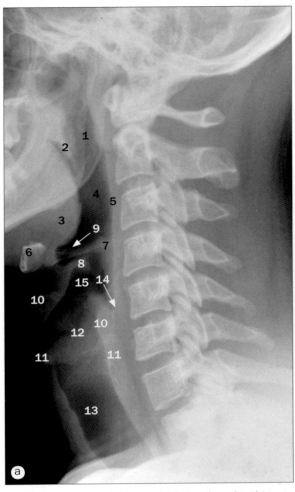

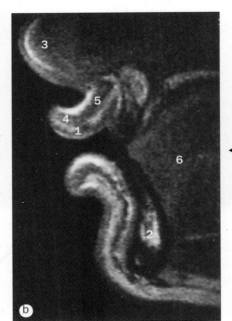

1 Nasopharynx
2 Soft palate
3 Base of tongue
4 Oropharynx
5 Retropharyngeal soft tissues
6 Body of hyoid
7 Greater horn of hyoid
8 Epiglottis
9 Vallecula
10 Thyroid cartilage
11 Cricoid cartilage
12 Larygneal space
13 Trachea
14 Entrance to oesophagus
15 Hypopharynx

1 Deltoid insertion of levator muscle
2 Mandible
3 Nose
4 Pars marginalis of orbicularis oris muscle
5 Pars peripheralis of orbicularis oris muscle
6 Tongue

(a) Soft tissues of the neck, lateral projection.

(b) The kiss, sagittal MR image.

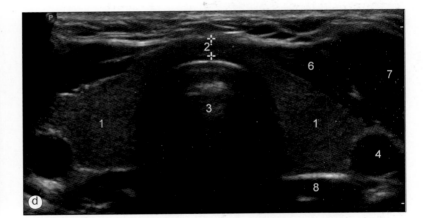

(c) and (d) Thyroid ultrasound, axial projection.

1 Thyroid gland lobe
2 Thyroid gland isthmus
3 Trachea
4 Common carotid artery
5 Internal jugular vein
6 Infrahyoid strap muscle
7 Sternocleidomastoid muscle
8 Prevertebral muscle

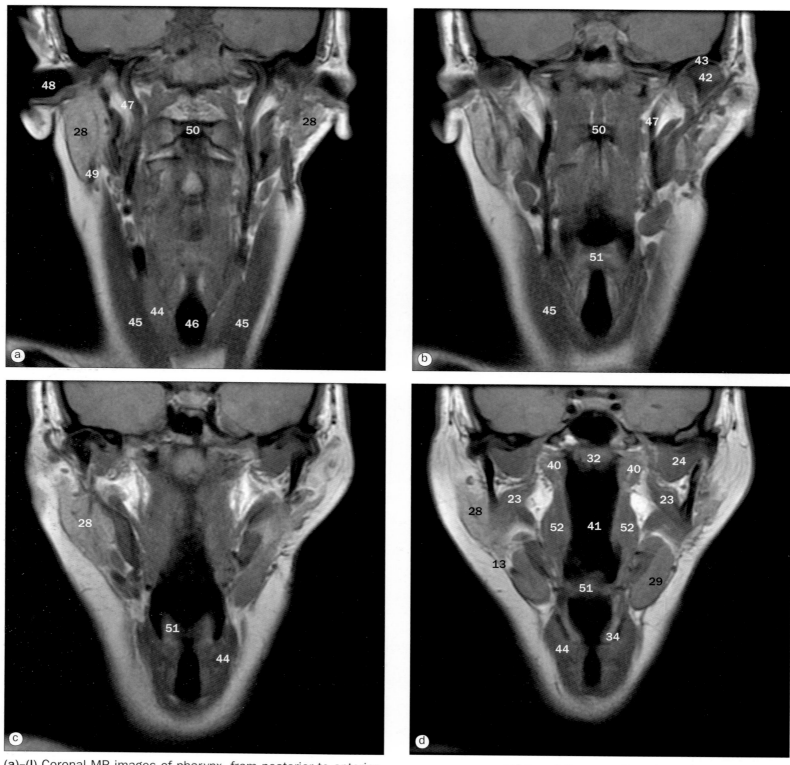

(a)–(l) Coronal MR images of pharynx, from posterior to anterior.

1 Maxillary sinus (antrum)	**8** Nasal septum
2 Hard palate	**9** Genioglossus muscle
3 Mandible	**10** Geniohyoid muscle
4 Alveolar ridge of maxilla	**11** Anterior belly of digastric muscle
5 Oral cavity	**12** Lingual septum
6 Inferior turbinate	**13** Platysmus muscle
7 Middle turbinate	**14** Hypoglossus muscle

The legends for pages 30–32 are common for all 3 pages.

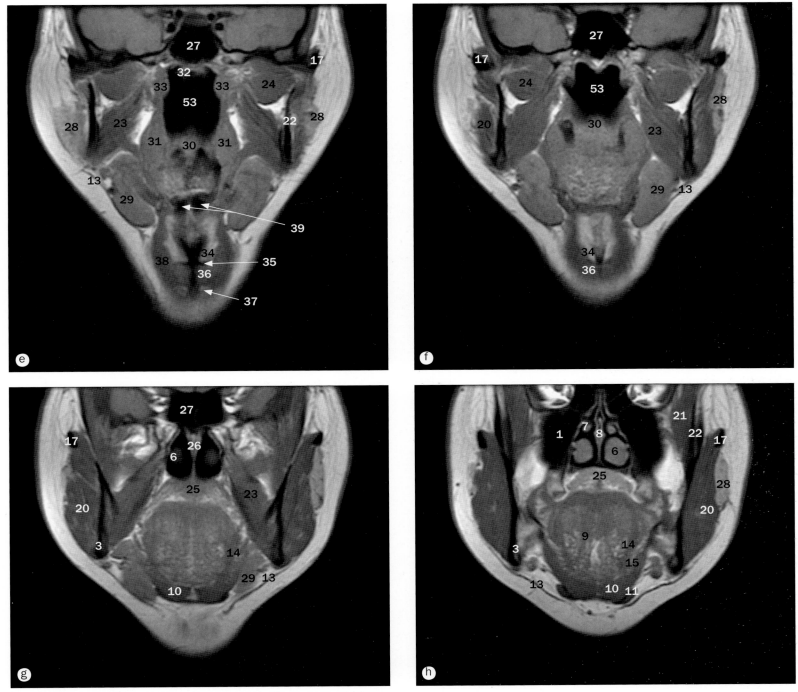

(a)–(l) Coronal MR images of pharynx, from posterior to anterior.

15 Mylohyoid muscle
16 Zygomatic bone
17 Zygomatic arch
18 Transverse muscle of tongue
19 Longitudinal muscle of tongue
20 Masseter muscle
21 Temporal muscle
22 Ramus of mandible
23 Medial pterygoid muscle

24 Lateral pterygoid muscle
25 Soft palate
26 Vomer
27 Sphenoid sinus (antrum)
28 Parotid gland
29 Submandibular gland
30 Uvula
31 Palatopharyngeus muscle
32 Pharyngeal tonsils

The legends for pages 30–32 are common for all 3 pages.

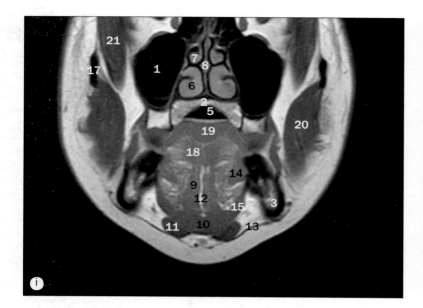

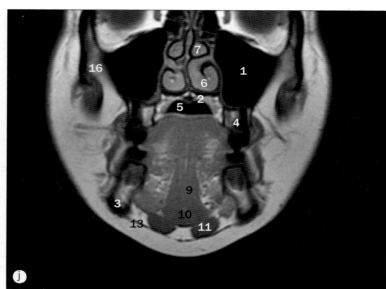

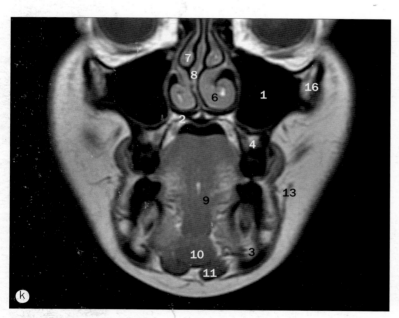

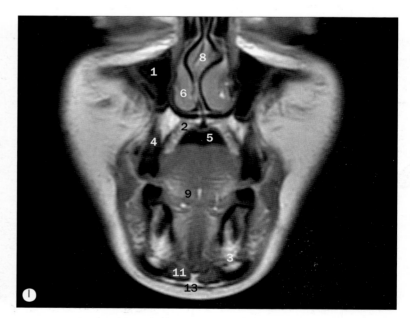

(a)–(l) Coronal MR images of pharynx, from posterior to anterior.

33 Levator veli palatini muscle
34 Vestibular fold
35 Larygneal ventricle
36 Vocalis muscle
37 Cricoid cartilage
38 Thyrohyoid muscle
39 Vallecula
40 Eustachian tubes
41 Oropharynx
42 Mandibular condyles
43 Temporomandibular joint

44 Thyroid gland
45 Sternocleidomastoid muscle
46 Trachea
47 Internal carotid artery
48 External auditory canal
49 Retromandibular vein
50 Anterior arch of C1
51 Epiglottis
52 Palatine tonsils
53 Nasopharynx

The legends for pages 30–32 are common for all 3 pages.

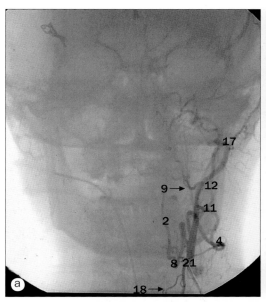

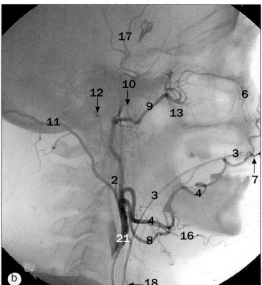

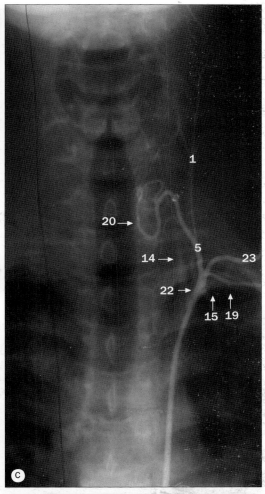

Digitally subtracted arteriograms of the external carotid artery, (a) anteróposterior projection, (b) lateral projection. (c) Thyroid arteriogram.

1 Ascending cervical artery	10 Middle meningeal artery	18 Superior thyroid artery
2 Ascending pharyngeal artery	11 Occipital artery	19 Suprascapular artery
	12 Posterior auricular artery	20 Thyroid branches of inferior thyroid artery
3 Endotracheal tube	13 Posterior superior alveolar artery	21 Tip of catheter in external carotid artery
4 Facial artery		
5 Inferior thyroid artery	14 Reflux of contrast into vertebral artery	
6 Infra-orbital artery		22 Tip of catheter in thyrocervical trunk
7 Labial branch of facial artery	15 Subclavian artery	
	16 Submental artery	23 Transverse cervical artery
8 Lingual artery	17 Superficial temporal artery	
9 Maxillary artery		

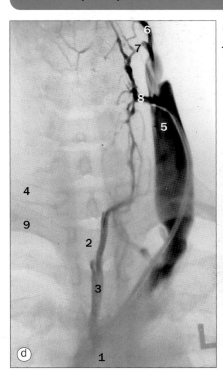

1 Left brachiocephalic vein	5 Internal jugular vein
2 Trachea	6 Lingual vein
3 Inferior thyroid vein	7 Superior thyroid vein
4 Transverse process of C7	8 Tip of catheter in middle thyroid vein
	9 Right first rib

1 Aortic arch	11 Right common carotid artery
2 Brachiocephalic artery	12 Left vertebral artery
3 Left common carotid artery	13 Superior vena cava
4 Left subclavian artery	14 External carotid artery
5 Left internal thoracic artery	15 Internal carotid artery
6 Right internal thoracic artery	16 Basilar artery
7 Right brachio-cephalic vein	17 Sigmoid sinus
8 Right lobe of the thyroid gland	18 Internal jugular vein
9 Costocervical trunk	19 Right subclavian vein
10 Right vertebral artery	20 Petrous portion of the internal carotid artery
	21 Right subclavian artery
	22 Jugular bulb

(d) Neck venogram.
(e) MR angiogram of neck vessels.

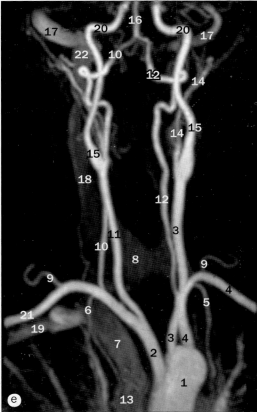

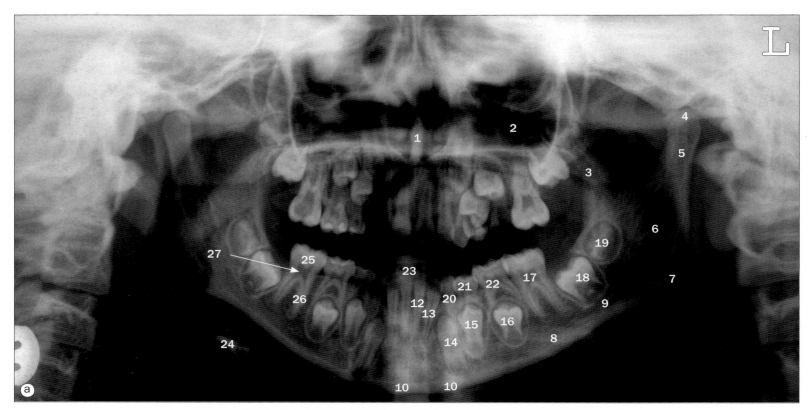

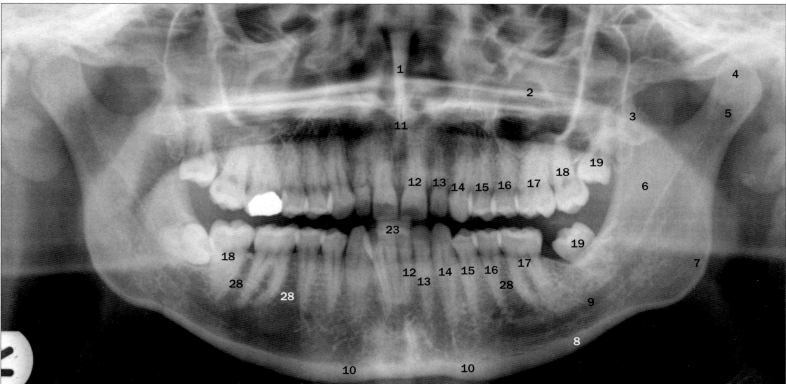

Dental panoramic tomogram (orthopantomogram) of (a) a 6-year-old child, (b) an adult.

1 Nasal septum	8 Mandibular body	15 Anterior premolar	22 Deciduous posterior premolar
2 Maxillary sinus (antrum)	9 Mandibular canal	16 Posterior premolar	23 Bite block
3 Coronoid process of mandible	10 Mental tubercle	17 First molar	24 Hyoid bone
4 Mandibular condylar head	11 Anterior nasal spine	18 Second molar	25 Crown of tooth
5 Mandibular condylar neck	12 Medial incisor	19 Third molar (wisdom tooth)	26 Root of tooth
6 Mandibular ramus	13 Lateral incisor	20 Deciduous canine tooth	27 Pulp chamber of tooth
7 Angle of mandible	14 Canine tooth	21 Deciduous anterior premolar	28 Alveolar bone

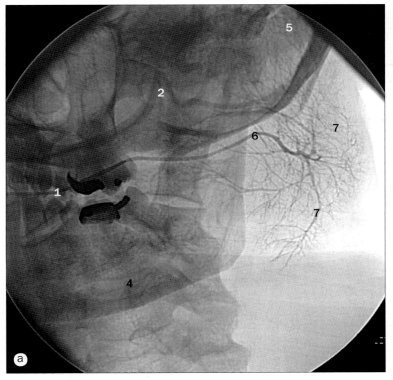

(a) Parotid sialogram.

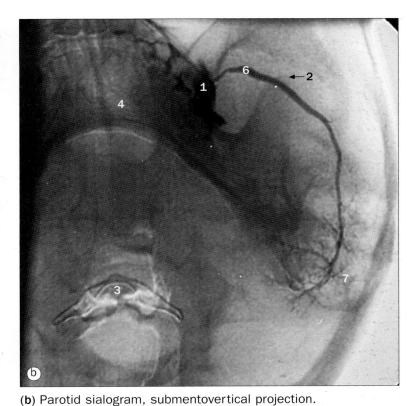

(b) Parotid sialogram, submentovertical projection.

1 Catheter
2 Coronoid process of mandible
3 Hyoid bone
4 Mandible
5 Mastoid process
6 Parotid (Stensen's) duct
7 Secondary ductules

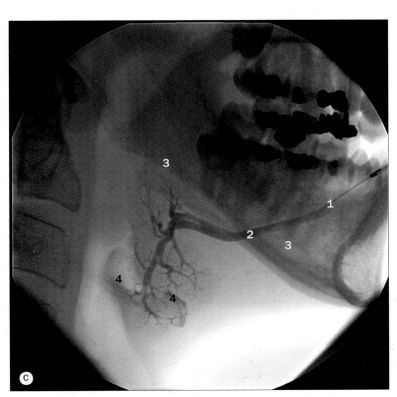

(c) Submandibular sialogram.

1 Catheter
2 Main submandibular (Wharton's) duct
3 Mandible
4 Secondary ductules

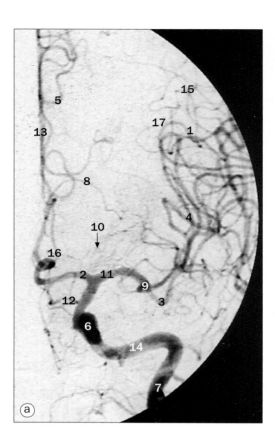

1 Angular branches of middle cerebral artery
2 Anterior cerebral artery
3 Anterior temporal branches of middle cerebral artery
4 Branches (in insula) of middle cerebral artery
5 Callosomarginal artery
6 Cavernous portion of internal carotid artery
7 Cervical portion of internal carotid artery
8 Frontopolar artery
9 Genu of middle cerebral artery
10 Lenticulostriate arteries
11 Middle cerebral artery
12 Orbitofrontal branch of pericallosal artery
13 Pericallosal artery
14 Petrous portion of internal carotid artery
15 Posterior parietal branches of middle cerebral artery
16 Recurrent artery of Heubner
17 Sylvian point

Digitally subtracted arterial phase of carotid arteriograms,
(a) anteroposterior projection, (b) lateral projection, (c) oblique
projection.

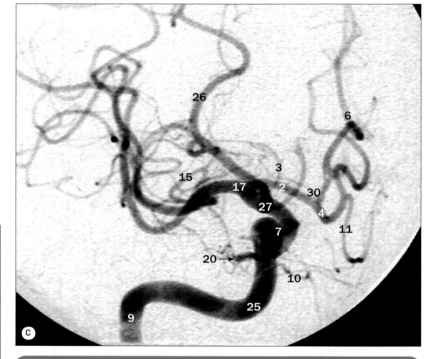

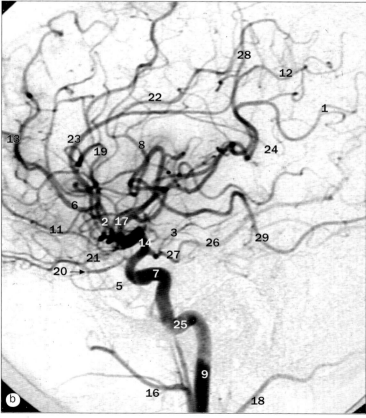

1 Angular artery
2 Anterior cerebral artery
3 Anterior choroidal artery
4 Anterior communicating artery
5 Anterior temporal artery
6 Callosomarginal artery
7 Cavernous portion of internal carotid artery
8 Central sulcus artery
9 Cervical portion of internal carotid artery
10 Ethmoidal branch of ophthalmic artery
11 Frontopolar artery
12 Inferior internal parietal artery
13 Internal frontal branch of anterior cerebral artery
14 Intracranial (supraclinoid) internal carotid artery
15 Lenticulostriate artery
16 Maxillary artery
17 Middle cerebral artery
18 Occipital artery
19 Operculofrontal artery
20 Ophthalmic artery
21 Orbitofrontal artery
22 Paracentral artery
23 Pericallosal artery
24 Pericallosal artery extending around corpus callosum
25 Petrous portion of internal carotid artery
26 Posterior cerebral artery
27 Posterior communicating artery
28 Posterior parietal artery
29 Posterior temporal artery
30 Recurrent artery of Heubner

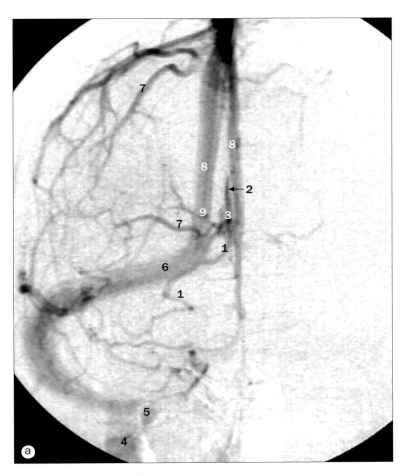

(a) Digitally subtracted venous phase of carotid arteriogram, anteroposterior projection.

1 Basal vein of Rosenthal
2 Inferior sagittal sinus
3 Internal cerebral vein
4 Internal jugular vein
5 Jugular bulb
6 Right transverse sinus
7 Superficial cortical veins
8 Superior sagittal sinus
9 Thalamostriate vein

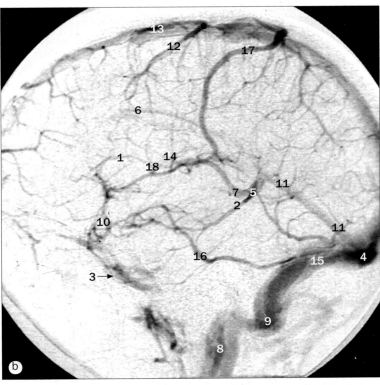

(b) Digitally subtracted venous phase of carotid arteriogram, lateral projection.

1 Anterior caudate vein
2 Basal vein of Rosenthal
3 Cavernous sinus
4 Confluence of venous sinuses (torcular Herophili)
5 Great cerebral vein of Galen
6 Inferior sagittal sinus
7 Internal cerebral vein
8 Internal jugular vein
9 Sigmoid sinus
10 Sphenoparietal sinus
11 Straight sinus
12 Superficial cerebral veins
13 Superior sagittal sinus
14 Thalamostriate vein
15 Transverse sinus
16 Vein of Labbé
17 Vein of Trolard
18 Venous angle

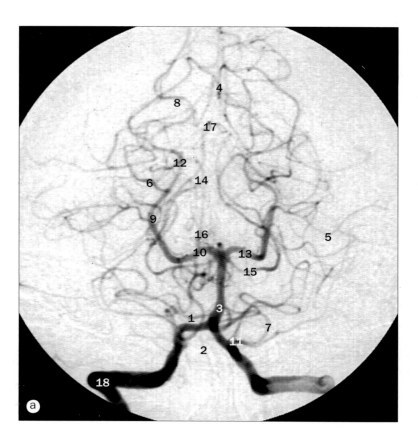

(a) Digitally subtracted arterial phase of vertebral arteriogram, anteroposterior projection.

1 Anterior inferior cerebellar artery
2 Anterior spinal artery
3 Basilar artery
4 Calcarine artery
5 Hemispheric branch of superior cerebellar artery
6 Inferior temporal artery
7 Medullary segment of posterior inferior cerebellar artery
8 Parieto-occipital artery
9 Posterior cerebral artery in ambient cistern
10 Posterior cerebral artery in interpeduncular cistern
11 Posterior inferior cerebellar artery
12 Quadrigeminal portion of posterior cerebral artery
13 Site of junction with posterior communicating artery
14 Superior cerebellar arteries behind brainstem
15 Superior cerebellar artery
16 Thalamoperforating branches of superior cerebellar artery
17 Vermian branch of superior cerebellar artery
18 Vertebral artery exiting transverse foramen of atlas (first cervical vertebra)

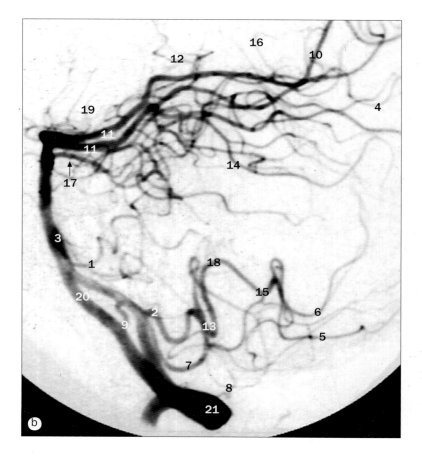

(b) Digitally subtracted arterial phase of vertebral arteriogram, lateral projection.

1 Anterior inferior cerebellar artery
2 Anterior medullary segment of posterior inferior cerebellar artery
3 Basilar artery
4 Calcarine artery
5 Hemispheric branches of posterior inferior cerebellar artery
6 Inferior vermian segment of posterior inferior cerebellar artery
7 Lateral medullary segment of posterior inferior cerebellar artery
8 Meningeal branch of vertebral artery
9 Origin of posterior inferior cerebellar artery
10 Parieto-occipital artery
11 Posterior cerebral artery
12 Posterior choroidal branches of posterior cerebral artery
13 Posterior medullary segment of posterior inferior cerebellar artery
14 Posterior temporal artery
15 Retrotonsillar segment of posterior inferior cerebellar artery
16 Splenial branches of posterior cerebral artery
17 Superior cerebellar artery
18 Supratonsillar segment of posterior inferior cerebellar artery
19 Thalamoperforate branches of posterior cerebral artery
20 Vertebral artery
21 Vertebral artery exiting transverse foramen of atlas (first cervical vertebra)

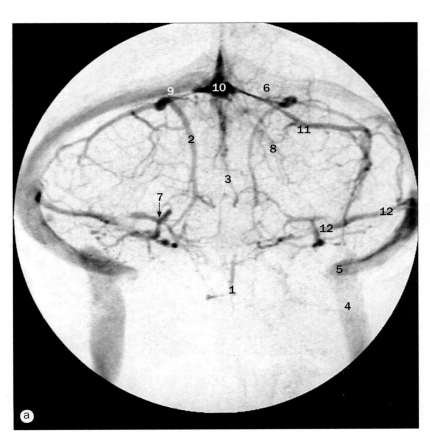

(a) Digitally subtracted venous phase of vertebral arteriogram, anteroposterior projection.

 1 Anterior pontomesencephalic vein
 2 Inferior hemispheric vein
 3 Inferior vermian vein
 4 Internal jugular vein
 5 Jugular bulb
 6 Left transverse sinus
 7 Petrosal vein
 8 Posterior mesencephalic vein
 9 Right transverse sinus
10 Straight sinus
11 Superior hemispheric vein
12 Superior petrosal sinus

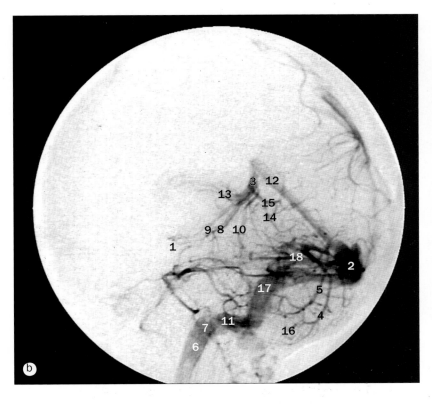

(b) Digitally subtracted venous phase of vertebral arteriogram, lateral projection.

 1 Anterior pontomesencephalic vein
 2 Confluence of venous sinuses (torcular Herophili)
 3 Great cerebral vein of Galen
 4 Inferior hemispheric vein
 5 Inferior vermian vein
 6 Internal jugular vein
 7 Jugular bulb
 8 Lateral mesencephalic vein
 9 Posterior mesencephalic vein
10 Precentral cerebellar vein
11 Sigmoid sinus
12 Straight sinus
13 Superior choroidal vein
14 Superior hemispheric vein
15 Superior vermian vein
16 Tonsillar vein
17 Transverse sinus
18 Vein of the great horizontal fissure

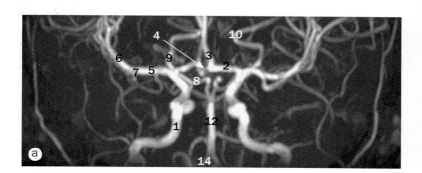

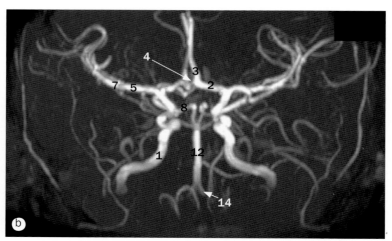

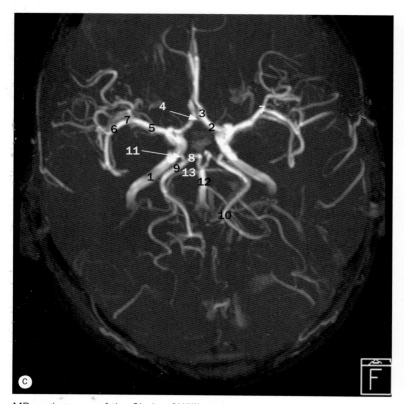

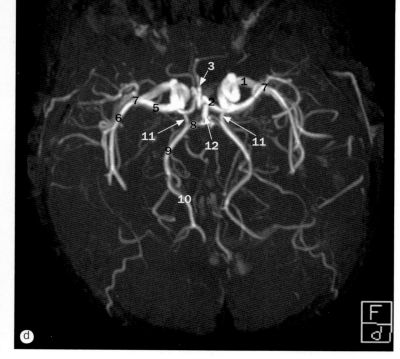

MR angiograms of the Circle of Willis, (**a**) and (**b**) coronal, (**c**) and (**d**) axial.

1 Internal carotid artery	**8** Precommunicating (P1) posterior cerebral artery (PCA) segment
2 Horizontal (A1) anterior cerebral artery (ACA) segment	**9** Ambient (P2) PCA segment
3 Vertical (A2) ACA segment	**10** Quadrigeminal (P3) PCA segment
4 Anterior communicating artery	**11** Posterior communicating artery
5 Horizontal (M1) middle cerebral artery (MCA) segment	**12** Basilar artery
6 Insular (M2) MCA segment	**13** Superior cerebellar artery
7 MCA genu (bifurcation)	**14** Vertebral artery

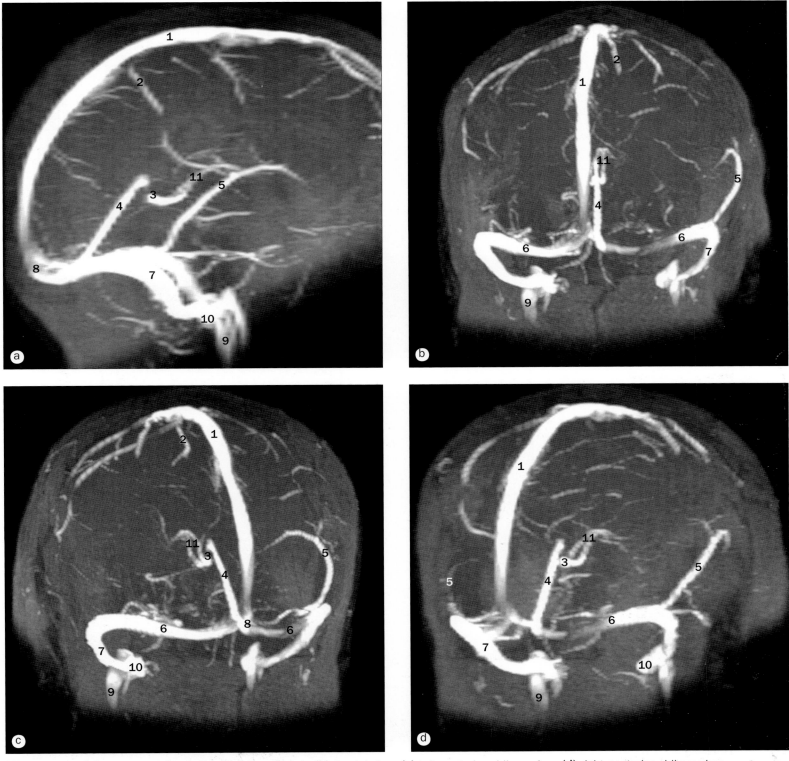

MR images of the venous circulation, (a) lateral view, (b) frontal view, (c) left posterior oblique view, (d) right posterior oblique view.

1 Superior sagittal sinus
2 Superficial cerebral veins
3 Vein of Galen
4 Straight sinus
5 Vein of Labbe'
6 Transverse sinus

7 Sigmoid sinus
8 Sinus confluence (torcular Herophilli)
9 Internal jugular vein
10 Jugular bulb
11 Internal cerebral vein

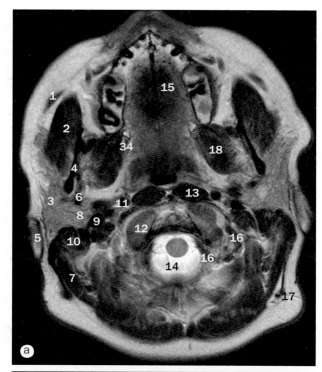

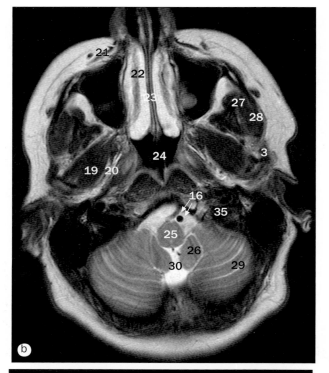

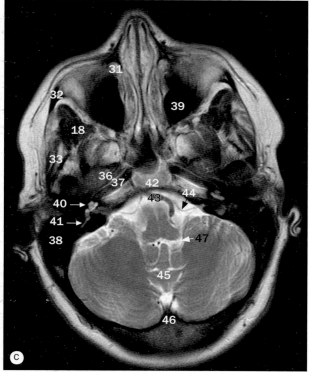

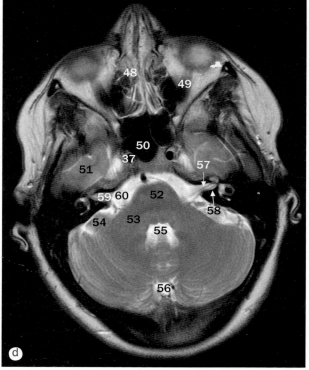

(a)–(n) Brain axial T2 images, from inferior to superior.

1 Parotid duct	**9** Internal jugular vein	**17** Occipital vessels	**24** Nasopharynx
2 Masseter muscle	**10** Mastoid process	**18** Medial pterygoid muscle	**25** Medulla oblongata
3 Parotid gland (superficial lobe)	**11** Internal carotid artery	**19** Lateral pterygoid muscle	**26** Cerebellar tonsil
4 Ramus of mandible	**12** Occipital condyle	**20** Lateral pterygoid plate	**27** Coronoid process of mandible
5 Pinna of ear	**13** Longus capitis muscle	**21** Levator labii superioris	**28** Temporalis muscle
6 Retromandibular vein	**14** Foramen magnum	alaeque nasi muscle	**29** Folia of cerebellar hemisphere
7 Sternocleidomastoid muscle	**15** Hard palate	**22** Inferior turbinate	**30** Foramen of Magendie
8 Parotid gland (deep lobe)	**16** Vertebral artery	**23** Nasal septum	

Numbers 1–161 are common to pages 42–45.

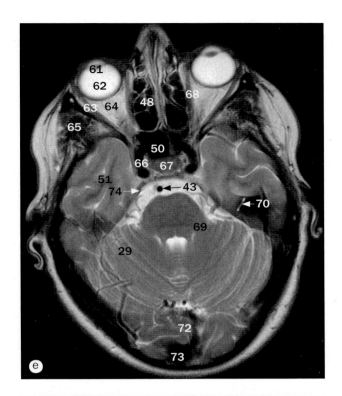

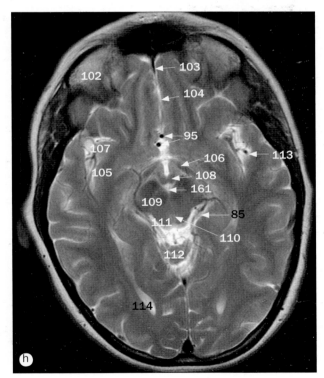

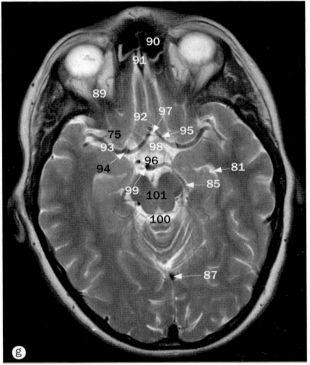

(a)–(n) Brain axial T2 images, from inferior to superior.

31 Nasolacrimal duct	**40** Cochlear	**48** Ethmoid air cells	**56** Cisterna magna
32 Zygomatic arch	**41** Posterior semicircular canal	**49** Inferior rectus muscle	**57** Facial nerve (seventh cranial nerve)
33 Head of mandible	**42** Clivus	**50** Sphenoid sinus	
34 Medial pterygoid plate	**43** Basilar artery	**51** Temporal lobe	**58** Vestibulocochlear nerve (eighth cranial nerve)
35 Jugular foramen	**44** Labyrinthine artery	**52** Pons	
36 Petrous temporal bone	**45** Inferior cerebellar vermis	**53** Middle cerebellar peduncle	**59** Internal auditory meatus
37 Internal carotid artery	**46** Inion (internal occipital protuberance)	**54** Flocculonodular lobe of cerebellum	**60** Cerebellopontine angle
38 Mastoid air cells		**55** Fourth ventricle	
39 Maxillary sinus (antrum)	**47** Foramen of Lushka		

Numbers 1–161 are common to pages 42–45.

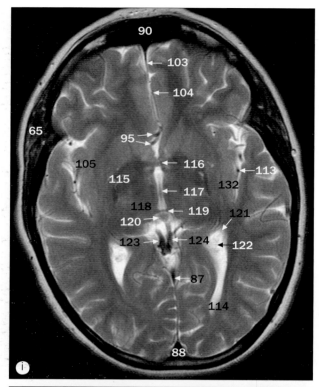

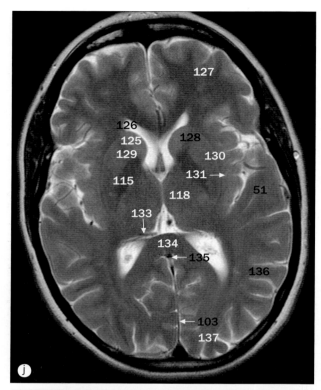

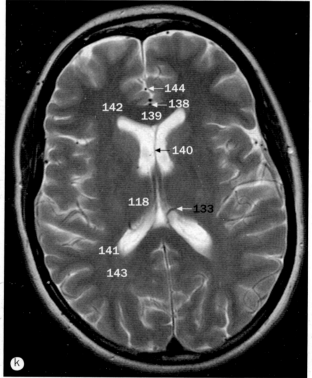

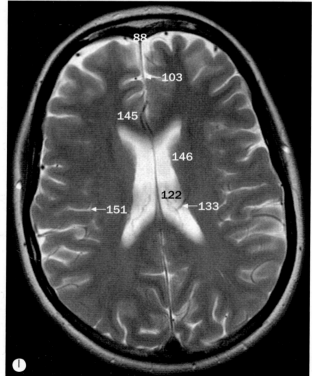

(a)–(n) Brain axial T2 images, from inferior to superior.

61 Lens	**67** Body of sphenoid	**73** Torcula herophili (confluence of venous sinuses)
62 Vitreous humour	**68** Medial rectus muscle	**74** Petroclinoid ligament
63 Lateral rectus muscle	**69** Superior cerebellar peduncle	**75** Optic nerve (second cranial nerve)
64 Retro-orbital fat	**70** Superior semicircular canal	**76** Infundibulum of frontal sinus
65 Temporalis muscle	**71** Superior cerebellar vermis	**77** Lacrimal gland
66 Internal carotid artery (cavernous part)	**72** Calcarine cortex of occipital lobe	

78 Superior ophthalmic vein
79 Pituitary gland
80 Internal carotid artery (supraclinoid part)
81 Temporal horn of lateral ventricle
82 Uncus of temporal lobe

Numbers 1–161 are common to pages 42–45.

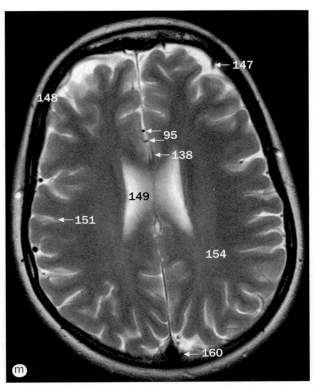

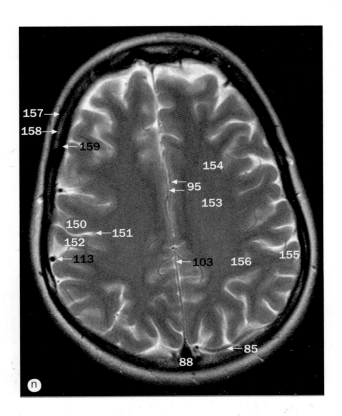

(a)-(n) Brain axial T2 images, from inferior to superior.

83 Hippocampus	103 Falx cerebri	121 Trigone of lateral ventricle	140 Septum pellucidum
84 Ambient cistern	104 Interhemispheric fissure	122 Choroid plexus	141 Optic radiation
85 Posterior cerebral artery	105 Insular gyri	123 Basal vein (of Rosenthal)	142 Forceps minor
86 Inferior colliculus	106 Optic tract	124 Internal cerebral vein (of Galen)	143 Forceps major
87 Straight sinus	107 Sylvian fissure (lateral sulcus)	125 Head of caudate nucleus	144 Frontopolar artery
88 Superior sagittal sinus	108 Mamillary body (of hypothalamus)	126 Frontal horn of lateral ventricle	145 Cingulate gyrus
89 Superior rectus muscle	109 Cerebral peduncle	127 Frontal lobe	146 Body of caudate nucleus
90 Frontal sinus	110 Aqueduct of Sylvius	128 Anterior limb of internal capsule	147 Cortical vein
91 Crista gali	111 Superior colliculus	129 Globus pallidus	148 Calvarium of skull
92 Olfactory nerve (first cranial nerve)	112 Folia of cerebellum	130 Putamen	149 Body (atrium) of lateral ventricle
93 Middle cerebral artery	113 Middle cerebral artery (second order branch)	131 External capsule	150 Precentral gyrus
94 Bifurcation of internal carotid artery	114 Occipital horn of lateral ventricle	132 Claustrum	151 Central sulcus of Rolando
95 Anterior cerebral artery	115 Posterior limb of internal capsule	133 Choroidal vessels	152 Post central gyrus
96 Suprasellar cistern	116 Anterior commisure	134 Splenium of corpus callosum	153 Centrum semiovale
97 Anterior communicating artery	117 Third ventricle	135 Inferior sagittal sinus	154 Corona radiata
98 Optic chiasma	118 Thalamus	136 Parietal lobe	155 Grey matter
99 Basilar artery bifurcation	119 Posterior commisure	137 Occipital lobe	156 White matter
100 Quadrigeminal cistern	120 Pineal gland	138 Callosomarginal artery	157 Outer table of calvarium
101 Midbrain (mesencephalon)		139 Genu of corpus callosum	158 Diploe
102 Orbital plate of frontal bone			159 Inner table of calvarium
			160 Arachnoid granulation
			161 Interpeduncular cistern

Numbers 1–161 are common to pages 42–45.

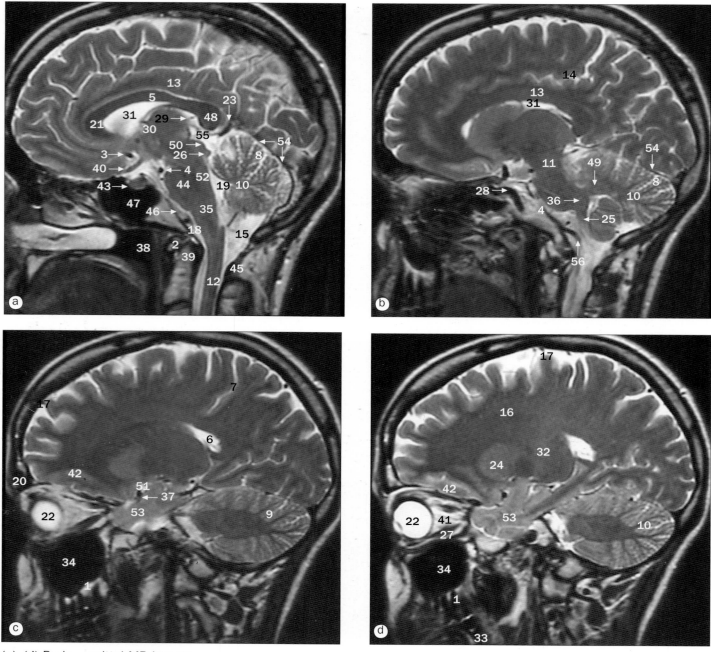

(a)–(d) Brain, sagittal MR images.

1 Alveolar ridge
2 Anterior arch of atlas (first cervical vertebra)
3 Anterior cerebral artery
4 Basilar artery
5 Body of corpus callosum
6 Body of lateral ventricle
7 Central sulcus of Rolando
8 Cerebellar folia
9 Cerebellar hemisphere
10 Cerebellum
11 Cerebral peduncle
12 Cervical spinal cord
13 Cingulate gyrus
14 Cingulate sulcus
15 Cisterna magna (cerebellomedullary cistern)
16 Corona radiata
17 Cortical vein
18 Foramen magnum
19 Fourth ventricle
20 Frontal sinus
21 Genu of corpus callosum
22 Globe
23 Great cerebral vein of Galen
24 Head of caudate nucleus
25 Inferior cerebellar peduncle
26 Inferior colliculus
27 Inferior rectus muscle
28 Internal carotid artery (in cavernous sinus)
29 Internal cerebral vein
30 Interventricular foramen of Monro
31 Lateral ventricle
32 Lentiform nucleus
33 Mandible
34 Maxillary sinus (antrum)
35 Medulla oblongata
36 Middle cerebellar peduncle
37 Middle cerebral artery
38 Nasopharynx
39 Odontoid process (dens)
40 Optic chiasma in suprasellar cistern
41 Optic nerve
42 Orbital cortex of frontal lobe
43 Pituitary gland
44 Pons
45 Posterior arch of atlas
46 Prepontine cistern
47 Sphenoidal sinus
48 Splenium of corpus callosum
49 Superior cerebellar peduncle
50 Superior colliculus
51 Sylvian fissure
52 Tegmentum of pons
53 Temporal lobe of brain
54 Tentorium cerebelli
55 Pineal gland
56 Vertebral artery

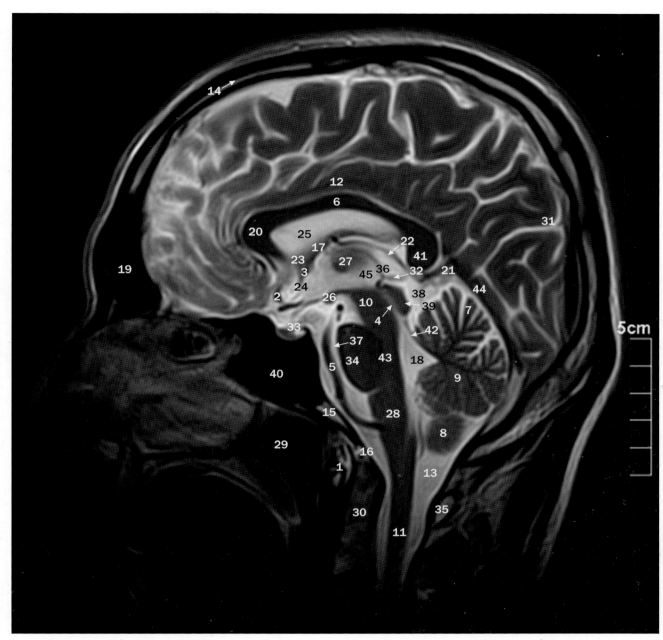

Brain, sagittal MR midline image.

1 Anterior arch of atlas (first cervical vertebra)
2 Anterior cerebral artery
3 Anterior commissure
4 Aqueduct of Sylvius
5 Basilar artery
6 Body of corpus callosum
7 Cerebellar folia
8 Cerebellar tonsil
9 Cerebellum
10 Cerebral peduncle of midbrain
11 Cervical spinal cord
12 Cingulate gyrus
13 Cisterna magna (cerebellomedullary cistern)
14 Diploe of calvarium

15 Fat in marrow of clivus
16 Foramen magnum
17 Fornix
18 Fourth ventricle
19 Frontal sinus
20 Genu of corpus callosum
21 Great cerebral vein of Galen
22 Internal cerebral vein
23 Interventricular foramen of Monro
24 Lamina terminalis
25 Lateral ventricle
26 Mammillary body
27 Massa intermedia of thalamus
28 Medulla oblongata
29 Nasopharynx
30 Odontoid process (dens)

31 Parieto-occipital fissure
32 Pineal gland
33 Pituitary gland
34 Pons
35 Posterior arch of atlas
36 Posterior commissure
37 Prepontine cistern
38 Quadrigeminal cistern
39 Quadrigeminal plate (tectum) of midbrain
40 Sphenoidal sinus
41 Splenium of corpus callosum
42 Superior medullary velum
43 Tegmentum of pons
44 Tentorium cerebelli
45 Third ventricle

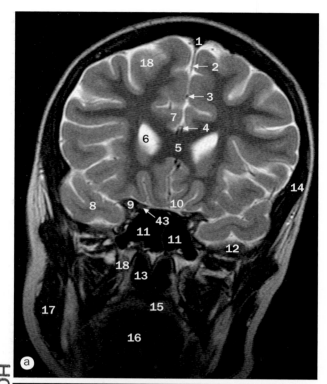

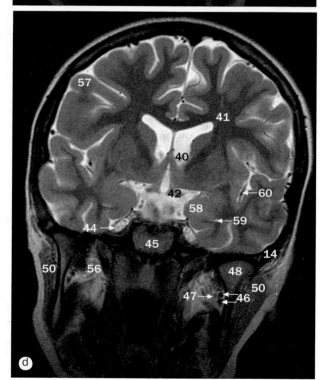

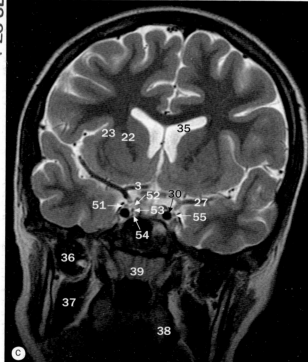

(a)–(p) Brain, coronal T2w MR images, from anterior to posterior.

1	Superior sagittal sinus	9	Anterior clinoid process	18	Frontal lobe
2	Falx cerebri	10	Olfactory cortex	19	Body of corpus callosum
3	Anterior cerebral artery	11	Sphenoidal sinus	20	Septum pellucidum
4	Callosomarginal artery	12	Greater wing of sphenoid	21	Head of caudate nucleus
5	Genu of corpus callosum	13	Nasopharynx	22	Anterior limb of internal capsule
6	Frontal horn of lateral ventricle	14	Temporalis muscle	23	External capsule
7	Cingulate gyrus	15	Hard palate	24	Insula gyrus
8	Temporal lobe	16	Oropharynx	25	Sylvian fissure (lateral sulcus)
		17	Masseter muscle		

26	Putamen
27	Middle cerebral artery
28	Supraclinoid part of internal carotid artery
29	Dural lateral wall of cavernous sinus
30	Internal carotid artery
31	Pituitary gland
32	Optic chiasma

Numbers 1–130 are common to pages 48–51.

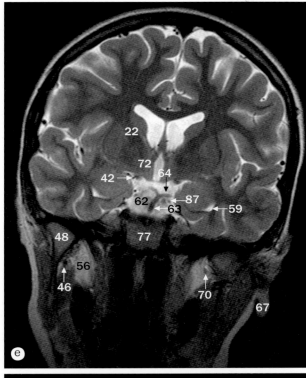

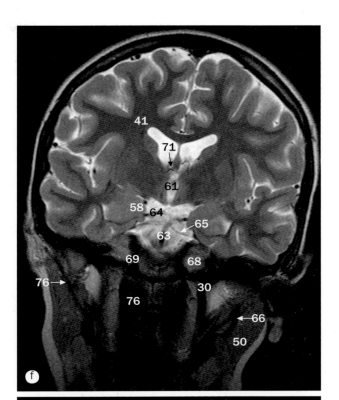

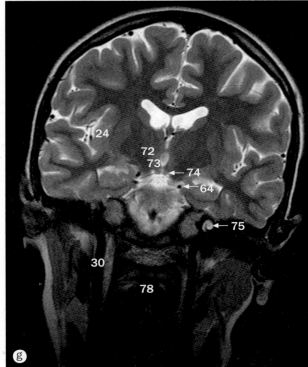

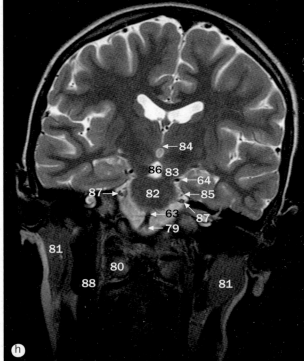

(a)–(p) Brain, coronal T2w MR images, from anterior to posterior.

33 Suprasellar cistern	**42** Optic tract
34 Globus pallidus	**43** Optic nerve (second cranial nerve)
35 Body (atrium) of lateral ventricle	**44** Trigeminal ganglion in Meckel's cave
36 Lateral pterygoid muscle	**45** Body of sphenoid
37 Medial pterygoid muscle	**46** Inferior alveolar vessels
38 Tongue	**47** Inferior alveolar nerve
39 Soft palate	**48** Head of mandible
40 Choroid plexus	**49** Coronoid process of mandible
41 Corona radiata	

50 Parotid gland	**55** Abducens nerve (sixth cranial nerve)
51 Occulomotor nerve (third cranial nerve)	**56** Infratemporal fossa
52 Trochlear nerve (fourth cranial nerve)	**57** Parietal lobe
53 Ophthalmic nerve (fifth cranial nerve, first division)	**58** Hippocampus
54 Maxillary nerve (fifth cranial nerve, second division)	**59** Temporal horn of lateral ventricle
	60 Middle cerebral artery (second order branch)
	61 Third ventricle

Numbers 1–130 are common to pages 48–51.

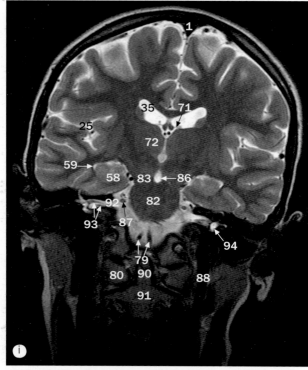

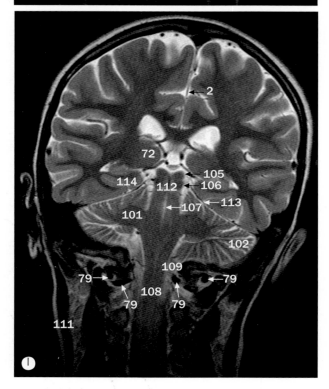

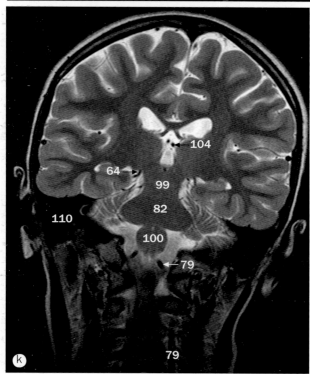

(a)–(p) Brain, coronal T2w MR images, from anterior to posterior.

62 Prepontine cistern	72 Thalamus	82 Pons	90 Odontoid peg of C2
63 Basilar artery	73 Hypothalamus	83 Cerebral peduncle	91 Body of C2
64 Posterior cerebral artery	74 Mamillary body (of	84 Massa intermedia of	92 Internal auditory meatus
65 Superior cerebellar artery	hypothalamus)	thalamus	93 Facial (seventh) and
66 Retromandibular vein	75 Cochlea	85 Abducens nerve (sixth cranial	vestibulocochlear (eighth)
67 Tragus of external ear	76 Pharyngobasilar raphe	nerve) in ambient cistern	nerves
68 Basiocciput	77 Basisphenoid	86 Interpeduncular cistern	94 Vestibule of vestibular
69 Spheno-occipital	78 Anterior arch of C1	87 Trigeminal nerve (fifth cranial	apparatus
synchondrosis	79 Vertebral artery	nerve)	95 Arcuate eminence of petrous
70 Auriculotemporal nerve	80 Lateral mass of C1	88 Internal jugular vein	temporal bone
71 Foramen of Monro	81 Sternocleidomastoid muscle	89 Body of caudate nucleus	96 Superior semicircular canal

Numbers 1–130 are common to pages 48–51.

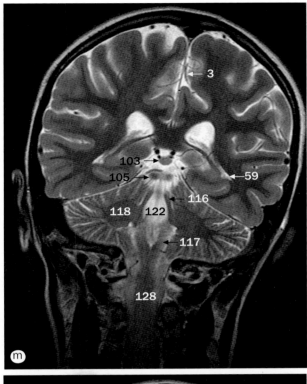

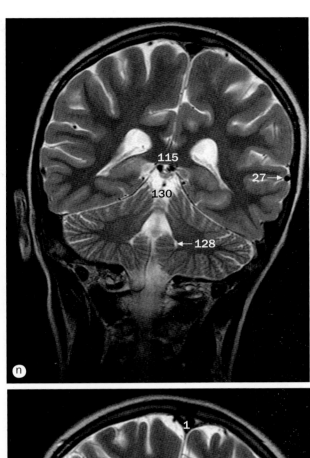

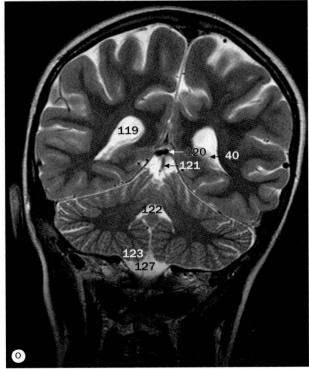

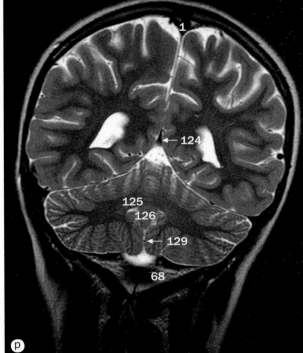

(a)–(p) Brain, coronal T2w MR images, from anterior to posterior.

97 Horizontal (lateral) semicircular canal	106 Inferior colliculus	115 Splenium of corpus callosum	123 Cerebellar tonsil
98 Posterior semicircular canal	107 Aqueduct of Sylvius	116 Superior cerebellar peduncle	124 Inferior sagittal sinus
99 Midbrain (mesencephalon)	108 Spinal cord	117 Inferior cerebellar peduncle	125 Dentate nucleus of cerebellum
100 Medulla oblongata	109 Foramen magnum	118 Cerebellar hemisphere	126 Nodule of cerebellum
101 Middle cerebellar peduncle	110 Mastoid air cells	119 Trigone of lateral ventricle	127 Cisterna magna
102 Cerebellar folia	111 Trapezius muscle	120 Internal cerebral vein (of Galen)	128 Lateral foramen (of Lushka)
103 Pineal gland	112 Tectum (quadrigeminal plate) of midbrain	121 Basal vein (of Rosenthal)	129 Medial foramen (of Magendie)
104 Internal cerebral veins	113 Tentorium cerebelli	122 Fourth ventricle	130 Quadrigeminal cistern
105 Superior colliculus	114 Uncus of temporal lobe		

Numbers 1–130 are common to pages 48–51.

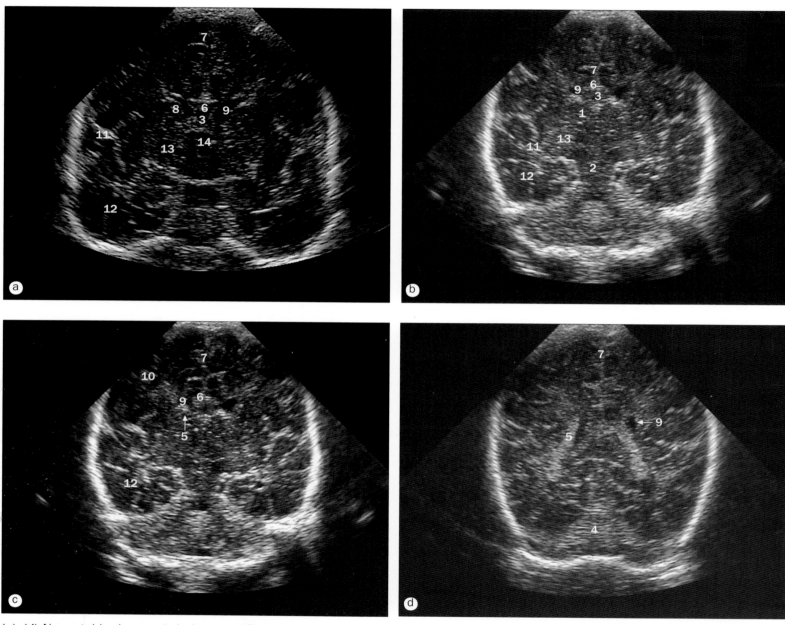

(a)–(d) Neonatal brain, coronal ultrasound images.

1 Body of caudate nucleus
2 Brainstem
3 Cavum septum pellucidum
4 Cerebellum
5 Choroid plexus
6 Corpus callosum
7 Falx cerebri
8 Head of caudate nucleus
9 Lateral ventricle
10 Parietal lobe of brain
11 Sylvian fissure
12 Temporal lobe
13 Thalamus
14 Third ventricle

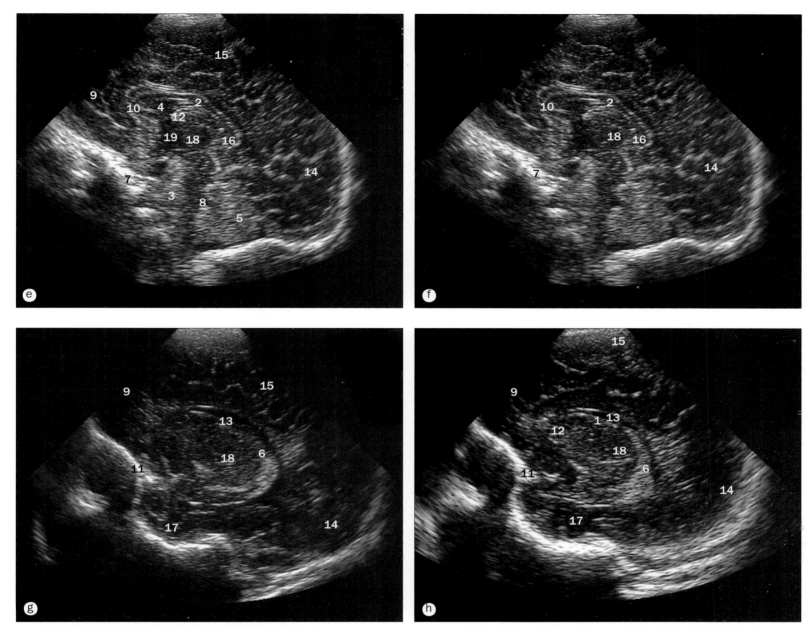

(e)–(h) Neonatal brain, sagittal ultrasound images.

1 Body of caudate nucleus	**11** Greater wing of sphenoid
2 Body of corpus callosum	**12** Head of caudate nucleus
3 Brainstem	**13** Lateral ventricle
4 Cavum septum pellucidum	**14** Occipital lobe
5 Cerebellum	**15** Parietal lobe of brain
6 Choroid plexus	**16** Splenium of corpus callosum
7 Clivus	**17** Temporal lobe
8 Fourth ventricle	**18** Thalamus
9 Frontal lobe	**19** Third ventricle
10 Genu of corpus callosum	

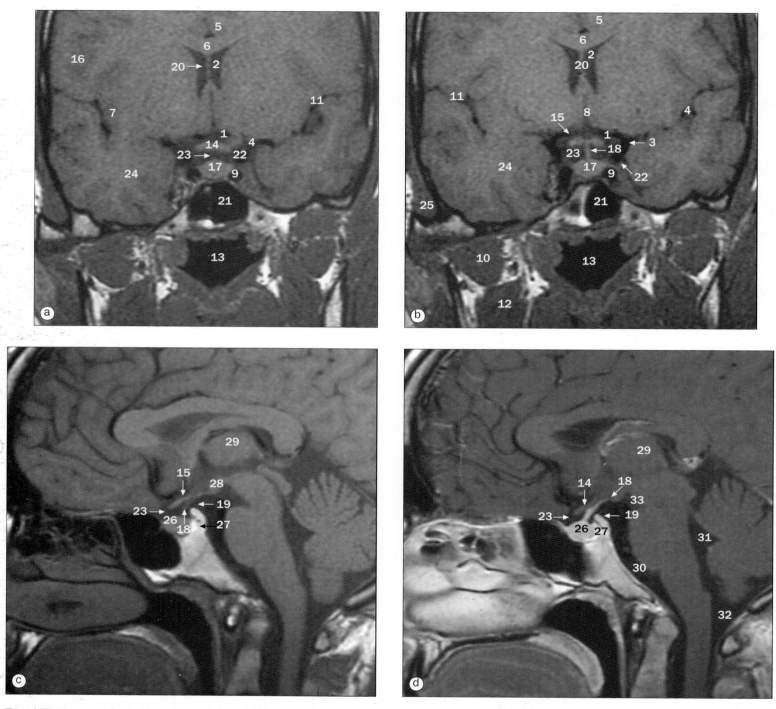

T1w MR images of pituitary fossa (**a**) and (**b**) coronal, (**c**) sagittal, (**d**) sagittal post gadolinium.

1 Anterior cerebral artery	7 Insula	15 Optic tract	25 Temporalis muscle
2 Anterior horn of lateral ventricle	8 Interhemispheric fissure	16 Parietal lobe of brain	26 Anterior pituitary gland
3 Bifurcation of internal carotid artery	9 Internal carotid artery in cavernous sinus	17 Pituitary gland	27 Posterior pituitary gland
	10 Lateral pterygoid muscle	18 Pituitary stalk	28 Mammillary body
4 Branch of middle cerebral artery in lateral sulcus (Sylvian fissure)	11 Lateral sulcus (Sylvian fissure)	19 Posterior clinoid process	29 Thalamus
	12 Medial pterygoid muscle	20 Septum pellucidum	30 Prepontine cistern
	13 Nasopharynx	21 Sphenoidal sinus	31 Fourth ventricle
5 Cingulate gyrus	14 Optic chiasma	22 Supraclinoid carotid artery	32 Cisterna magna
6 Corpus callosum		23 Suprasellar cistern	33 Interpeduncular cistern
		24 Temporal lobe of brain	

2 Vertebral column and spinal cord

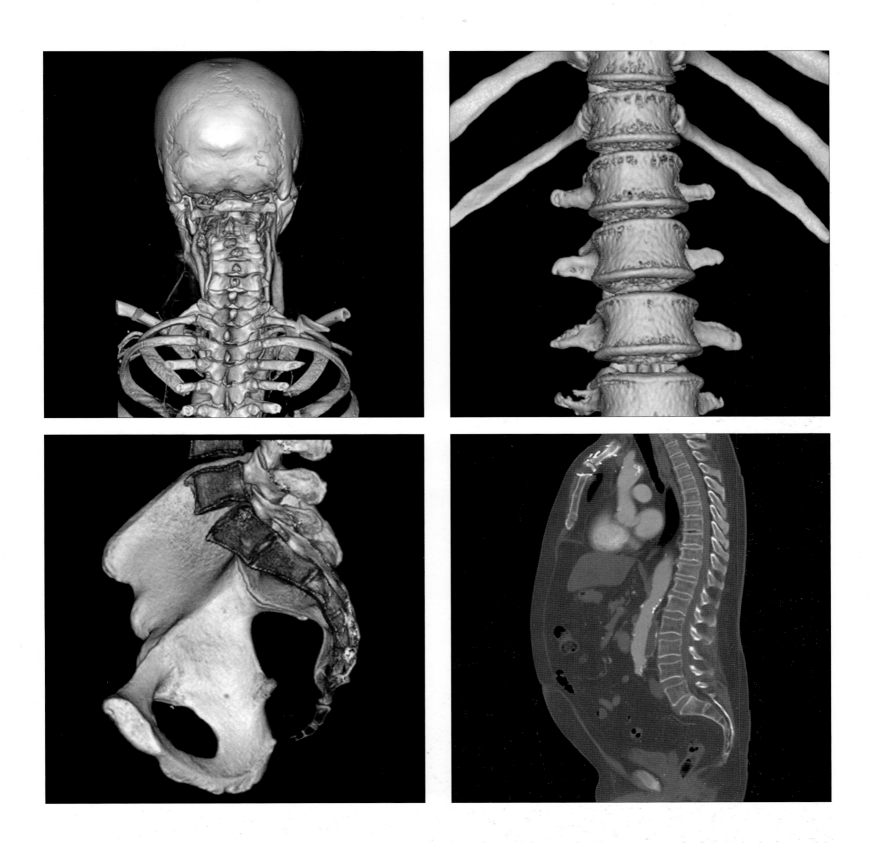

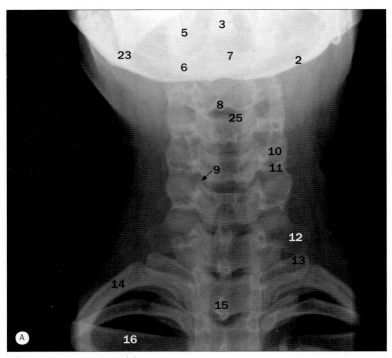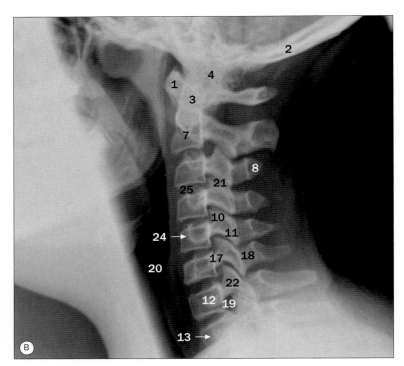

(a) Cervical spine, anteroposterior projection, (b) cervical spine, lateral projection.

1 Anterior arch of atlas	9 Uncovertebral joint (Lushka) of	15 Spinous process of T1	21 Facet (zygaphophyseal joint) of
2 Basiocciput	C5/6	16 Clavicle	C3/4
3 Odontoid peg (of axis)	10 Superior articular process of	17 Pedicle of C6	22 Pars interarticularis of C7
4 Occipital condyle	C5	18 Lamina of C6	23 Angle of mandible
5 Lateral mass of atlas (C1)	11 Inferior articular process of C5	19 Intervertebral foramen of C7/	24 Transverse process of C5
6 Lateral mass of axis (C2)	12 Transverse process of C7	T1 (for C8 root)	25 Intervertebral disc at C3/4
7 Body of axis (C2)	13 Transverse process of T1	20 Epiglottis	
8 Spinous process of C3	14 First rib		

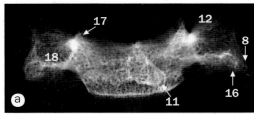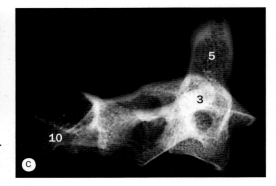

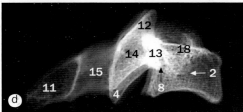

X-ray films of dessicated cervical vertebrae.
(a) AP view C4.
(b) Lateral view C1.
(c) Lateral view C2.
(d) Lateral view C4.

1 Anterior arch of atlas (first cervical vertebra)	vertebra)	12 Superior articular process (facet) of fourth cervical vertebra
2 Anterior tubercle of transverse process of fourth cervical vertebra	7 Body of atlas (first cervical vertebra)	13 Pedicle of C4
3 Body of axis (second cervical vertebra)	8 Posterior tubercle of transverse process of fourth cervical vertebra	14 Pars interarticularis of C4
4 Inferior articular process (facet) of fourth cervical vertebra	9 Posterior tubercle of atlas (first cervical vertebra)	15 Lamina of C4
5 Odontoid process (dens) of axis (second cervical vertebra)	10 Spinous process of axis (second cervical vertebra)	16 Intertubercular lamella of C4 transverse process
6 Posterior arch of atlas (first cervical	11 Spinous process of fourth cervical vertebra	17 Posterolateral lip (uncus) of C4
		18 Body of transverse process of C4

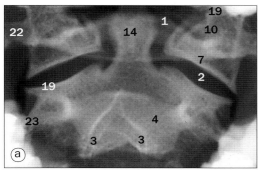

(a)

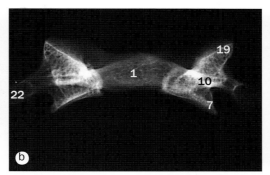

(b)

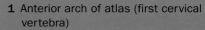

(c)

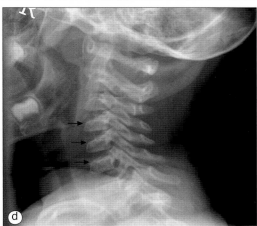

(d)

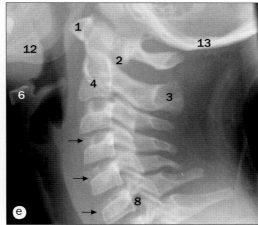

(e)

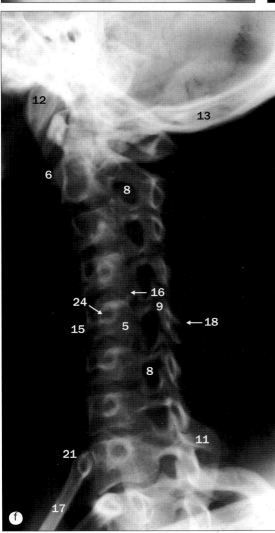

(f)

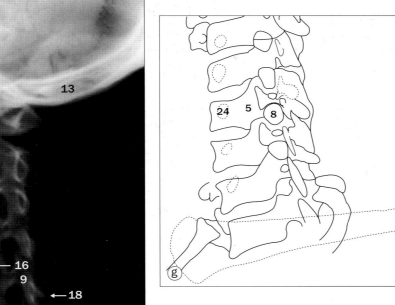

(g)

1 Anterior arch of atlas (first cervical vertebra)
2 Atlanto-axial joint
3 Bifid spinous process of axis (second cervical vertebra)
4 Body of axis (second cervical vertebra)
5 Body of fifth cervical vertebra
6 Hyoid bone
7 Inferior articular process (facet) of atlas (first cervical vertebra)
8 Intervertebral foramen
9 Lamina of fifth cervical vertebra
10 Lateral mass of atlas (first cervical vertebra)
11 Left first rib
12 Mandible
13 Occipital bone
14 Odontoid process (dens) of axis (second cervical vertebra)
15 Posterior tubercle of transverse process of fifth cervical vertebra
16 Posterolateral lip (uncus) of fifth cervical vertebra
17 Right first rib
18 Spinous process of fifth cervical vertebra
19 Superior articular process (facet) of atlas (first cervical vertebra)
20 Superior articular process (facet) of axis (second cervical vertebra)
21 Trachea
22 Transverse process of atlas (first cervical vertebra)
23 Transverse process of axis (second cervical vertebra)
24 Transverse process of fifth cervical vertebra

(a) Atlas (first cervical vertebra) and axis (second cervical vertebra), 'open mouth' anteroposterior projection.
(b) Dried atlas (first cervical vertebra), anteroposterior projection.
(c) Dried axis (second cervical vertebra), anteroposterior projection.
(d) Cervical spine X-ray of a 3 year old, lateral projection. The atlanto-axial joint can normally be up to 5 mm (up to 3 mm in adults).
(e) Cervical spine X-ray of a 9 year old, lateral projection. Note normal physiological wedging of the vertebral bodies (arrows) due to unossified superior endplate apophyses.
(f) Oblique X-ray of adult cervical spine.
(g) Line drawing of (f).

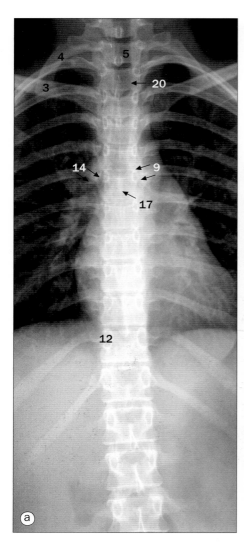

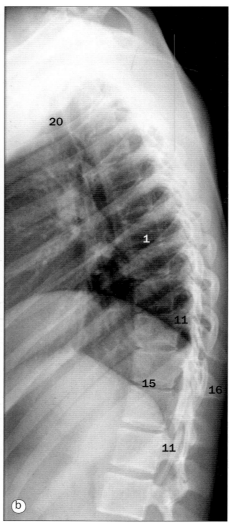

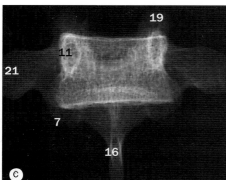

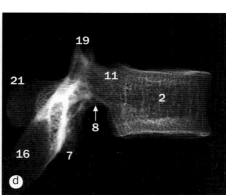

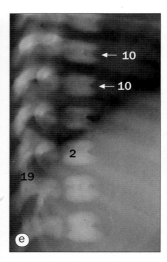

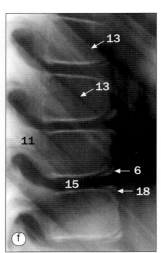

1   Body of sixth thoracic vertebra
2   Body of vertebra
3   Clavicle
4   First rib
5   First thoracic vertebra
6   Inferior annular epiphysial discs for vertebral body
7   Inferior articular process (facet)
8   Inferior vertebral notch
9   Left main bronchus
10 Natal cleft
11 Pedicle
12 Pedicle of eleventh thoracic vertebra
13 Ribs
14 Right main bronchus
15 Site of intervertebral disc
16 Spinous process
17 Spinous process of sixth thoracic vertebra
18 Superior annular epiphysial discs for vertebral body
19 Superior articular process (facet)
20 Trachea
21 Transverse process

(a) Thoracic spine, anteroposterior projection.

(b) Thoracic spine, lateral projection.

(c) Dried thoracic vertebra, anteroposterior projection.

(d) Dried sixth thoracic vertebra, lateral projection.

Thoracic spine, (e) of a 7-day-old neonate, (f) of a 12-year-old child, lateral projections.

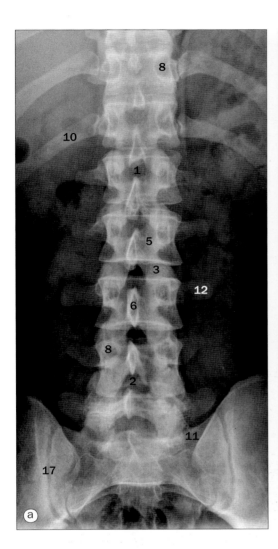

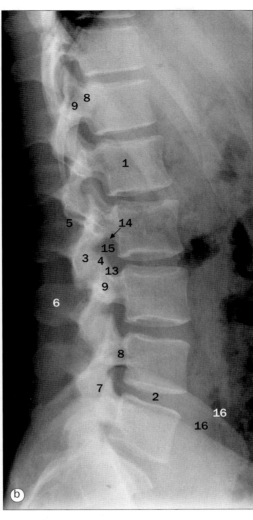

(a) Lumbar spine, anteroposterior radiograph.

(b) Lumbar spine, lateral projection.

(c) Dried second lumbar vertebra, anteroposterior projection.

(d) Dried second lumbar vertebra, lateral projection.

(e) Lumbar spine, oblique projection.

1 Body of first lumbar vertebra
2 Intervertebral disc L4/5
3 Inferior articular process (facet) of L2
4 Superior articular process (facet) L3
5 Lamina of L2
6 Spinous process of L3
7 Facet (zygapophyseal joint) of L4/5
8 Pedicle
9 Pars interarticularis
10 Right twelfth rib
11 Sacral promontory
12 Transverse process of L3
13 Mamillary process
14 Inferior vertebral notch of L2
15 Neural foramen of L2/3 (for L2 root)
16 Iliac crest
17 Sacroiliac joint

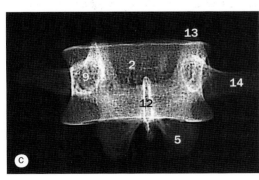

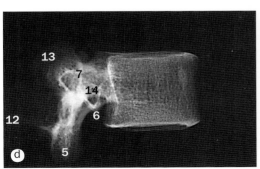

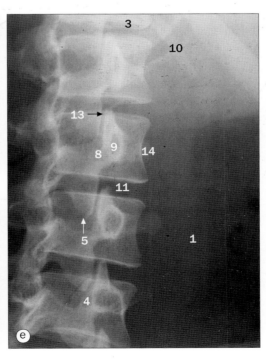

1 Psoas muscle outline
2 Body of second lumbar vertebra
3 Body of twelfth thoracic vertebra
4 Body of fourth lumbar vertebra
5 Inferior articular process (facet) of second lumbar vertebra
6 Inferior vertebral notch of second lumbar vertebra
7 Mamillary process of second lumbar vertebra
8 Pars interarticularis
9 Pedicle of second lumbar vertebra
10 Twelfth rib
11 Intervertebral disc space between L2 and L3
12 Spinous process of second lumbar vertebra
13 Superior articular process (facet) of second lumbar vertebra
14 Transverse process of second lumbar vertebra

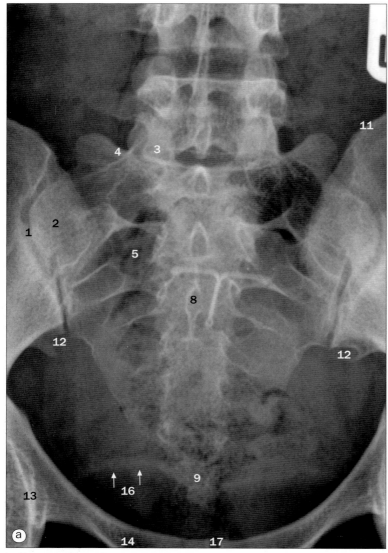

(a) Sacrum, anteroposterior projection.

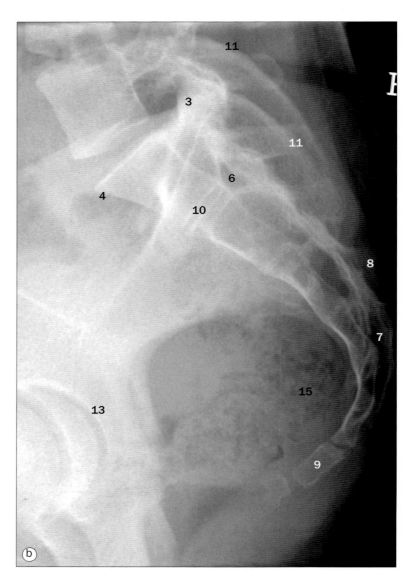

(b) Sacrum and coccyx, lateral projection.

1 Sacroiliac joint
2 Ala of sacrum
3 Superior articular process of sacrum
4 Sacral promontory
5 Sacral foramen (S1/2 for right S1 root)
6 Upper part of sacral canal
7 Lower part of sacral canal
8 Spinous tubercle on median sacral crest
9 Coccyx
10 Rudimentary S1/2 disc space
11 Iliac crest
12 Preauricular (paraglenoid) sulcus
13 Acetabular roof
14 Superior pubic ramus
15 Rectum
16 Levator ani (outlined by fat in ischioanal fossa)
17 Symphysis pubis

The preauricular (paraglenoid) sulcus is a characteristic of the female pelvis and is due to bone resorption at the insertion of the anterior sacroiliac ligament. It is prominent in parous women.

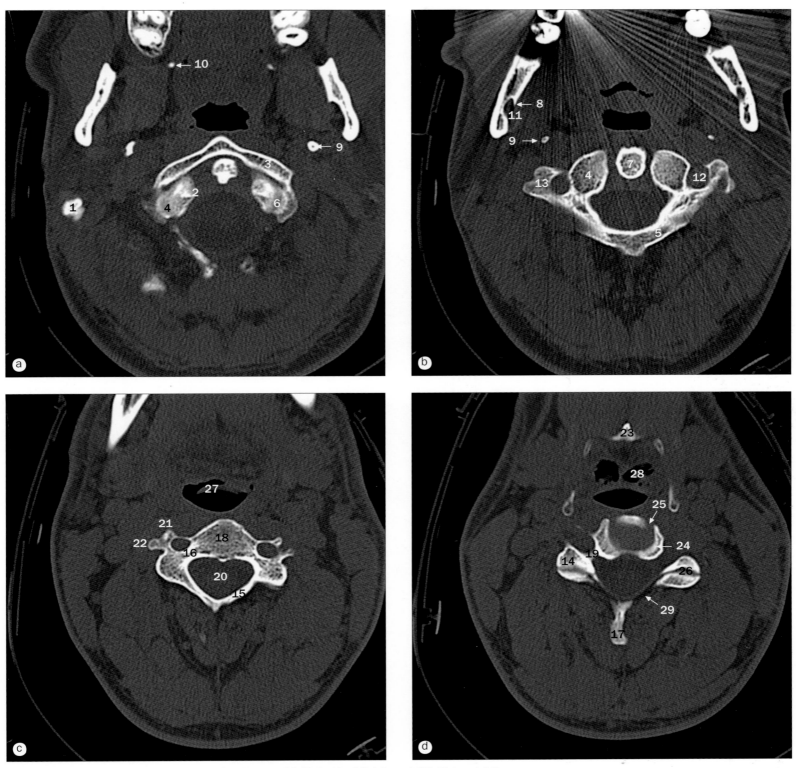

Axial CT images of the upper cervical spine at C1/2 (**a,b**), C2 (**c**) and C2/3 level (**d**).

1 Mastoid process (tip)	**11** Inferior alveolar foramen of mandibular ramus
2 Transverse ligament (attachment)	**12** Foramen transversarium of C1
3 Anterior arch of atlas (C1)	**13** Transverse process of C1
4 Lateral mass of atlas	**14** Inferior articular process of C2
5 Posterior arch of C1	**15** Lamina of C2
6 Groove for vertebral artery	**16** Pedicle of C2
7 Odontoid process (dens) of axis (C2)	**17** Spinous process of C2
8 Lingula of mandible	**18** Body of C2
9 Styloid process	**19** Intervertebral foramen of C2/3
10 Hamulus of medial pterygoid plate	**20** Spinal cord

21 Anterior tubercle of transverse process of C2
22 Posterior tubercle of transverse process of C2
23 Thyroid cartilage
24 Uncus of C3 vertebral body
25 Uncovertebral joint (of Luschka) at C2/3
26 Facet (zygapophyseal) joint at C2/3
27 Epiglottis
28 Vallecula
29 Ligamentum flavum

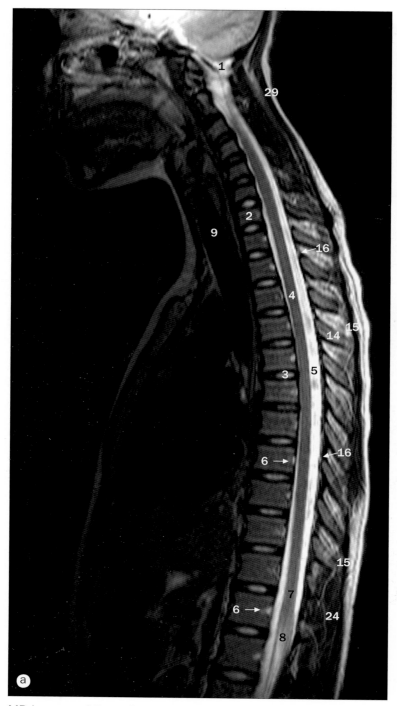

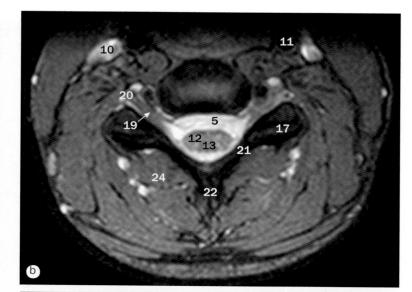

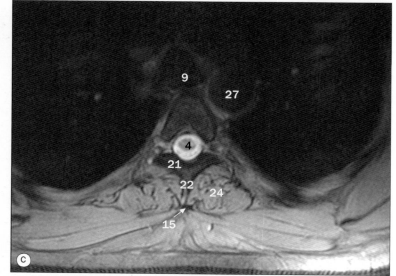

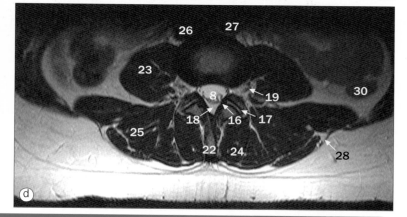

MR images of the spine, (a) sagittal T2 wide field of view and axial T2 sections from the (b) cervical, (c) thoracic and (d) lumbar regions.

1 Foramen magnum
2 Body of C7
3 Nucleus pulposus of T5/6 intervertebral disc
4 Spinal cord
5 CSF in subarachnoid space (flow void artefact)
6 Basivertebral vein

7 Conus medullaris
8 Cauda equina
9 Trachea
10 Internal jugular vein
11 Common carotid artery
12 Grey matter of spinal cord
13 White matter of spinal cord

14 Spinous process of T4
15 Supraspinous ligament
16 Ligamentum flavum
17 Facet (zygapophyseal) joint
18 Epidural fat
19 Dorsal root ganglion
20 Spinal nerve root
21 Lamina
22 Spinous process

23 Psoas major muscle
24 Erector spinae muscle
25 Multifidus muscle
26 Inferior vena cava
27 Aorta
28 Thoracolumbar fascia
29 Ligamentum nuchae
30 Descending colon

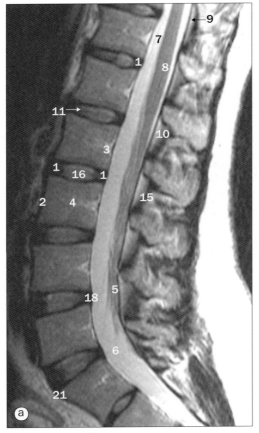

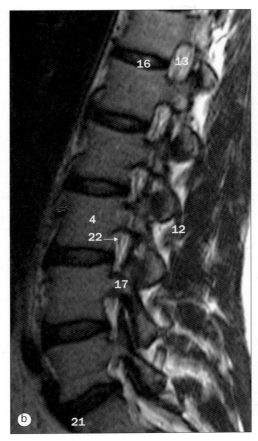

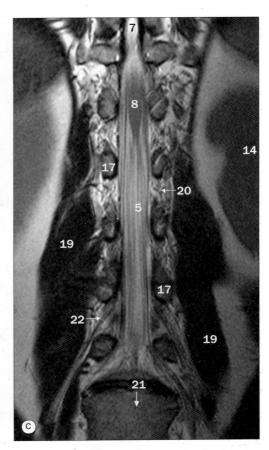

Lumbosacral spine, (a) sagittal MR image, (b) parasagittal MR image, (c) coronal MR image.

1 Annulus fibrosus	**9** Dural sac
2 Anterior longitudinal ligament	**10** Epidural space (fat filled)
3 Basivertebral vein	**11** Internuclear cleft
4 Body of third lumbar vertebra	**12** Interspinous ligament
5 Cauda equina	**13** Intervertebral foramen
6 Caudal lumbar thecal sac	**14** Kidney
7 Cerebrospinal fluid	**15** Ligamentum flavum
8 Conus medullaris	**16** Nucleus pulposus

17 Pedicle
18 Posterior longitudinal ligament and
annulus fibrosus
19 Psoas muscle
20 Radicular vessels
21 Sacral promontory
22 Spinal nerve root in intervertebral
foramen

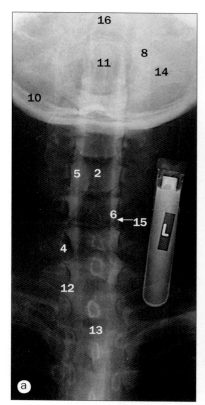

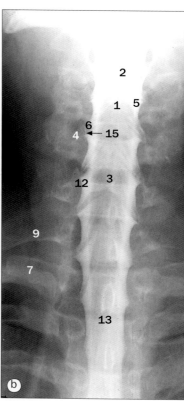

Cervical myelogram, (a) with the neck extended, (b) with the neck slightly flexed, anteroposterior projections.

Non-ionic water-soluble contrast medium is introduced into the lumbar subarachnoid space via a lumbar puncture. The patient is positioned prone, with the neck hyperextended, and strapped onto a tilting table. The contrast medium is then run up into the cervical region to demonstrate the cervical spinal cord and exiting nerve roots. There are eight cervical nerve roots: the roots of the eighth cervical nerve exit through the intervertebral foramina between the seventh cervical vertebra and the first thoracic vertebra. The normal cervical cord enlargement (3) (for the brachial plexus) extends from the third cervical vertebra to the second thoracic vertebra. It is maximal at the fifth cervical vertebra and should not be mistaken for an intramedullary lesion.

1 Anterior spinal artery
2 Cervical cord
3 Cervical cord enlargement
4 Cervical spinal nerve exiting through intervertebral foramen
5 Contrast medium in cervical subarachnoid space
6 Dorsal root of spinal nerve
7 First rib
8 Lateral mass of atlas (first cervical vertebra)
9 Normal large transverse process of seventh cervical vertebra
10 Occiput
11 Odontoid process (dens)
12 Root of eighth cervical nerve
13 Thoracic cord
14 Transverse foramen
15 Ventral root of spinal nerve
16 Vertebral artery

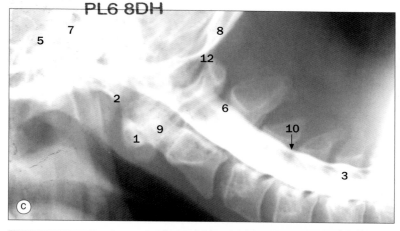

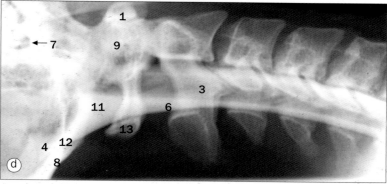

Cervical myelogram, (c) with the patient prone, (d) with the patient supine, lateral projections.

1 Anterior arch of atlas (first cervical vertebra)
2 Anterior rim of foramen magnum
3 Cervical cord
4 Cisterna magna (cerebellomedullary cistern)
5 Clivus
6 Contrast medium in cervical subarachnoid space
7 External acoustic meatus
8 Occiput
9 Odontoid (process) dens
10 Posterior indentation on theca from ligamentum flavum
11 Posterior inferior cerebellar artery
12 Posterior rim of foramen magnum
13 Posterior tubercle of atlas (first cervical vertebra)

Lumbar radiculogram, (**a**) lateral projection, (**b**) oblique projection, (**c**) anteroposterior projection.

Non-ionic water-soluble contrast medium is introduced into the lumbar subarachnoid space via a lumbar puncture. The nerve roots of the cauda equina are well demonstrated and exit through the intervertebral foramina. The nerve roots extending from the conus to the terminal thecal sac pass below the pedicle of the corresponding vertebra. The thecal sac terminates at the level of the first/second sacral vertebrae. The filum terminale may be seen. Tilting the prone patient slightly head down allows the contrast to flow cranially and outlines the conus and lower thoracic cord. The cord is uniform in size from the second to the tenth thoracic vertebra, at which point its second, smaller expansion (for the lumbosacral plexus) extends from the tenth thoracic vertebra to the level of the first lumbar vertebra. The conus medullaris usually terminates at the first/second lumbar vertebrae, but may be seen at a level above and below as a normal variant.

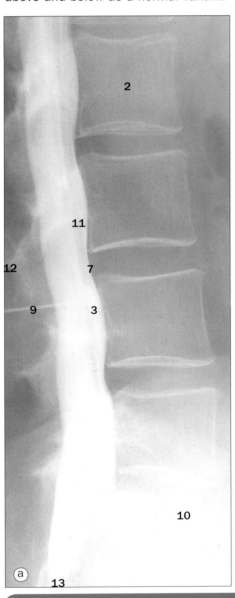
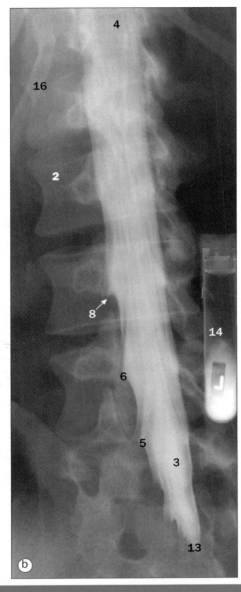
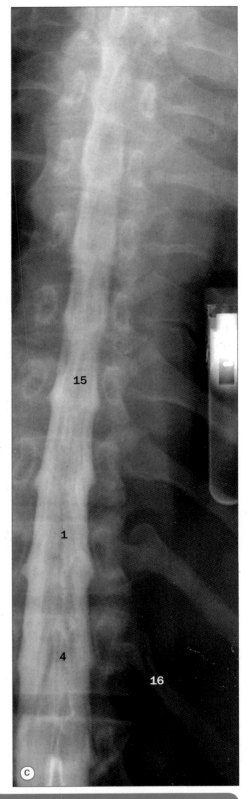

1 Anterior median fissure	**8** Lateral extension of subarachnoid space around spinal nerve roots	**12** Spinous process of third lumbar vertebra
2 Body of second lumbar vertebra	**9** Lumbar puncture needle in space between third and fourth lumbar vertebrae	**13** Terminal theca at first/second sacral vertebra
3 Contrast medium in subarachnoid space		**14** Test tube containing contrast medium to indicate tilt of patient
4 Conus medullaris	**10** Sacral promontory	**15** Thoracic cord
5 Fifth lumbar spinal nerve	**11** Spinal nerves within subarachnoid space (cauda equina)	**16** Twelfth rib
6 Fourth lumbar spinal nerve		
7 Intervertebral disc indentations in anterior thecal margin		

(a) Subtracted lumbar venogram.

Since the advent of CT and MR imaging techniques, lumbar venography is rarely performed. However, the anatomy of the vertebral veins is optimally demonstrated by this technique. Venous drainage of the spinal cord is longitudinally arranged via plexi, which anastomose freely with the internal (6) and external (1 and 4) vertebral venous plexi, which also communicate (4 and 2). Note how the internal veins bend laterally at the level of the disc interspace and medially at the level of pedicles, where they unite via a connecting vein (2).

1 Ascending lumbar veins
2 Basivertebral veins
3 Catheter in common iliac vein
4 Intervertebral veins
5 Lateral sacral veins
6 Longitudinal vertebral venous plexi
7 Sacral venous plexus
8 Tip of catheter in intravertebral vein

(b) Spinal arteriogram.

1 Anterior spinal artery
2 Arteria radicularis magna (Adamkiewicz)
3 Normal transdural stenosis of the arteria radicularis magna
4 Selective catheterisation of left eleventh intercostal artery

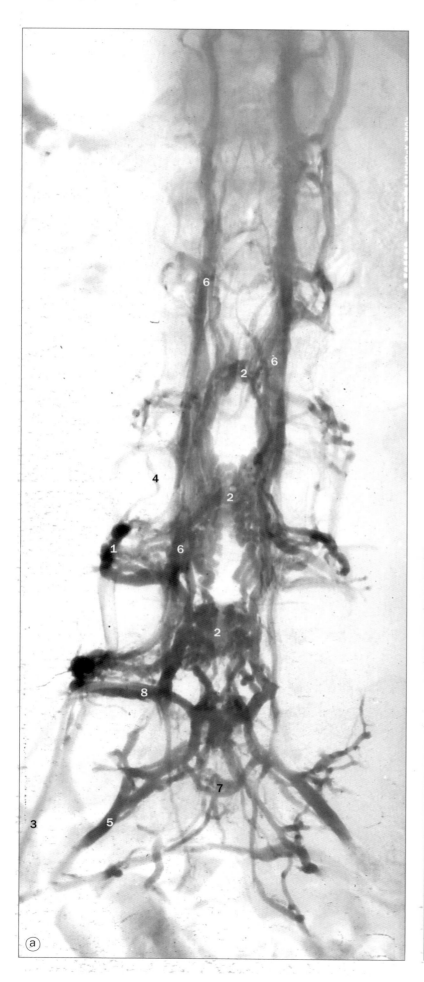

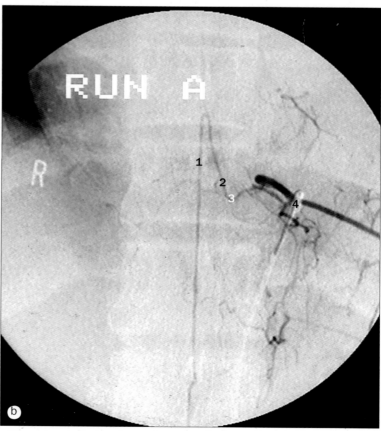

3 Upper limb

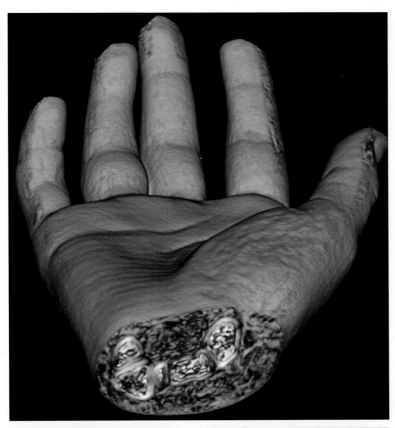

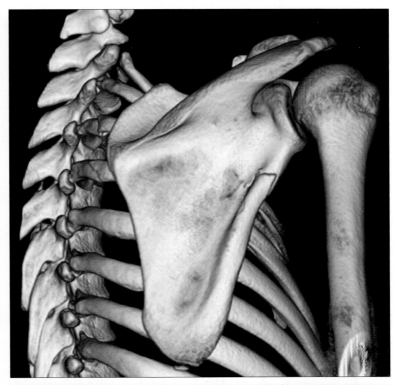

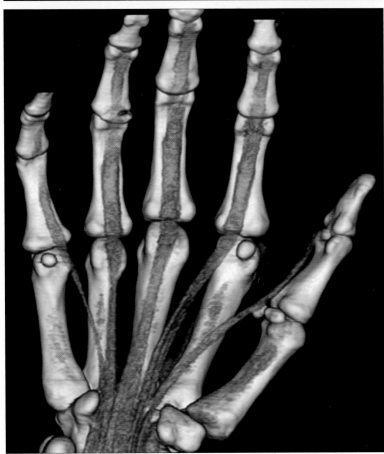

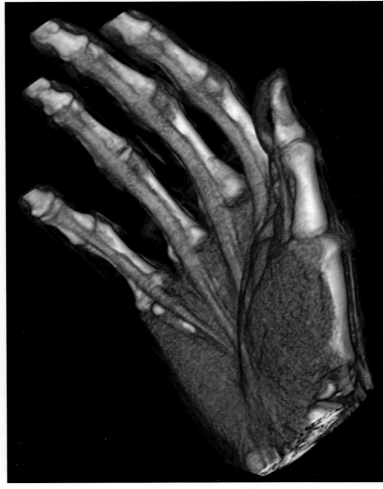

(a) Shoulder, anteroposterior radiograph.

1 Acromion of scapula
2 Anatomical neck
3 Clavicle
4 Coracoid process of scapula
5 Glenoid fossa of scapula
6 Greater tubercle (tuberosity) of
  humerus
7 Head of humerus
8 Lesser tubercle (tuberosity) of
  humerus
9 Scapula
10 Surgical neck

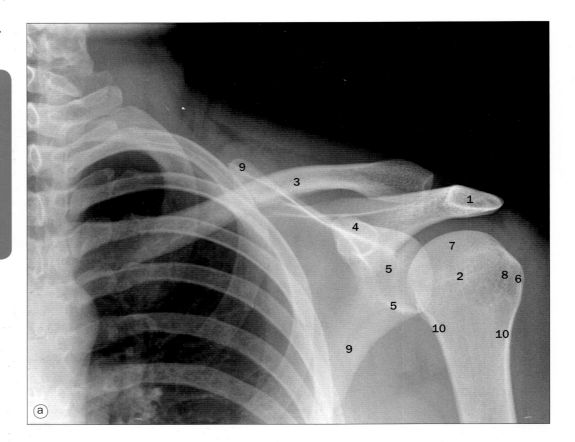

(b) Shoulder, axial (supero-inferior) projection.

1 Acromion of scapula
2 Clavicle
3 Coracoid process of scapula
4 Glenoid fossa of scapula
5 Greater tubercle (tuberosity) of
  humerus
6 Head of humerus
7 Intertubercular groove of humerus
8 Lesser tubercle (tuberosity) of
  humerus
9 Spine of scapula

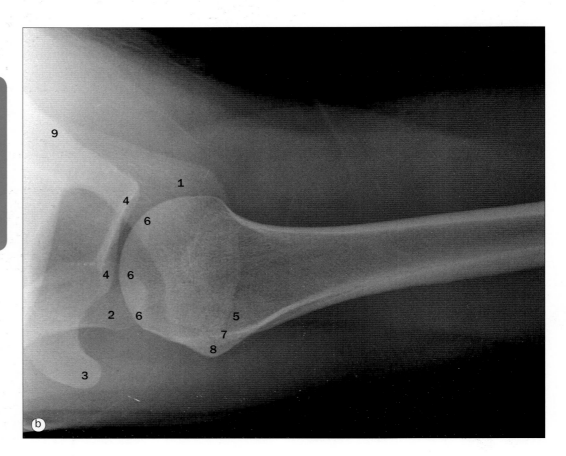

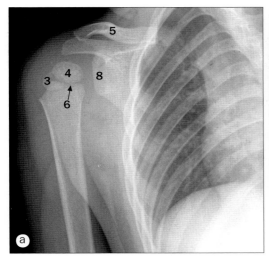

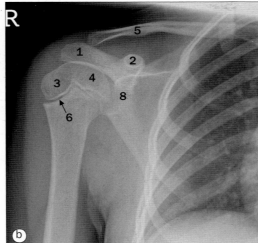

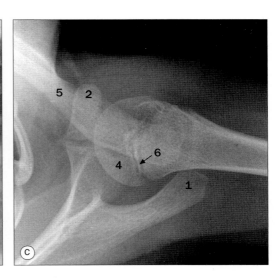

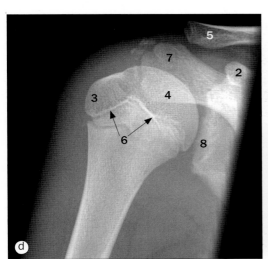

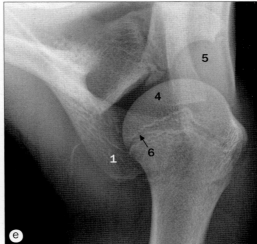

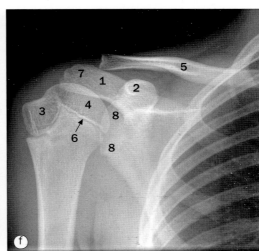

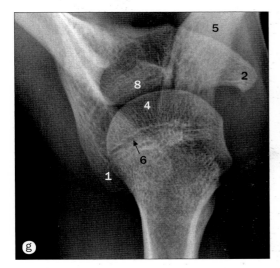

Shoulder, **(a)** (anteroposterior) of a 1-year-old child, **(b)** (anteroposterior) and **(c)** (axial) of a 6-year-old child, **(d)** (anteroposterior) and **(e)** (axial) of a 12-year-old child **(f)** (anteroposterior) and **(g)** (axial) of a 14-year-old child.

1	Acromion of scapula	5	Clavicle
2	Centre for coracoid process	6	Epiphysial line
3	Centre for greater tubercle (tuberosity) of humerus	7	Centre for acromion
4	Centre for head of humerus	8	Glenoid fossa of scapula

CLAVICLE (m)	Appears	Fused
Lateral end	5 wiu	20+ yrs
Medial end	15 yrs	20+ yrs
SCAPULA (c)		
Body	8 wiu	15 yrs
Coracoid	<1 yr	20 yrs
Coracoid base	Puberty	15–20 yrs
Acromion	Puberty	15–20 yrs

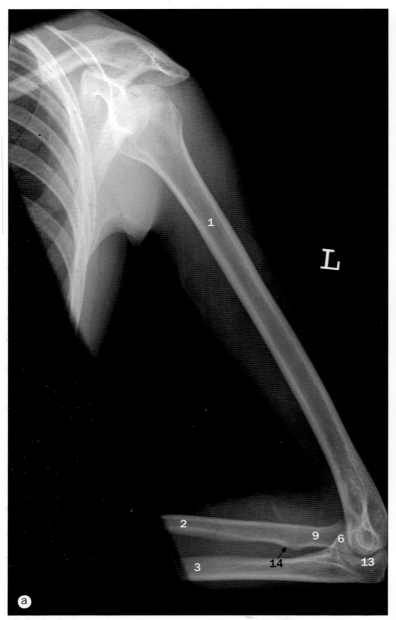

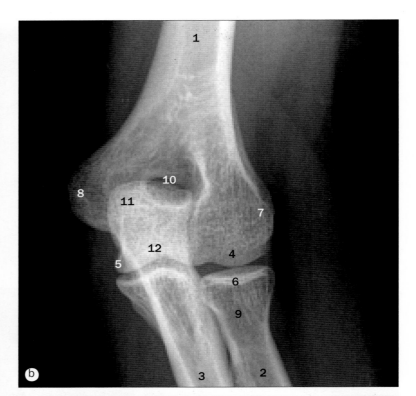

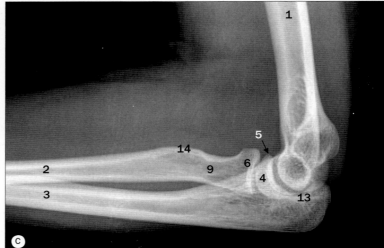

(a) Humerus, lateral projection, (b) elbow, anteroposterior projection, (c) elbow, lateral projection.

1	Humerus	8	Medial epicondyle of humerus
2	Radius	9	Neck of radius
3	Ulna	10	Olecranon fossa of humerus
4	Capitulum of humerus	11	Olecranon of ulna
5	Coronoid process of ulna	12	Trochlea of humerus
6	Head of radius	13	Trochlear notch of ulna
7	Lateral epicondyle of humerus	14	Tuberosity of radius

HUMERUS (c)	Appears	Fused
Shaft	8 wiu	15–20 yrs
Head	1–6 mths	15–20 yrs
Greater tubercle	6 mths–1 yr	15–20 yrs
Lesser tubercle	3–5 yrs	18–20 yrs
Capitulum	4 mths–1 yr	13–16 yrs
Medial trochlea	10 yrs	13–16 yrs
Medial epicondyle	3–6 yrs	13–16 yrs
Lateral epicondyle	9–12 yrs	13–16 yrs

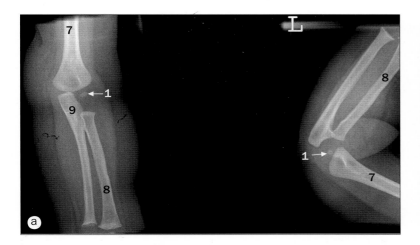

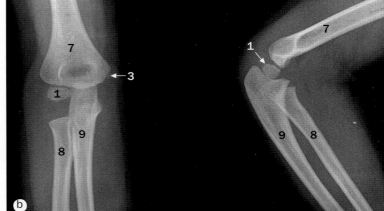

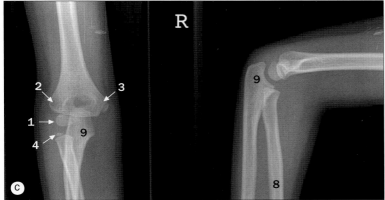

Elbow images, (**a**) 7-month-old child, (**b**) 3-year-old child, (**c**) 6-year-old child, (**d**) 9-year-old child.

RADIUS (c)		
Shaft	8 wiu	
Proximal	4–6 yrs	13–16 yrs
Distal	1 yr	16–18 yrs
ULNA (c)		
Shaft	8 wiu	
Proximal	8–10 yrs	13–15 yrs
Distal	5–7 yrs	16–18 yrs

1 Centre for capitulum
2 Centre for lateral epicondyle
3 Centre for medial epicondyle
4 Centre for radial head
5 Centre for trochlea
6 Epiphysial line
7 Humerus
8 Radius
9 Ulna
10 Centre for olecranon

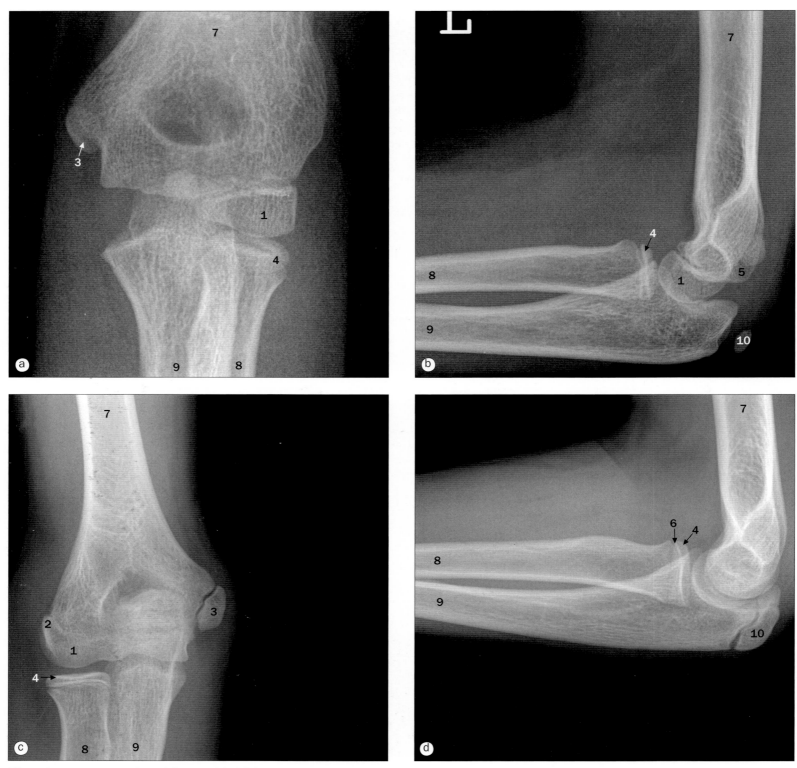

Elbow images, **(a)** and **(b)** 11-year-old child, **(c)** and **(d)** 14-year-old child.

1 Centre for capitulum	**6** Epiphyseal line
2 Centre for lateral epicondyle	**7** Humerus
3 Centre for medial epicondyle	**8** Radius
4 Centre for radial head	**9** Ulna
5 Centre for trochlea	**10** Centre for olecranon

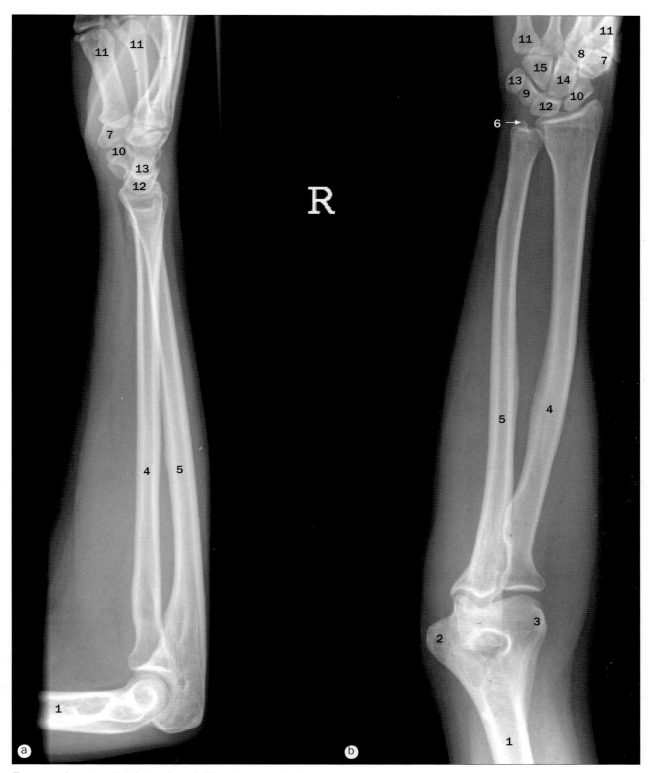

Forearm images, (a) lateral and (b) anteroposterior.

1 Humerus	5 Ulna	10 Scaphoid
2 Medial epicondyle of humerus	6 Styloid of ulna	11 Metacarpals
3 Lateral epicondyle of humerus	7 Trapezium	12 Lunate
4 Radius	8 Trapezoid	13 Pisiform
	9 Triquetral	14 Capitate
		15 Hamate

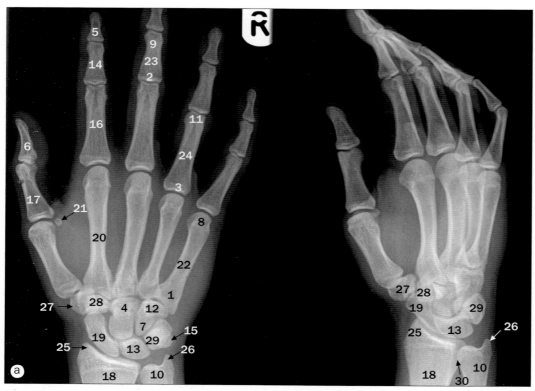

(a) Bones of the hand, dorsopalmar and oblique projection.

1 Base of fifth metacarpal	**12** Hook of hamate	**22** Shaft of fifth metacarpal
2 Base of middle phalanx of middle finger	**13** Lunate	**23** Shaft of middle phalanx of middle finger
3 Base of proximal phalanx of ring finger	**14** Middle phalanx of index finger	**24** Shaft of proximal phalanx of ring finger
4 Capitate	**15** Pisiform	**25** Styloid process of radius
5 Distal phalanx of index finger	**16** Proximal phalanx of index finger	**26** Styloid process of ulna
6 Distal phalanx of thumb	**17** Proximal phalanx of thumb	**27** Trapezium
7 Hamate	**18** Radius	**28** Trapezoid
8 Head of fifth metacarpal	**19** Scaphoid	**29** Triquetral
9 Head of middle phalanx of middle finger	**20** Second metacarpal	**30** Ulnar notch of radius
10 Head of ulna	**21** Sesamoid bone	**31** Base of metacarpal
11 Head of proximal phalanx of ring finger		

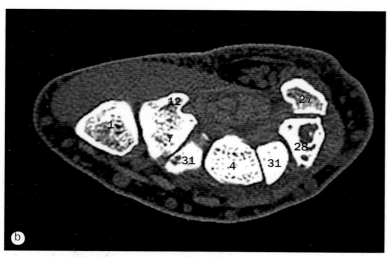

(b) Axial CT through carpal tunnel.

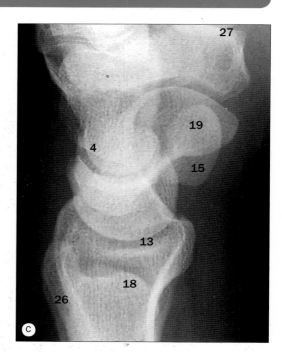

(c) Bones of the wrist, lateral projection.

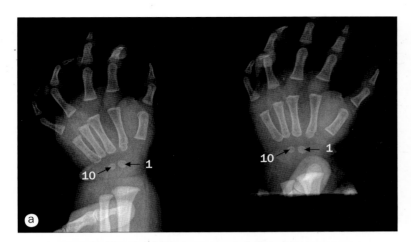

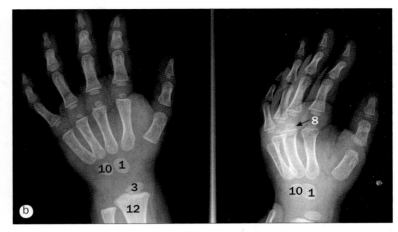

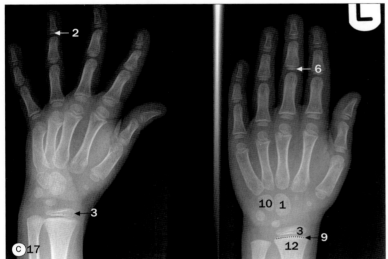

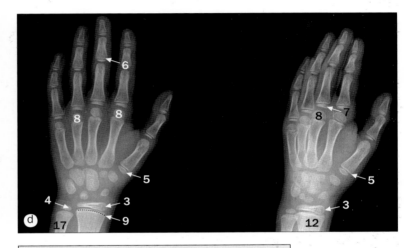

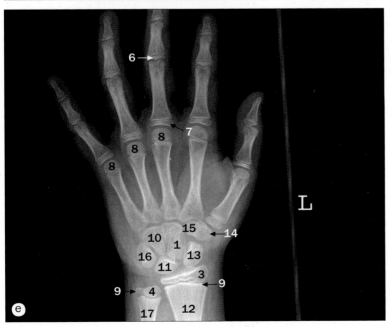

CARPUS (c)	Appears	Fused
Capitate	1–3 mths	
Hamate	2–4 mths	
Triquetral	2–3 yrs	
Lunate	2–4 yrs	
Scaphoid	4–6 yrs	
Trapezium	4–6 yrs	
Trapezoid	4–6 yrs	
Pisiform (sesamoid)	8–12 yrs	
METACARPALS (c)		
Shaft	9 wiu	
Head	1–2 yrs	14–19 yrs
PHALANGES (c)		
Shaft	8–12 wiu	
Base	1–3 yrs	14–18 yrs

Bones of the hand (dorsopalmar projections), **(a)** of a 10-month-old child, **(b)** of a 2-year-old child, **(c)** of a 6-year-old child, **(d)** of a 9-year-old child, to illustrate centres of ossification, **(e)** of an 11-year-old child.

1 Capitate	**5** Centre for first metacarpal	**8** Centre for second metacarpal (applies to second to fifth metacarpals)	**12** Radius
2 Centre for distal phalanx of ring finger	**6** Centre for middle phalanx of middle finger		**13** Scaphoid
3 Centre for distal radius	**7** Centre for proximal phalanx of middle finger	**9** Epiphysial line	**14** Trapezium
4 Centre for distal ulna		**10** Hamate	**15** Trapezoid
		11 Lunate	**16** Triquetral
			17 Ulna

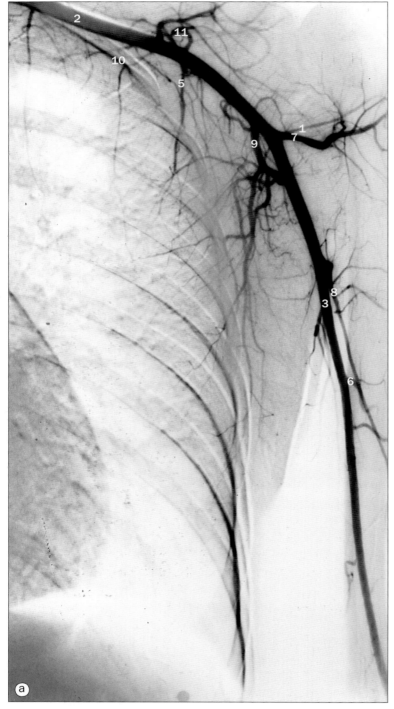

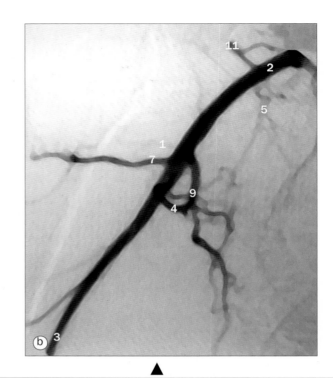

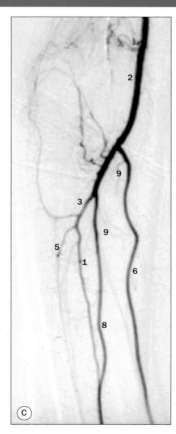

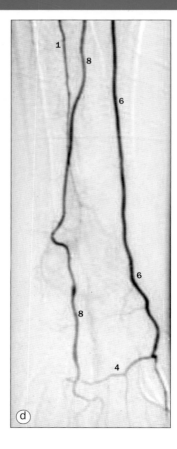

Axillary arteriograms, (**a**) subtracted, (**b**) digitally subtracted, (**c**) and (**d**) brachial arteriograms.

1 Anterior circumflex humeral artery	**7** Posterior circumflex humeral artery
2 Axillary artery	**8** Profunda brachii artery
3 Brachial artery	**9** Subscapular artery
4 Circumflex scapular artery	**10** Superior thoracic artery
5 Lateral thoracic artery	**11** Thoraco-acromial artery
6 Muscular branches of brachial artery	

1 Anterior interosseous artery	**5** Posterior interosseous artery
2 Brachial artery	**6** Radial artery
3 Common interosseous artery	**7** Radial recurrent artery
4 Deep palmar arch	**8** Ulnar artery
	9 Ulnar recurrent artery

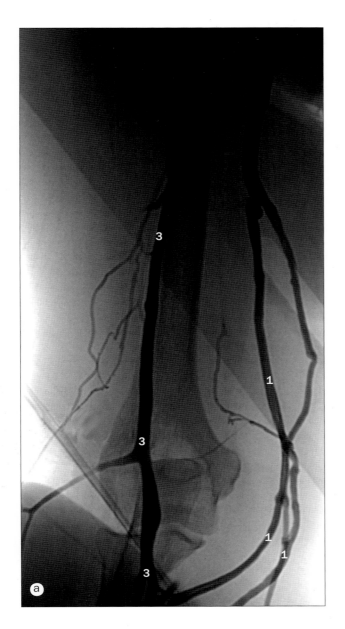

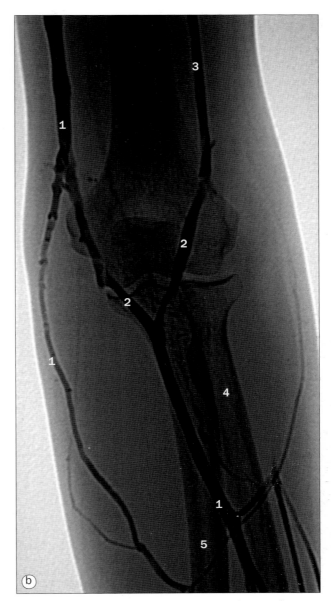

(a) and (b) Upper limbs venograms, (c) superior vena cavogram.

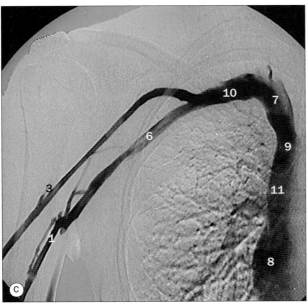

1 Basilic vein
2 Median cubital vein
3 Cephalic vein
4 Radius
5 Ulna
6 Axillary vein
7 Brachiocephalic vein
8 Right atrium
9 Site of entry of left brachiocephalic vein
10 Subclavian vein
11 Superior vena cava

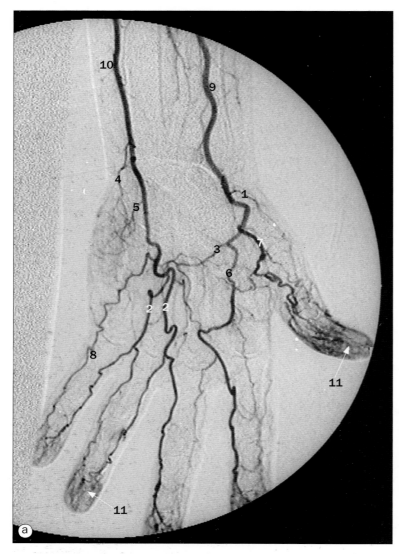

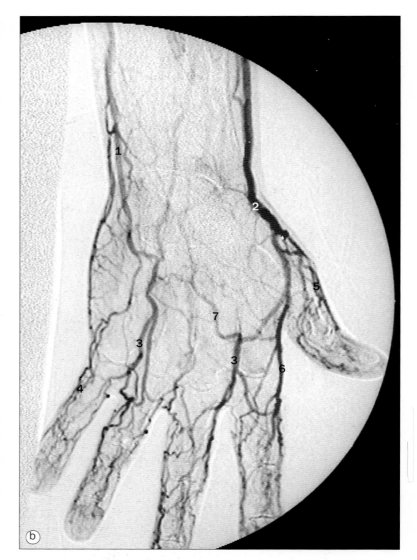

(a) Digitally subtracted hand arteriogram.
In this patient there is an incomplete superficial palmar arch.

(b) Venous phase of hand arteriogram.

1 Artery to radial aspects of thumb
2 Common palmar digital artery
3 Deep palmar arch
4 Deep palmar branch of ulnar artery
5 Palmar carpal branch of ulnar artery
6 Palmar metacarpal artery
7 Princeps pollicis artery
8 Proper palmar digital artery
9 Radial artery
10 Ulnar artery
11 Pulp anastomoses

1 Basilic vein
2 Cephalic vein
3 Common palmar digital vein
4 Palmar digital vein
5 Princeps pollicis vein
6 Radialis indicis vein
7 Superficial palmar venous arch

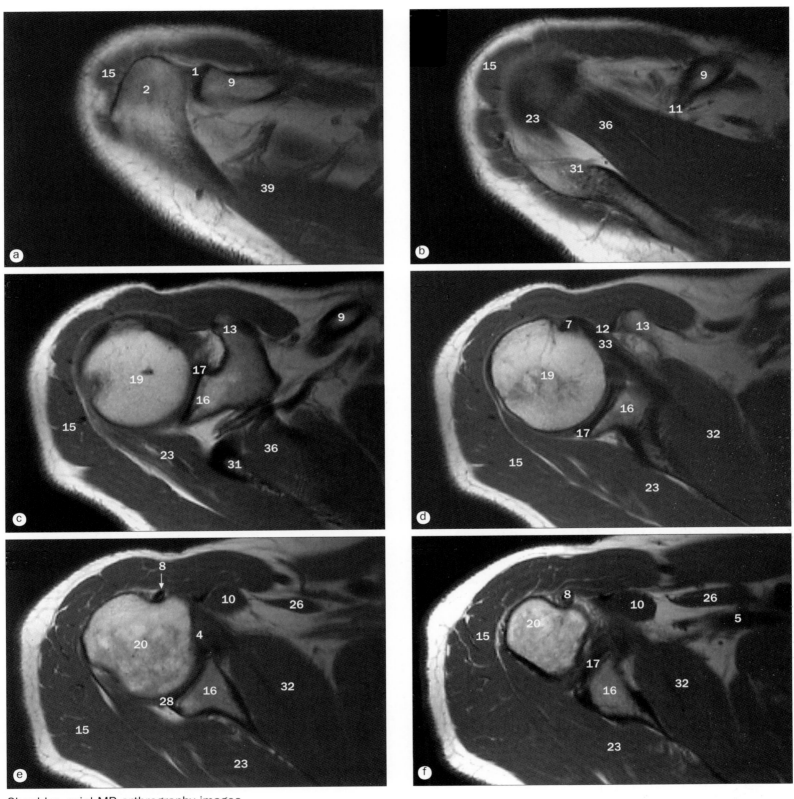

Shoulder, axial MR arthrography images.

1	Acromioclavicular joint	9	Clavicle	17	Glenoid labrum
2	Acromion	10	Coracobrachialis muscle	18	Greater tuberosity
3	Anterior capsule of shoulder joint	11	Coracoclavicular ligament	19	Head of humerus
4	Anterior labrum	12	Coracohumeral ligament	20	Humerus
5	Axillary artery and vein	13	Coracoid process	21	Inferior glenohumeral ligament
6	Axillary recess	14	Deltoid tendon	22	Inferior labrum
7	Biceps brachii tendon	15	Deltoid muscle	23	Infraspinatus muscle
8	Biceps brachii tendon (long head)	16	Glenoid	24	Infraspinatus tendon

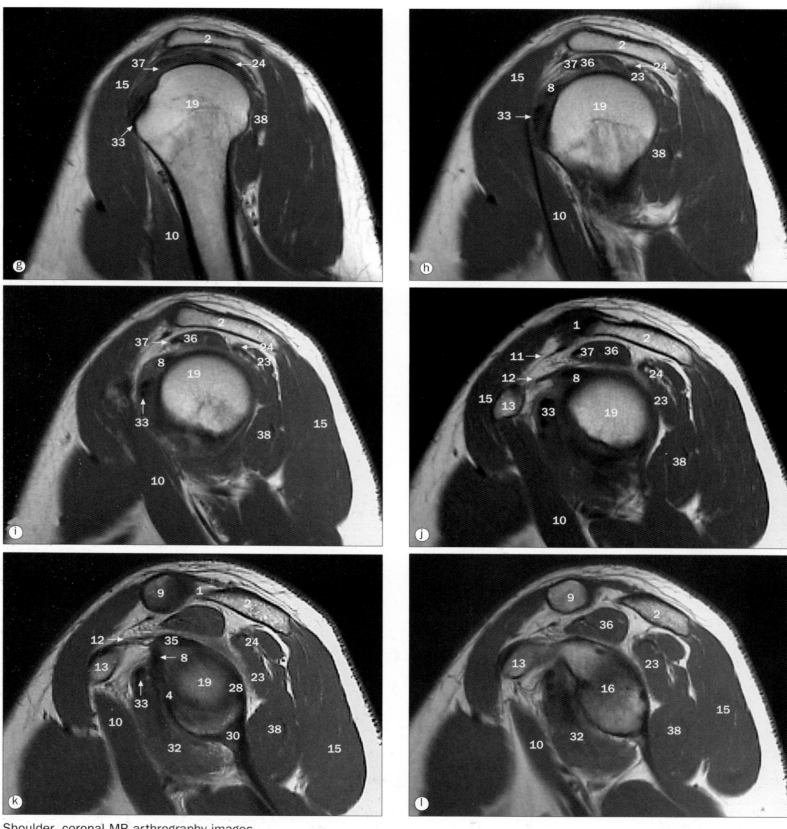

Shoulder, coronal MR arthrography images.

25 Middle glenohumeral ligament	**30** Scapula	**35** Superior labrum
26 Pectoralis minor muscle	**31** Spine of scapula	**36** Supraspinatus muscle
27 Posterior capsule of shoulder joint	**32** Subscapularis muscle	**37** Supraspinatus tendon
28 Posterior labrum	**33** Subscapularis tendon	**38** Teres minor muscle
29 Rotator cuff	**34** Superior glenohumeral ligament	**39** Trapezius muscle

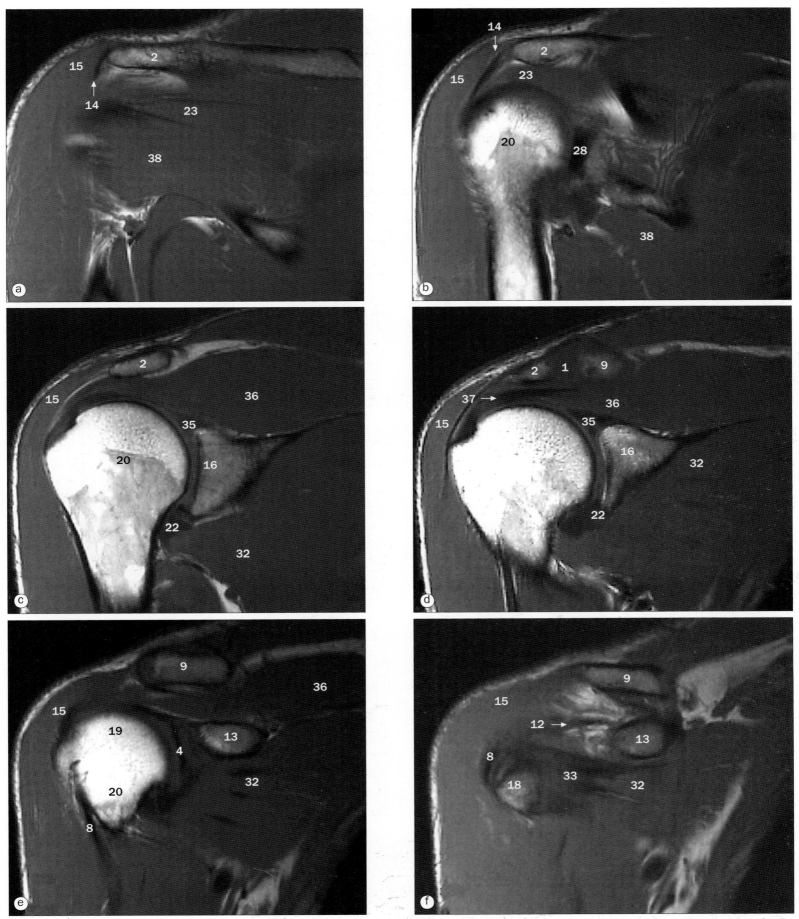

Shoulder, sagittal oblique MR arthrography images. See pages 79 and 80 for key to labels.

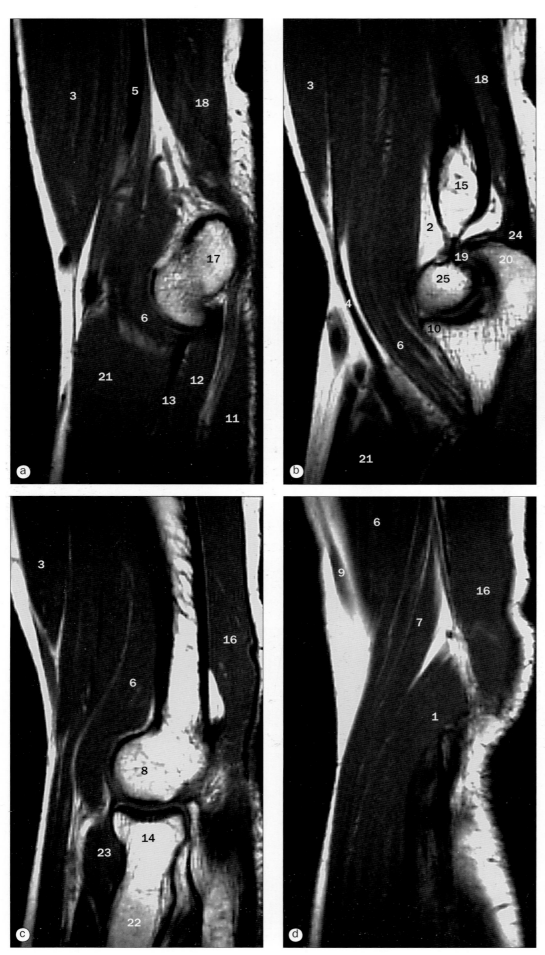

(a)–(d) Elbow, sagittal MR images.

1 Abductor pollicis longus muscle
2 Anterior fat pad
3 Biceps brachii muscle
4 Biceps brachii tendon
5 Brachial artery
6 Brachialis muscle
7 Brachioradialis muscle
8 Capitulum of humerus
9 Cephalic vein
10 Coronoid process of ulna
11 Flexor carpi ulnaris muscle
12 Flexor digitorum profundus muscle
13 Flexor digitorum superficialis muscle
14 Head of radius
15 Humerus
16 Lateral head of triceps muscle
17 Medial epicondyle
18 Medial head of triceps muscle
19 Olecranon fossa of humerus
20 Olecranon process of ulna
21 Pronator teres muscle
22 Radius
23 Supinator muscle
24 Tendon of triceps muscle
25 Trochlea of humerus

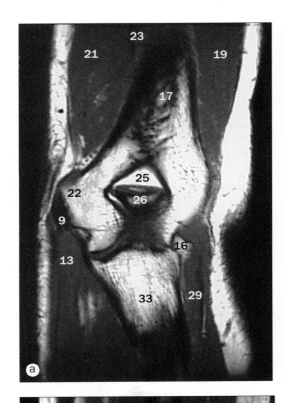

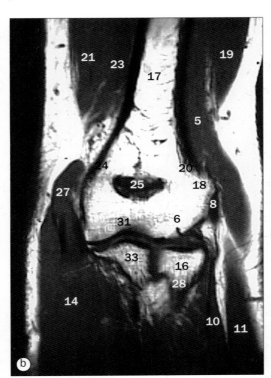

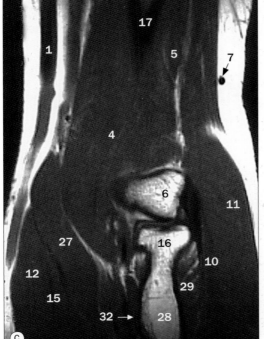

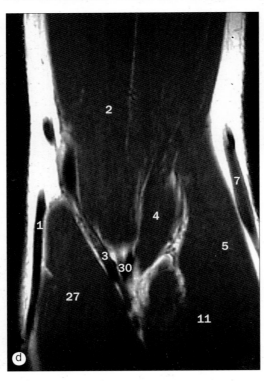

(a)–(d) Elbow, coronal MR images.

1 Basilic vein
2 Biceps brachii muscle
3 Brachial artery
4 Brachialis muscle
5 Brachioradialis muscle
6 Capitulum of humerus
7 Cephalic vein
8 Common extensor origin
9 Common flexor origin
10 Extensor carpi radialis brevis muscle
11 Extensor carpi radialis longus muscle
12 Flexor carpi radialis muscle
13 Flexor carpi ulnaris muscle
14 Flexor digitorum profundus muscle
15 Flexor digitorum superficialis muscle
16 Head of radius
17 Humerus
18 Lateral epicondyle
19 Lateral head of triceps muscle
20 Lateral supracondylar ridge
21 Long head of triceps muscle
22 Medial epicondyle
23 Medial head of triceps muscle
24 Medial supracondylar ridge
25 Olecranon fossa of humerus
26 Olecranon process of ulna
27 Pronator teres muscle
28 Radius
29 Supinator muscle
30 Tendon of biceps brachii muscle
31 Trochlea of humerus
32 Tuberosity of radius
33 Ulna

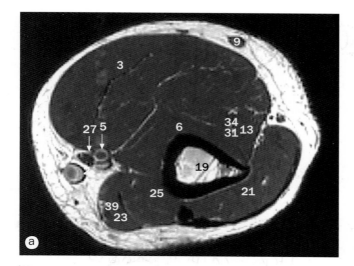

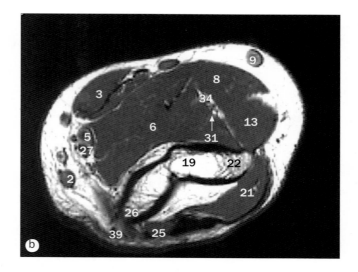

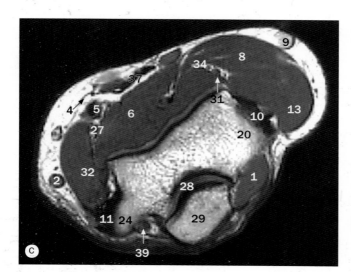

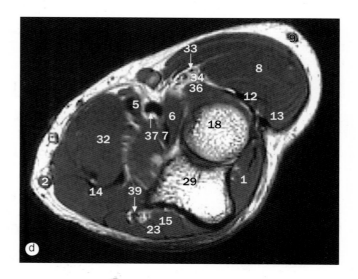

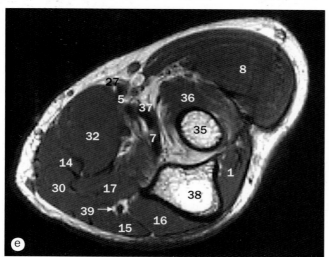

(a)–(e) Elbow, axial MR images.

1 Anconeus muscle	**20** Lateral epicondyle
2 Basilic vein	**21** Lateral head of triceps
3 Biceps brachii muscle	muscle
4 Bicipital aponeurosis	**22** Lateral supracondylar ridge
5 Brachial artery	**23** Long head of triceps muscle
6 Brachialis muscle	**24** Medial epicondyle
7 Brachialis tendon	**25** Medial head of triceps
8 Brachioradialis muscle	muscle
9 Cephalic vein	**26** Medial supracondylar ridge
10 Common extensor origin	**27** Median nerve
11 Common flexor origin	**28** Olecranon fossa of humerus
12 Extensor carpi radialis	**29** Olecranon process of ulna
brevis muscle	**30** Palmaris longus muscle
13 Extensor carpi radialis	**31** Profunda brachii artery
longus muscle	**32** Pronator teres muscle
14 Flexor carpi radialis muscle	**33** Radial artery
15 Flexor carpi ulnaris muscle	**34** Radial nerve
16 Flexor digitorum profundus	**35** Radius
muscle	**36** Supinator muscle
17 Flexor digitorum	**37** Tendon of biceps brachii
superficialis muscle	muscle
18 Head of radius	**38** Ulna
19 Humerus	**39** Ulnar nerve

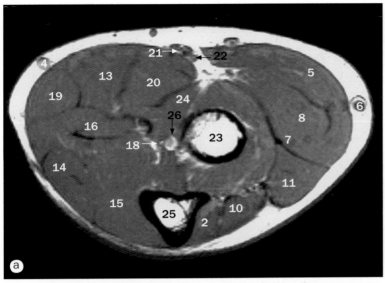

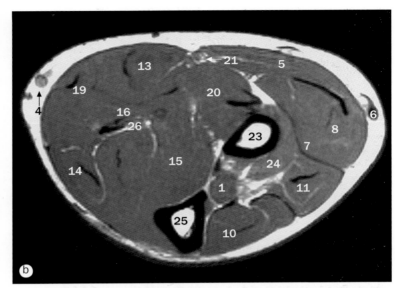

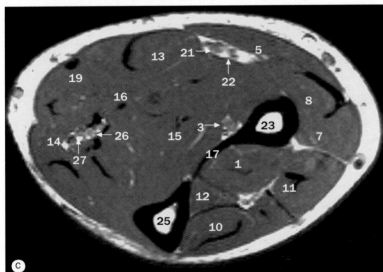

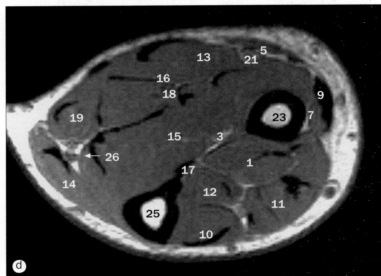

(a)–(d) Forearm, axial MR images.

1 Abductor pollicis longus muscle
2 Anconeus muscle
3 Anterior interosseous artery
4 Basilic vein
5 Brachioradialis muscle
6 Cephalic vein
7 Extensor carpi radialis brevis muscle
8 Extensor carpi radialis longus muscle
9 Extensor carpi radialis longus tendon

10 Extensor carpi ulnaris muscle
11 Extensor digitorum muscle
12 Extensor pollicis longus muscle
13 Flexor carpi radialis muscle
14 Flexor carpi ulnaris muscle
15 Flexor digitorum profundus muscle
16 Flexor digitorum superficialis muscle
17 Interosseous membrane
18 Median nerve

19 Palmaris longus muscle
20 Pronator teres muscle
21 Radial artery
22 Radial nerve
23 Radius
24 Supinator muscle
25 Ulna
26 Ulnar artery
27 Ulnar nerve

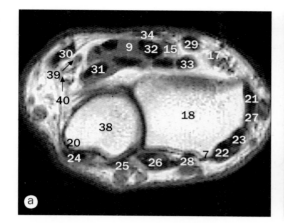
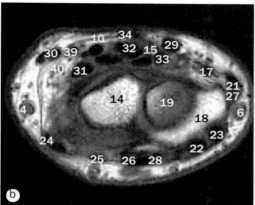
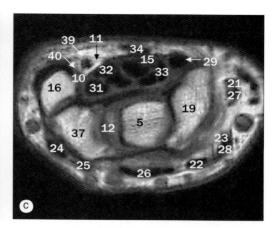
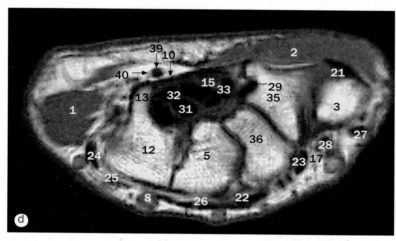
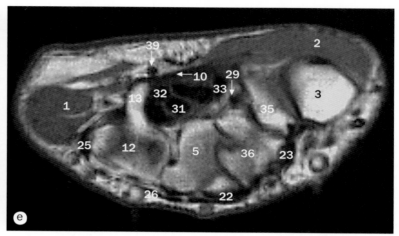

(a)–(e) Wrist, axial MR images.

1 Abductor digiti minimi muscle	**16** Pisiform	**29** Tendon of flexor carpi radialis muscle
2 Abductor pollicis brevis muscle	**17** Radial artery	**30** Tendon of flexor carpi ulnaris muscle
3 Base of first metacarpal	**18** Radius	**31** Tendon of flexor digitorum profundus muscle
4 Basilic vein	**19** Scaphoid	
5 Capitate	**20** Styloid process of ulna	**32** Tendon of flexor digitorum superficialis muscle
6 Cephalic vein	**21** Tendon of abductor pollicis longus muscle	
7 Dorsal tubercle of radius	**22** Tendon of extensor carpi radialis brevis muscle	**33** Tendon of flexor pollicis longus muscle
8 Dorsal venous arch		**34** Tendon of palmaris longus muscle
9 Flexor digitorum superficialis muscle	**23** Tendon of extensor carpi radialis longus muscle	**35** Trapezium
10 Flexor retinaculum		**36** Trapezoid
11 Guyon's canal	**24** Tendon of extensor carpi ulnaris muscle	**37** Triquetral
12 Hamate	**25** Tendon of extensor digiti minimi muscle	**38** Ulna
13 Hook of hamate	**26** Tendon of extensor digitorum muscle	**39** Ulnar artery
14 Lunate	**27** Tendon of extensor pollicis brevis muscle	**40** Ulnar nerve
15 Median nerve	**28** Tendon of extensor pollicis longus muscle	

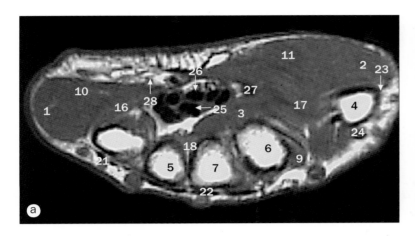

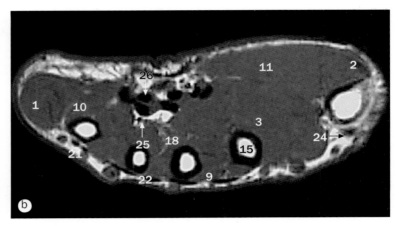

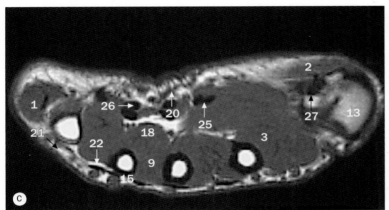

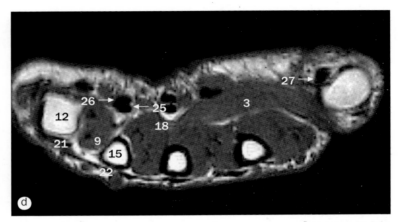

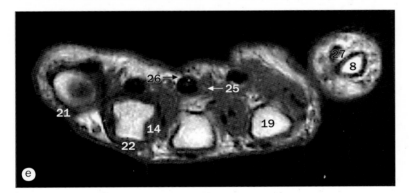

(a)–(e) Hand, axial MR images.

1 Abductor digiti minimi muscle	**18** Palmar interossei muscles
2 Abductor pollicis brevis muscle	**19** Proximal phalanx of index finger
3 Adductor pollicis muscle	**20** Superficial palmar arch
4 Base of first metacarpal	**21** Tendon of extensor digiti minimi muscle
5 Base of fourth metacarpal	**22** Tendon of extensor digitorum muscle
6 Base of second metacarpal	**23** Tendon of extensor pollicis brevis muscle
7 Base of third metacarpal	**24** Tendon of extensor pollicis longus muscle
8 Distal phalanx of thumb	**25** Tendon of flexor digitorum profundus muscle
9 Dorsal interossei muscles	**26** Tendon of flexor digitorum superficialis muscle
10 Flexor digiti minimi muscle	**27** Tendon of flexor pollicis longus muscle
11 Flexor pollicis brevis muscle	**28** Ulnar artery
12 Head of fifth metacarpal	
13 Head of first metacarpal	
14 Lumbrical muscle	
15 Metacarpal shaft	
16 Opponens digiti minimi muscle	
17 Opponens pollicis muscle	

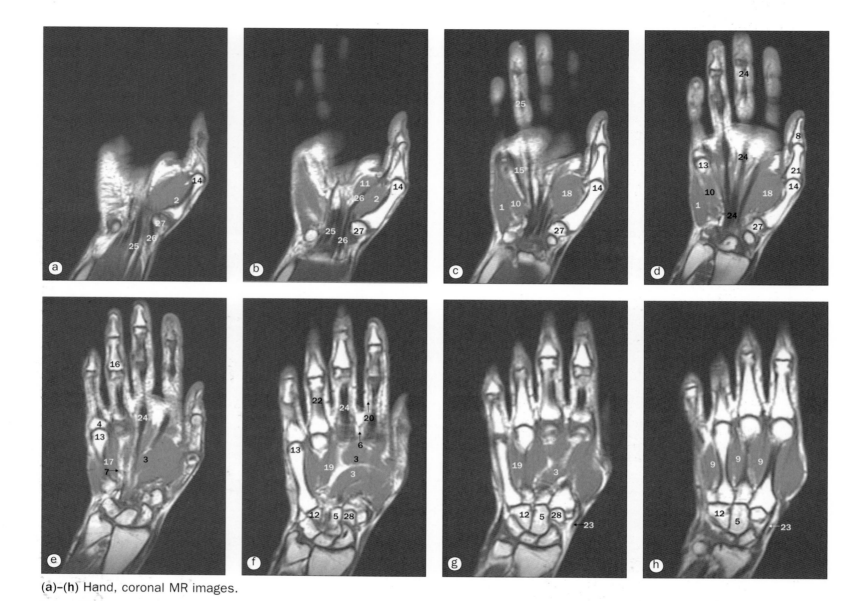

(a)–(h) Hand, coronal MR images.

1 Abductor digiti minimi muscle	**8** Distal phalanx of thumb	**17** Opponens digiti minimi muscle	**24** Tendon of flexor digitorum profundus muscle
2 Abductor pollicis brevis muscle	**9** Dorsal interossei muscles	**18** Opponens pollicis muscle	**25** Tendon of flexor digitorum superficialis muscle
3 Adductor pollicis muscle	**10** Flexor digiti minimi muscle	**19** Palmar interossei muscles	**26** Tendon of flexor pollicis longus muscle
4 Base of proximal phalanx	**11** Flexor pollicis brevis muscle	**20** Proper palmar digital artery	**27** Trapezium
5 Capitate	**12** Hamate	**21** Proximal phalanx of thumb	**28** Trapezoid
6 Common palmar digital artery	**13** Head of fifth metacarpal	**22** Shaft of proximal phalanx	
7 Deep palmar arch	**14** Head of first metacarpal	**23** Tendon of extensor pollicis longus muscle	
	15 Lumbrical muscle		
	16 Middle phalanx		

4 Thorax

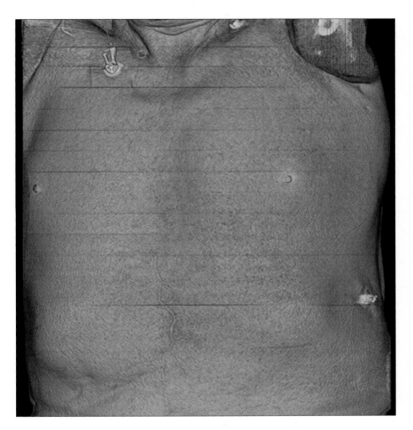

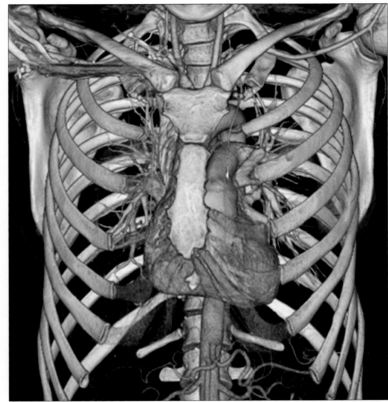

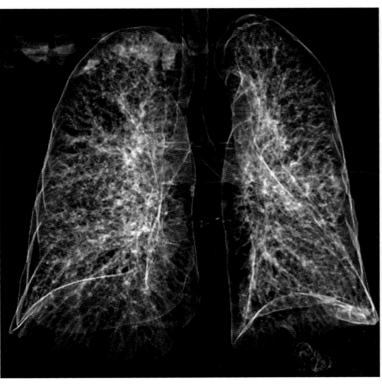

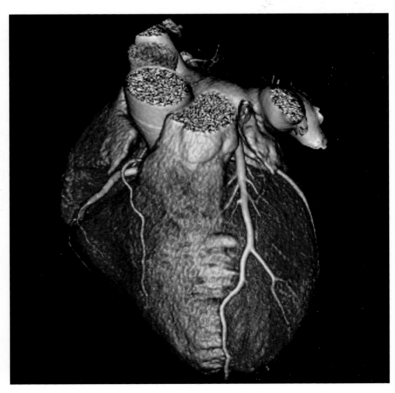

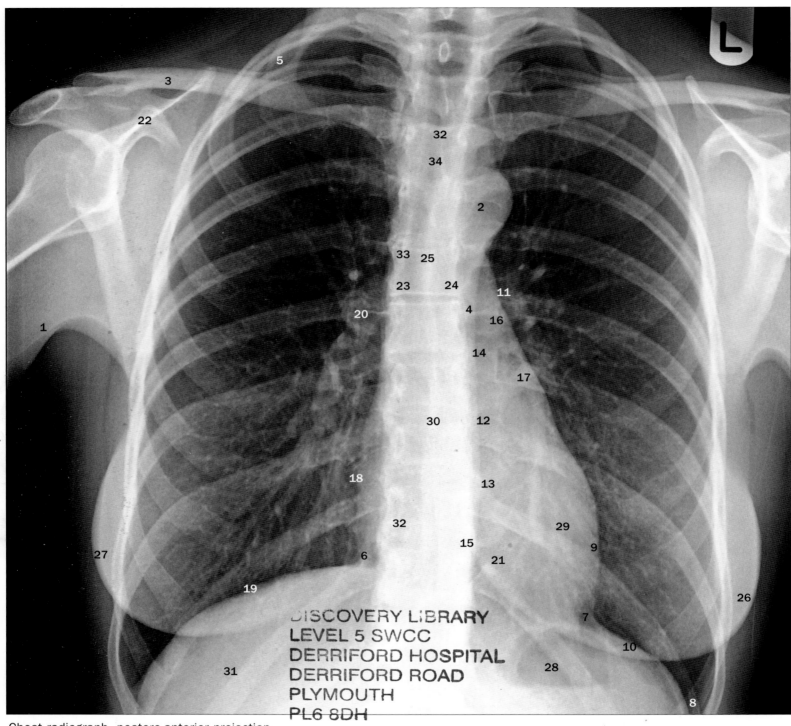

Chest radiograph, postero-anterior projection.

1 Anterior axillary fold	**10** Left dome of diaphragm	**18** Right atrial border	**27** Right breast outline
2 Arch of aorta (aortic knuckle or knob)	**11** Left pulmonary artery	**19** Right dome of diaphragm	**28** Gas in fundus of stomach
3 Clavicle	**12** Position of aortic valve	**20** Right pulmonary artery	**29** Position of left ventricle
4 Descending aorta	**13** Position of mitral valve	**21** Right ventricle	**30** Position of left atrium
5 First rib	**14** Position of pulmonary valve	**22** Spine of scapula	**31** Position of liver
6 Inferior vena cava	**15** Position of tricuspid valve	**23** Right main bronchus	**32** Manubrium
7 Left cardiophrenic angle	**16** Pulmonary trunk	**24** Left main bronchus	**33** Superior vena cava
8 Left costophrenic angle	**17** Region of tip of auricle of left atrium	**25** Carina	**34** Trachea
9 Left ventricular border		**26** Left breast outline	

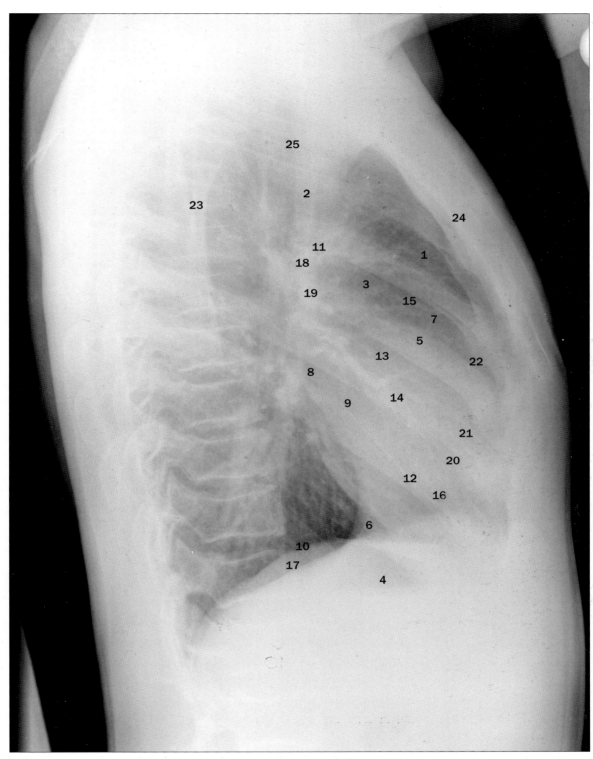

Chest radiograph, lateral projection.

1 Anterior mediastinal space	**7** Infundibulum of right ventricle (below) with pulmonary trunk (above)	**13** Position of aortic valve	**21** Right ventricle
2 Arch of aorta (aortic knuckle or knob)		**14** Position of mitral valve	**22** Right ventricular border of heart
		15 Position of pulmonary valve	
3 Ascending aorta	**8** Left atrial border of heart	**16** Position of tricuspid valve	**23** Scapula
4 Gas in fundus of stomach	**9** Left atrium	**17** Right dome of diaphragm	**24** Sternum
5 Horizontal fissure	**10** Left dome of diaphragm	**18** Right main bronchus	**25** Trachea
6 Inferior vena cava	**11** Left main pulmonary artery	**19** Right main pulmonary artery	
	12 Left oblique fissure	**20** Right oblique fissure	

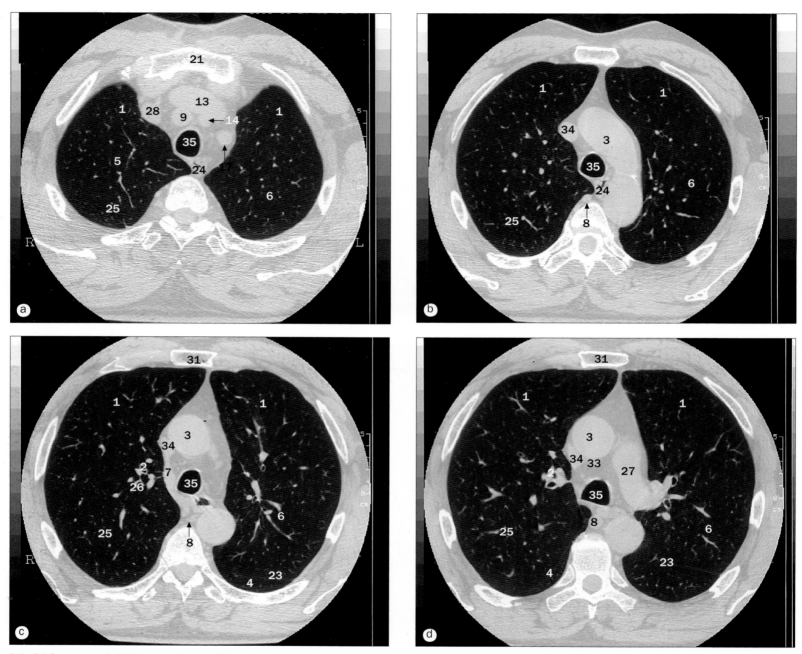

(a)–(h) Lungs, axial high-resolution CT images.

1 Anterior segment superior lobe	**8** Azygos vein	**15** Left inferior lobe bronchus
2 Anterior segmental bronchus	**9** Brachiocephalic trunk	**16** Left main bronchus
3 Aorta	**10** Bronchus intermedius	**17** Left subclavian artery
4 Apical segment inferior lobe	**11** Horizontal fissure	**18** Left superior lobe bronchus
5 Apical segment right superior lobe	**12** Lateral segment middle lobe	**19** Right superior pulmonary vein
6 Apicoposterior segment left superior lobe	**13** Left brachiocephalic vein	**20** Lingular segmental bronchus
7 Azygos arch	**14** Left common carotid artery	

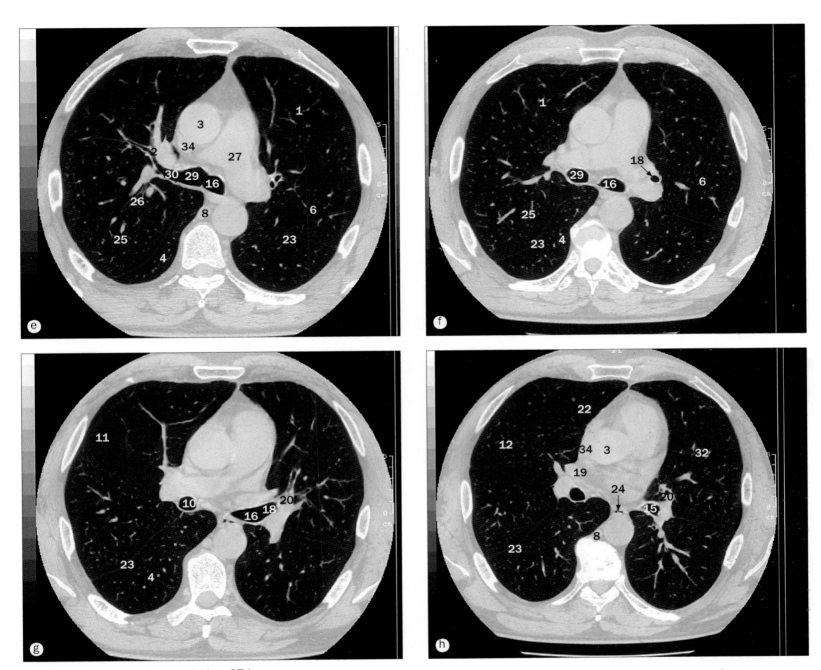

(a)–(h) Lungs, axial high-resolution CT images.

21 Manubrium of sternum
22 Medial segment middle lobe
23 Oblique fissure
24 Oesophagus
25 Posterior segment superior lobe

26 Posterior segmental bronchus
27 Pulmonary artery
28 Right brachiocephalic vein
29 Right main bronchus
30 Right superior lobe bronchus

31 Sternum
32 Superior lingular segment
33 Superior pericardial recess
34 Superior vena cava
35 Trachea

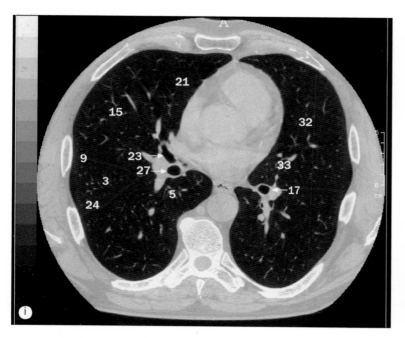
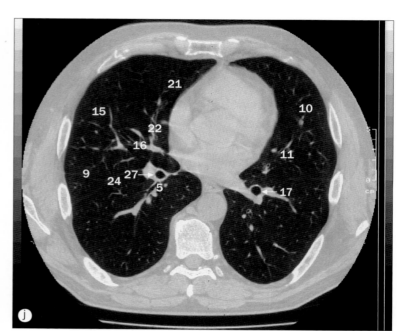
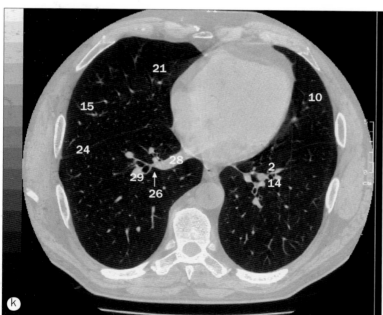
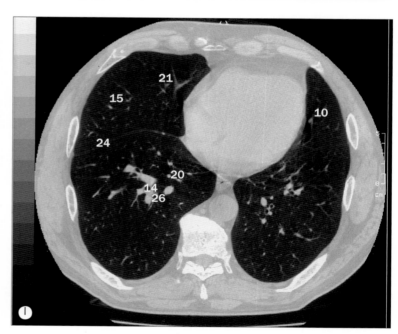

(i)–(p) Lungs, axial high-resolution CT images.

1 Anterior basal segment inferior lobe	**7** Heart	**13** Lateral basal segment inferior lobe
2 Anterior basal segmental bronchus	**8** Hemi-azygos vein	**14** Lateral basal segmental bronchus
3 Anterior segment superior lobe	**9** Horizontal fissure	**15** Lateral segment middle lobe
4 Aorta	**10** Inferior lingular segment	**16** Lateral segmental bronchus of middle lobe
5 Apical segment inferior lobe bronchus	**11** Inferior lingular segmental bronchus	
6 Azygos vein	**12** Inferior vena cava	**17** Left inferior lobe bronchus

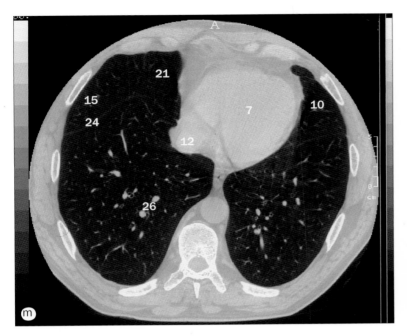

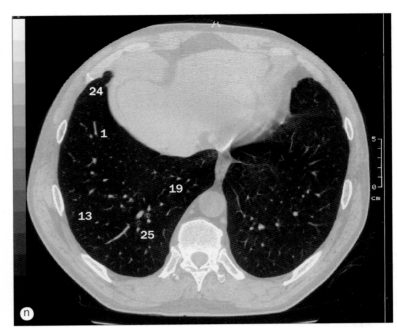

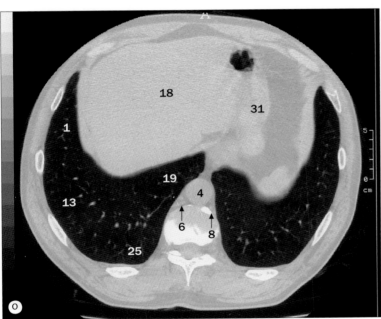

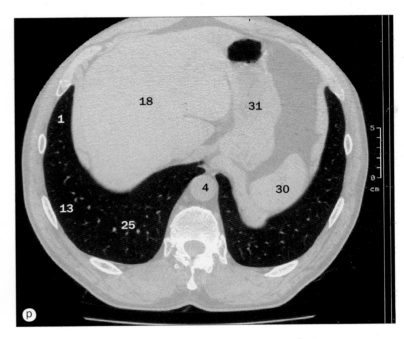

(i)–(p) Lungs, axial high-resolution CT images.

18 Liver	**23** Middle lobe bronchus	**29** Right lower lobe pulmonary artery
19 Medial basal segment inferior lobe	**24** Oblique fissure	**30** Spleen
20 Medial basal segmental bronchus	**25** Posterior basal segment inferior lobe	**31** Stomach
21 Medial segment middle lobe	**26** Posterior basal segmental bronchus	**32** Superior lingular segment
22 Medial segmental bronchus of middle lobe	**27** Right inferior lobe bronchus	**33** Superior lingular segmental bronchus
	28 Right inferior pulmonary vein	

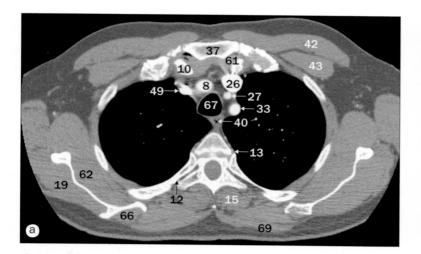

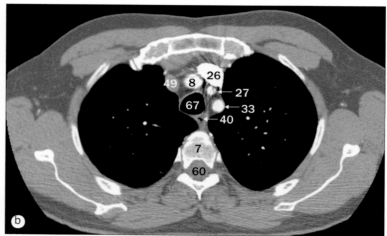

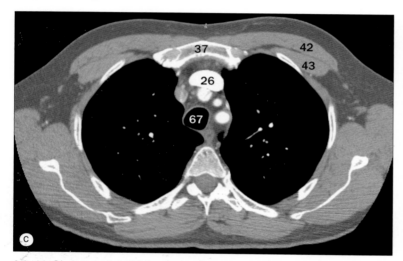

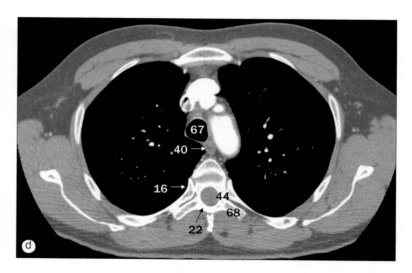

(a)–(t) Chest, axial CT images of mediastinum.

1 Anterior interventricular branch of left coronary artery	**12** Costotransverse joint	**24** Left atrial appendage (auricle)
2 Aortic valve	**13** Costovertebral joint	**25** Left atrium
3 Arch of aorta (aortic knuckle or knob)	**14** Descending aorta	**26** Left brachiocephalic vein
4 Ascending aorta	**15** Erector spinae muscle	**27** Left common carotid artery
5 Azygos vein	**16** Head of rib	**28** Left hemidiaphragm
6 Body of sternum	**17** Hemi-azygos vein	**29** Left inferior lobe bronchus
7 Body of vertebra	**18** Inferior vena cava	**30** Left inferior pulmonary vein
8 Brachiocephalic trunk	**19** Infraspinatus muscle	**31** Left main bronchus
9 Carina (bifurcation of trachea)	**20** Interatrial septum	**32** Left pulmonary artery
10 Clavicle	**21** Internal thoracic artery and vein	**33** Left subclavian artery
11 Coronary sinus	**22** Lamina	**34** Left superior lobe bronchus
	23 Latissimus dorsi muscle	**35** Left superior pulmonary vein

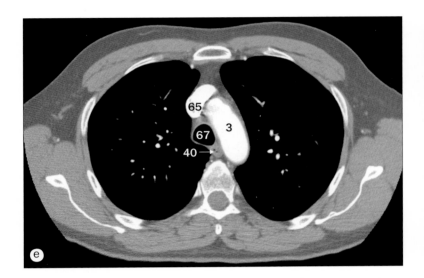

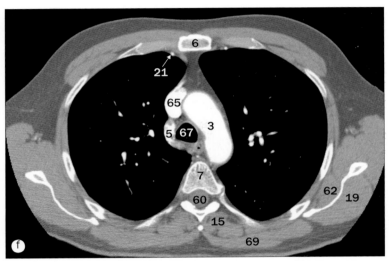

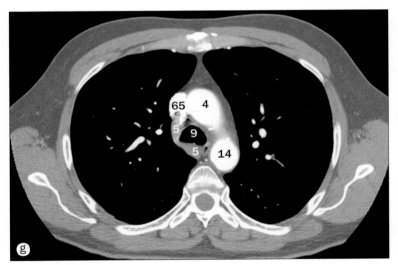

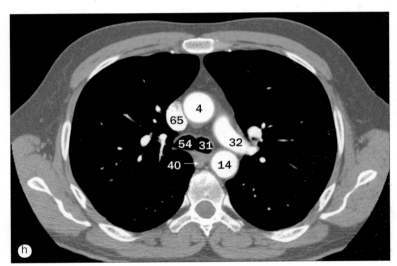

(a)–(t) Chest, axial CT images of mediastinum.

36 Left ventricular cavity	49 Right brachiocephalic vein	62 Subscapularis muscle
37 Manubrium of sternum	50 Right hemidiaphragm	63 Superior lobe branch of right pulmonary
38 Mitral valve	51 Right inferior lobe bronchus	artery
39 Muscular interventricular septum	52 Right inferior pulmonary vein	64 Superior pericardial recess
40 Oesophagus	53 Right lobe of liver	65 Superior vena cava
41 Papillary muscles	54 Right main bronchus	66 Supraspinatus muscle
42 Pectoralis major muscle	55 Right pulmonary artery	67 Trachea
43 Pectoralis minor muscle	56 Right superior lobe bronchus	68 Transverse process
44 Pedicle	57 Right superior pulmonary vein	69 Trapezius muscle
45 Pericardium	58 Right ventricular cavity	70 Tricuspid valve
46 Pulmonary trunk	59 Serratus anterior muscle	71 Xiphisternum
47 Right atrial appendage (auricle)	60 Spinal canal	
48 Right atrium	61 Sternoclavicular joint	

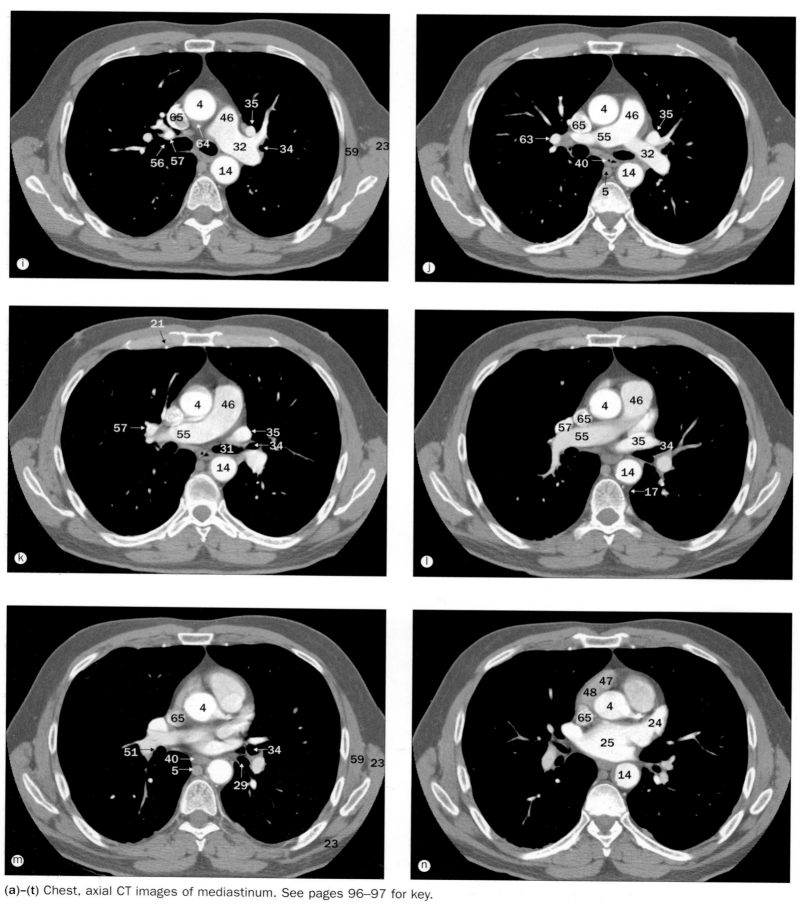

(a)–(t) Chest, axial CT images of mediastinum. See pages 96–97 for key.

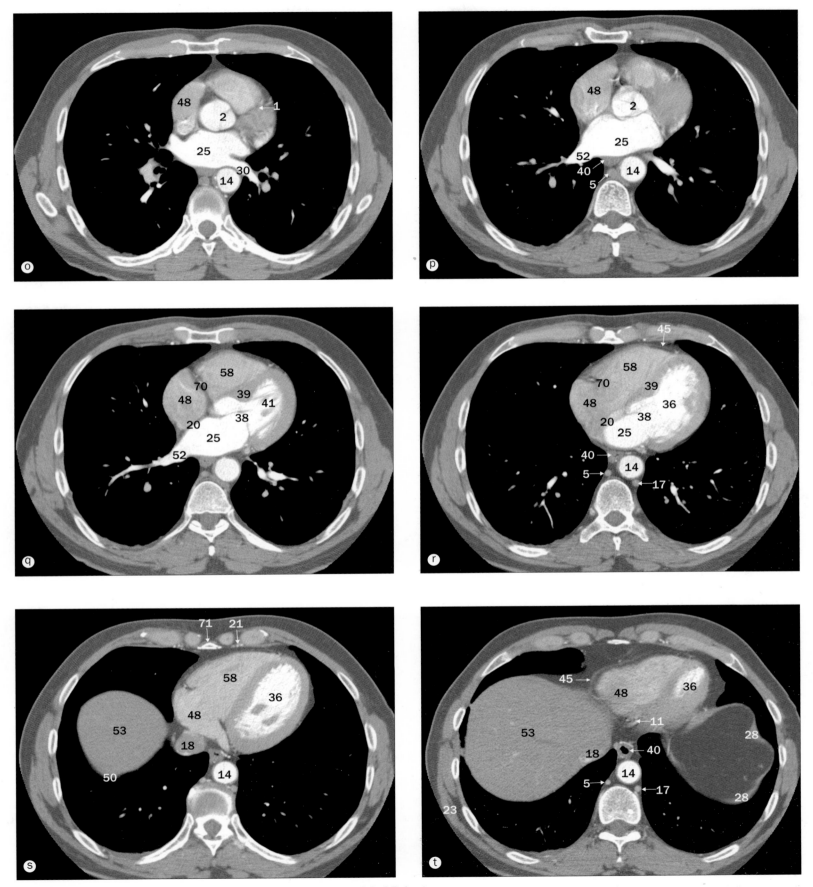

(a)–(t) Chest, axial CT images of mediastinum. See pages 96–97 for key.

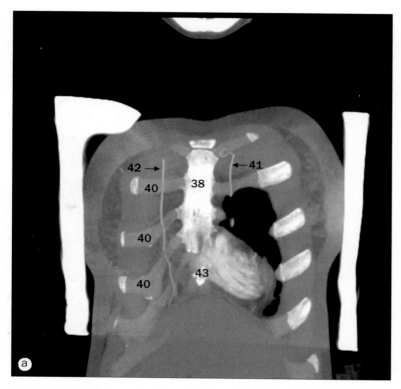

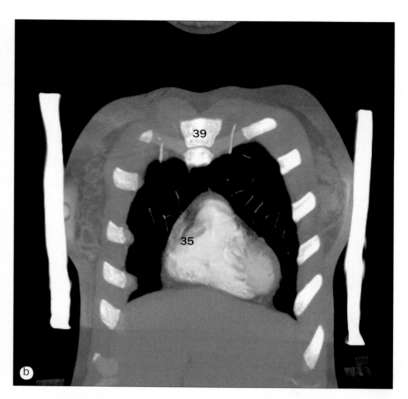

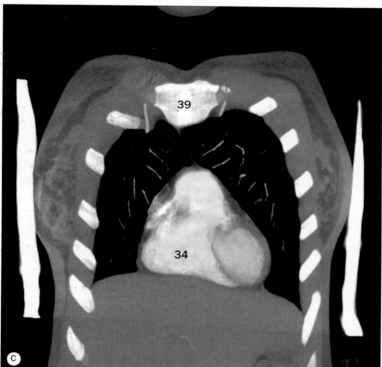

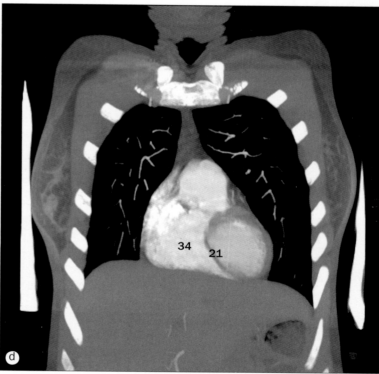

(a)–(p) Chest, coronal CT images, from anterior to posterior.

1 Aortic valve	9 Interatrial septum	17 Left superior pulmonary vein
2 Arch of aorta (aortic knuckle or knob)	10 Left atrial appendage (auricle)	18 Left ventricular cavity
3 Ascending aorta	11 Left atrium	19 Left ventricular wall
4 Brachiocephalic trunk	12 Left brachiocephalic vein	20 Membranous interventricular septum
5 Carina (bifurcation of trachea)	13 Left common carotid artery	21 Muscular interventricular septum
6 Clavicle	14 Left main bronchus	22 Papillary muscles
7 Descending aorta	15 Left pulmonary artery	23 Pericardium
8 Inferior vena cava	16 Left subclavian artery	24 Pulmonary trunk

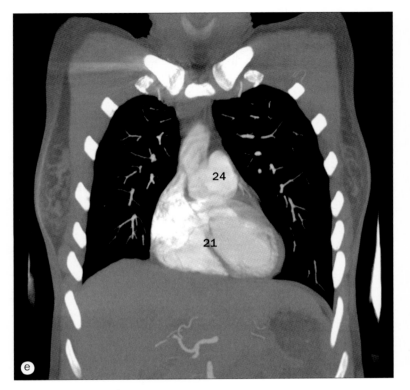

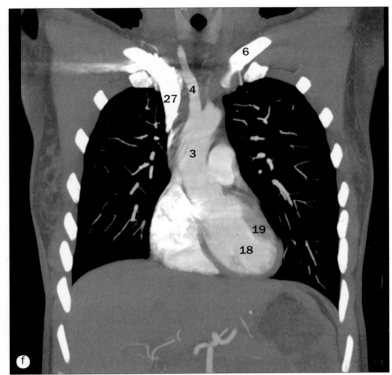

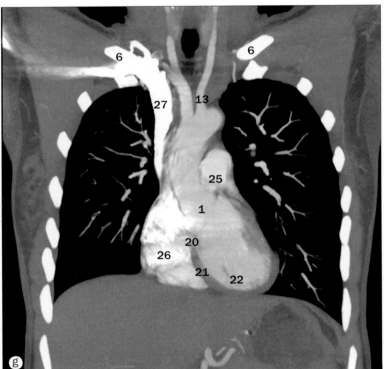

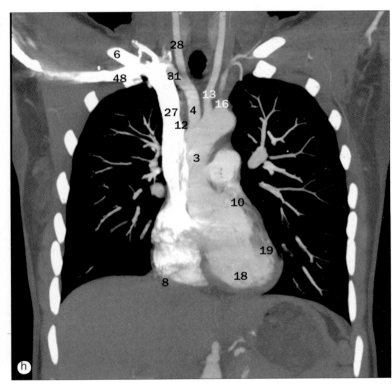

(a)–(p) Chest, coronal CT images, from anterior to posterior.

25 Pulmonary valve	**34** Right ventricular cavity	**43** Xiphisternum
26 Right atrium	**35** Right ventricular wall	**44** Tricuspid valve
27 Right brachiocephalic vein	**36** Superior vena cava	**45** Mitral valve
28 Right common carotid artery	**37** Trachea	**46** Left axillary artery
29 Right main bronchus	**38** Sternum	**47** Left subclavian artery
30 Right pulmonary artery	**39** Manubrium	**48** Right subclavian vein
31 Right subclavian artery	**40** Anterior costal cartilage	**49** Left inferior pulmonary vein
32 Right superior lobe pulmonary artery	**41** Left internal thoracic (mammary) artery	**50** Abdominal aorta
33 Right superior pulmonary vein	**42** Right internal thoracic (mammary) artery	**51** Right inferior pulmonary vein

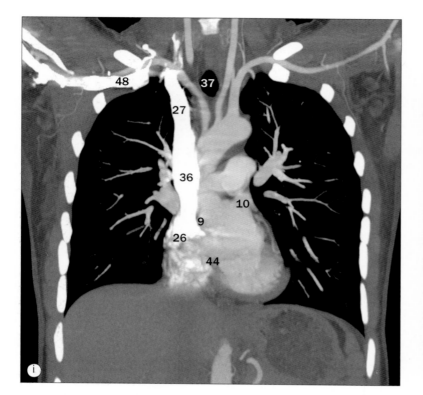

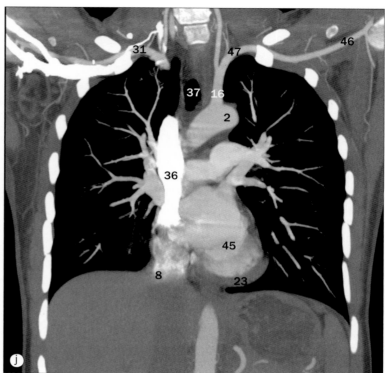

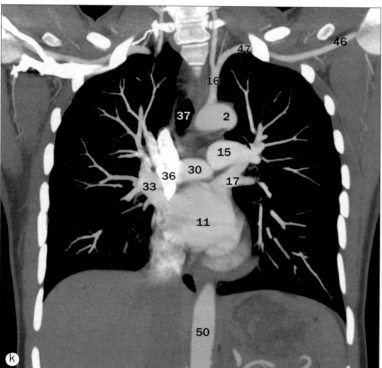

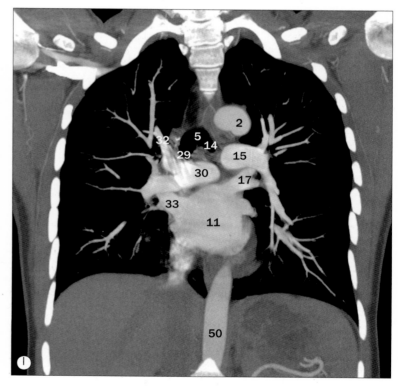

(a)–(p) Chest, coronal CT images, from anterior to posterior.

1 Aortic valve	**9** Interatrial septum	**17** Left superior pulmonary vein
2 Arch of aorta (aortic knuckle or knob)	**10** Left atrial appendage (auricle)	**18** Left ventricular cavity
3 Ascending aorta	**11** Left atrium	**19** Left ventricular wall
4 Brachiocephalic trunk	**12** Left brachiocephalic vein	**20** Membranous interventricular septum
5 Carina (bifurcation of trachea)	**13** Left common carotid artery	**21** Muscular interventricular septum
6 Clavicle	**14** Left main bronchus	**22** Papillary muscles
7 Descending aorta	**15** Left pulmonary artery	**23** Pericardium
8 Inferior vena cava	**16** Left subclavian artery	**24** Pulmonary trunk

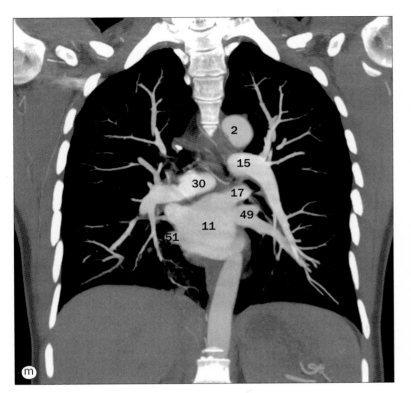

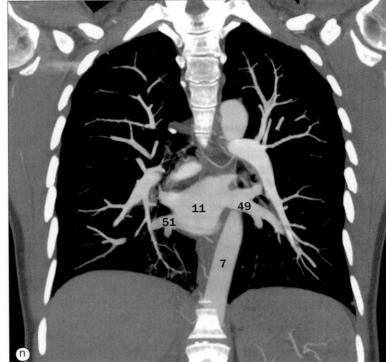

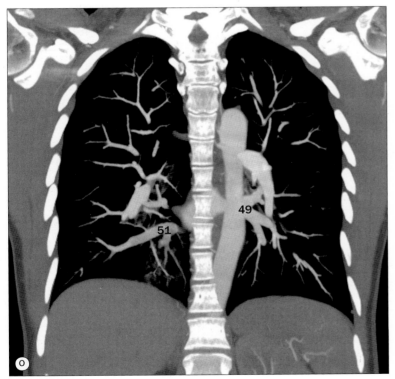

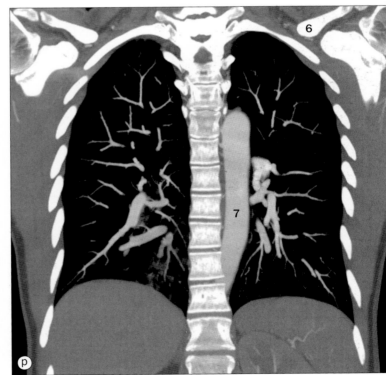

(a)–(p) Chest, coronal CT images, from anterior to posterior.

25 Pulmonary valve	34 Right ventricular cavity	43 Xiphisternum
26 Right atrium	35 Right ventricular wall	44 Tricuspid valve
27 Right brachiocephalic vein	36 Superior vena cava	45 Mitral valve
28 Right common carotid artery	37 Trachea	46 Left axillary artery
29 Right main bronchus	38 Sternum	47 Left subclavian artery
30 Right pulmonary artery	39 Manubrium	48 Right subclavian vein
31 Right subclavian artery	40 Anterior costal cartilage	49 Left inferior pulmonary vein
32 Right superior lobe pulmonary artery	41 Left internal thoracic (mammary) artery	50 Abdominal aorta
33 Right superior pulmonary vein	42 Right internal thoracic (mammary) artery	51 Right inferior pulmonary vein

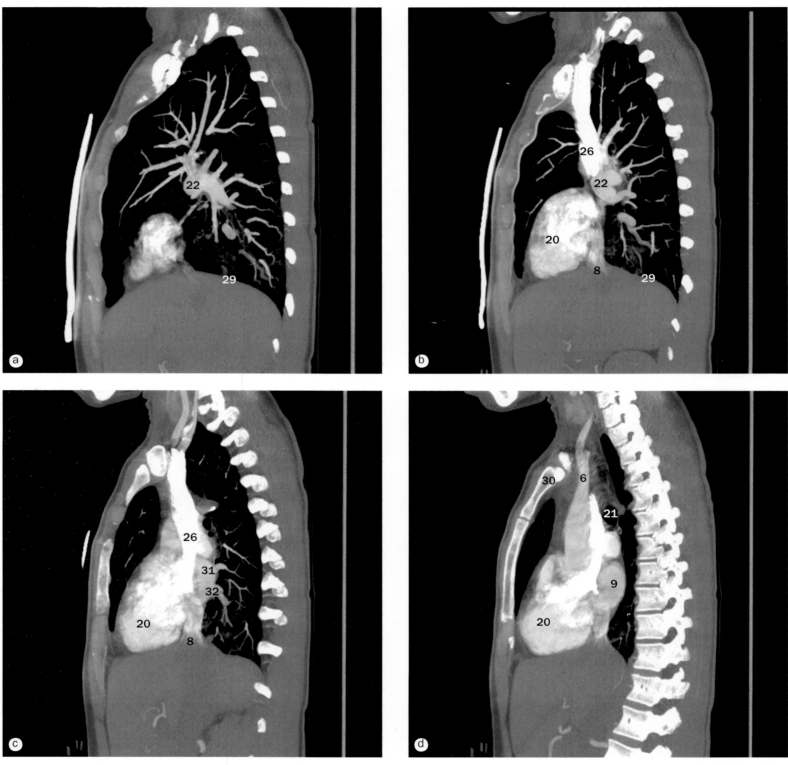

(a)–(p) Chest, sagittal CT images, from right to left.

1 Aortic valve	**8** Inferior vena cava	**15** Mitral valve
2 Arch of aorta (aortic knuckle or knob)	**9** Left atrium	**16** Muscular interventricular septum
3 Ascending aorta	**10** Left common carotid artery	**17** Pericardium
4 Body of sternum	**11** Left main bronchus	**18** Pulmonary trunk
5 Body of vertebra	**12** Left pulmonary artery	**19** Pulmonary valve
6 Brachiocephalic trunk	**13** Left subclavian artery	**20** Right atrium
7 Descending aorta	**14** Left ventricular cavity	**21** Right main bronchus

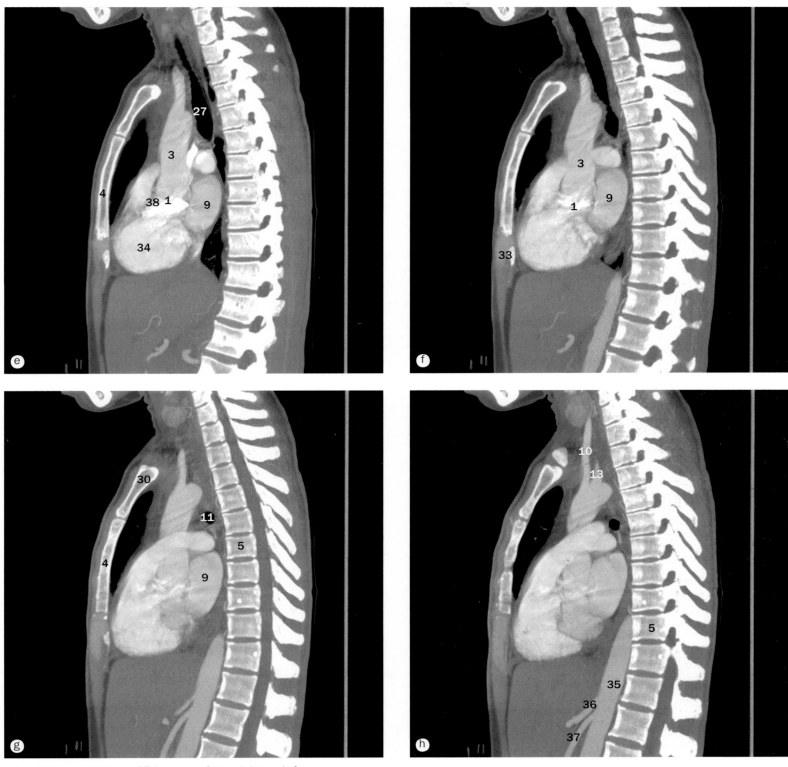

(a)–(p) Chest, sagittal CT images, from right to left.

22 Right pulmonary artery	**28** Left dome of diaphragm	**34** Tricuspid valve
23 Right ventricular cavity	**29** Right dome of diaphragm	**35** Abdominal aorta
24 Right ventricular outflow tract	**30** Manubrium	**36** Coeliac axis
25 Right ventricular wall	**31** Right superior pulmonary vein	**37** Superior mesenteric artery
26 Superior vena cava	**32** Right inferior pulmonary vein	**38** Right coronary artery
27 Trachea	**33** Xiphisternum	

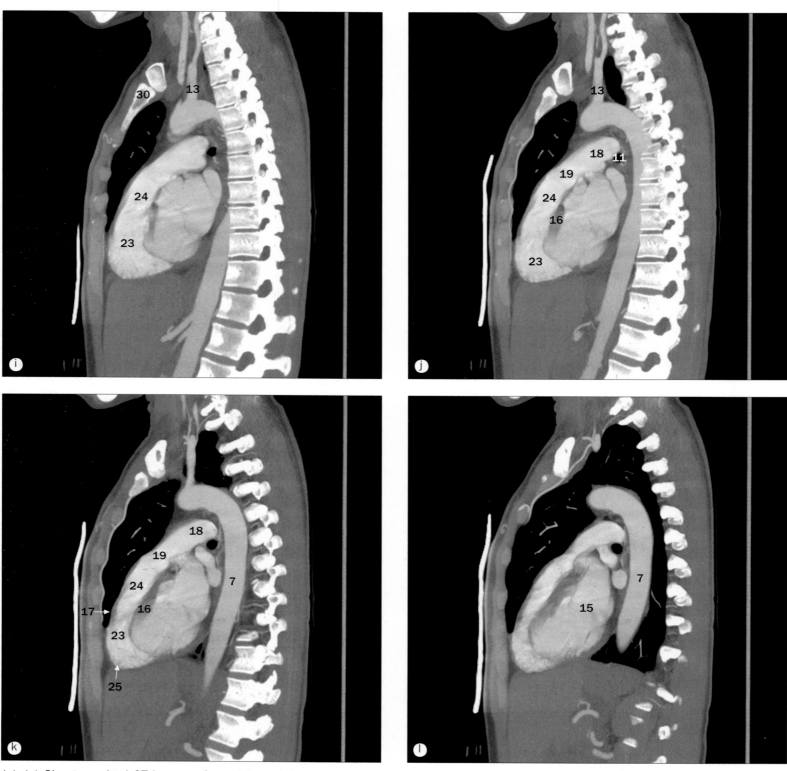

(a)–(p) Chest, sagittal CT images, from right to left.

1 Aortic valve	8 Inferior vena cava	15 Mitral valve
2 Arch of aorta (aortic knuckle or knob)	9 Left atrium	16 Muscular interventricular septum
3 Ascending aorta	10 Left common carotid artery	17 Pericardium
4 Body of sternum	11 Left main bronchus	18 Pulmonary trunk
5 Body of vertebra	12 Left pulmonary artery	19 Pulmonary valve
6 Brachiocephalic trunk	13 Left subclavian artery	20 Right atrium
7 Descending aorta	14 Left ventricular cavity	21 Right main bronchus

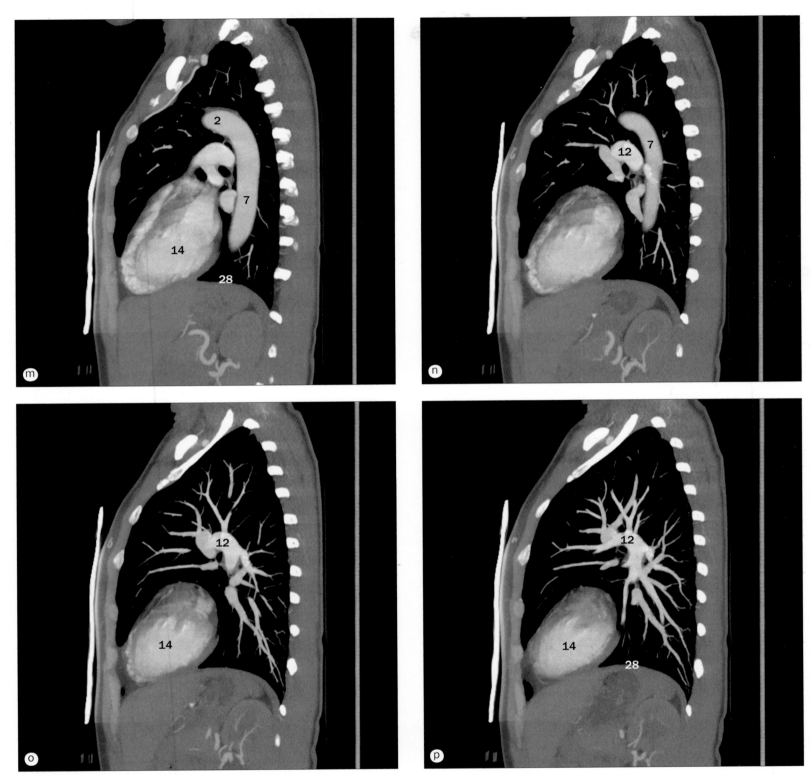

(a)–(p) Chest, sagittal CT images, from right to left.

22 Right pulmonary artery	**28** Left dome of diaphragm	**34** Tricuspid valve
23 Right ventricular cavity	**29** Right dome of diaphragm	**35** Abdominal aorta
24 Right ventricular outflow tract	**30** Manubrium	**36** Coeliac axis
25 Right ventricular wall	**31** Right superior pulmonary vein	**37** Superior mesenteric artery
26 Superior vena cava	**32** Right inferior pulmonary vein	**38** Right coronary artery
27 Trachea	**33** Xiphisternum	

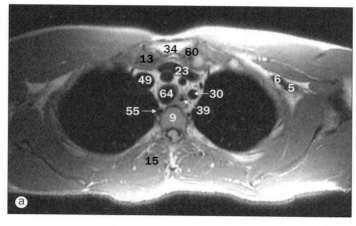

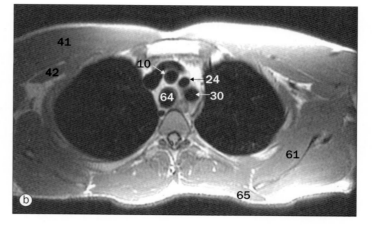

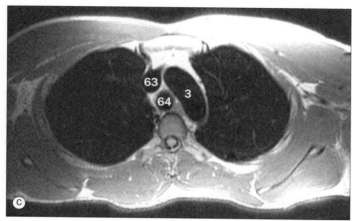

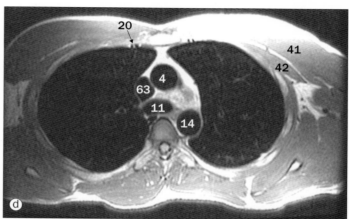

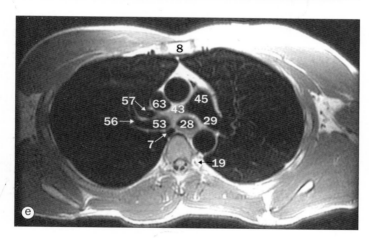

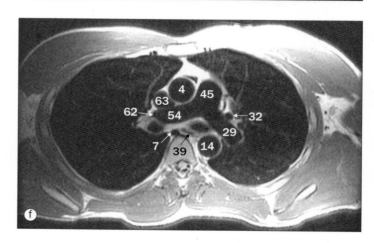

(a)–(l) Chest, axial MR images.

1 Anterior interventricular branch of left coronary artery	**12** Circumflex branch of left coronary artery	**24** Left common carotid artery
2 Aortic valve	**13** Clavicle	**25** Left coronary artery
3 Arch of aorta (aortic knuckle or knob)	**14** Descending aorta	**26** Left inferior lobe bronchus
4 Ascending aorta	**15** Erector spinae muscle	**27** Left inferior pulmonary vein
5 Axillary artery	**16** Hemi-azygos vein	**28** Left main bronchus
6 Axillary vein	**17** Inferior vena cava	**29** Left pulmonary artery
7 Azygos vein	**18** Interatrial septum	**30** Left subclavian artery
8 Body of sternum	**19** Intercostal artery	**31** Left superior lobe bronchus
9 Body of vertebra	**20** Internal thoracic artery and vein	**32** Left superior pulmonary vein
10 Brachiocephalic trunk	**21** Left atrial appendage (auricle)	**33** Left ventricular cavity
11 Carina (bifurcation of trachea)	**22** Left atrium	**34** Manubrium of sternum
	23 Left brachiocephalic vein	**35** Membranous interventricular septum

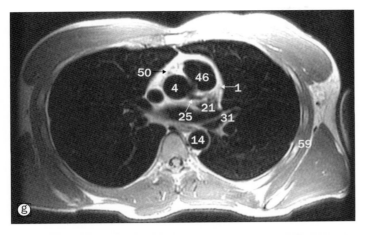

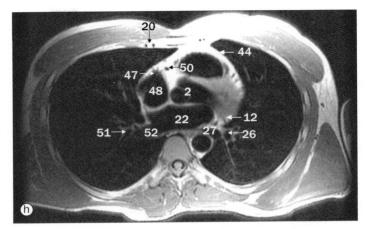

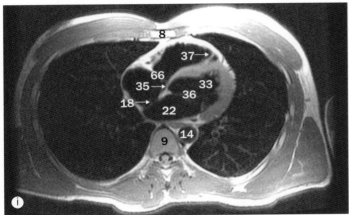

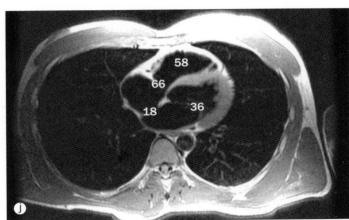

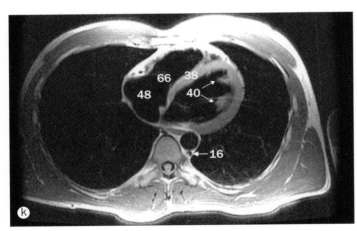

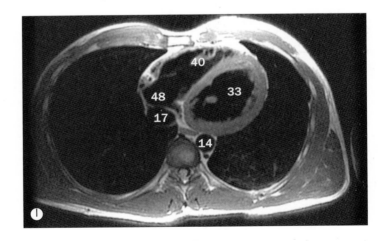

(a)–(l) Chest, axial MR images.

36 Mitral valve	**47** Right atrial appendage (auricle)	**58** Right ventricular cavity
37 Moderator band	**48** Right atrium	**59** Serratus anterior muscle
38 Muscular interventricular septum	**49** Right brachiocephalic vein	**60** Sternoclavicular joint
39 Oesophagus	**50** Right coronary artery	**61** Subscapularis muscle
40 Papillary muscles	**51** Right inferior lobe bronchus	**62** Superior lobe branch of
41 Pectoralis major muscle	**52** Right inferior pulmonary vein	right pulmonary artery
42 Pectoralis minor muscle	**53** Right main bronchus	**63** Superior vena cava
43 Pericardial recess	**54** Right pulmonary artery	**64** Trachea
44 Pericardium	**55** Right superior intercostal vein	**65** Trapezius muscle
45 Pulmonary trunk	**56** Right superior lobe bronchus	**66** Tricuspid valve
46 Pulmonary valve	**57** Right superior pulmonary vein	

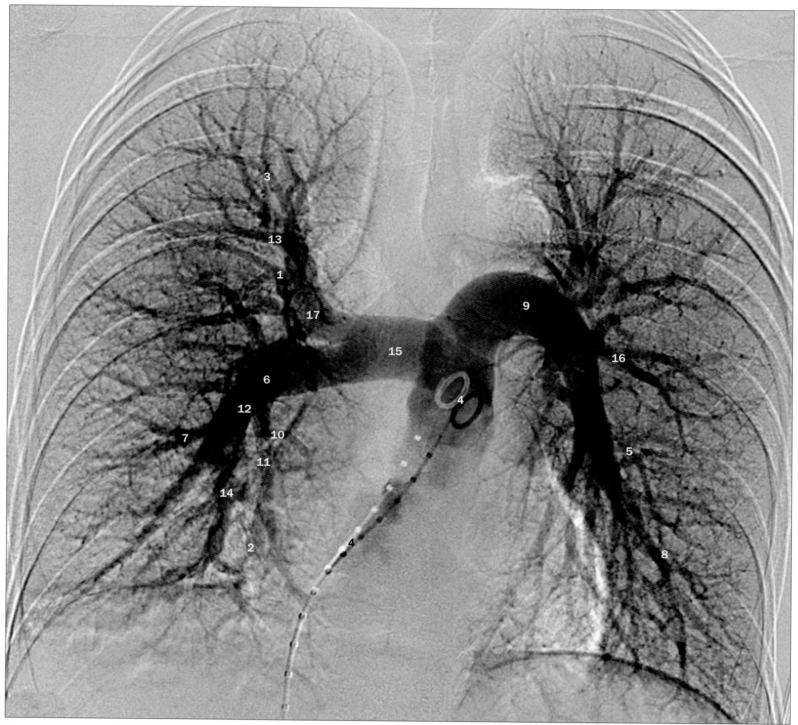

Pulmonary arteriogram, arterial phase.

1 Anterior artery (superior lobe)
2 Anterior basal artery
3 Apical artery (superior lobe)
4 Catheter in main pulmonary artery via
  a femoral vein, inferior vena cava, right
  atrium and right ventricle
5 Inferior lingular artery

6 Inferior lobe pulmonary artery
7 Lateral artery (middle lobe)
8 Lateral basal artery
9 Left pulmonary artery
10 Medial artery (middle lobe)
11 Medial basal artery
12 Middle lobe pulmonary artery

13 Posterior artery (superior lobe)
14 Posterior basal artery
15 Right pulmonary artery
16 Superior lingular artery
17 Superior lobe pulmonary artery

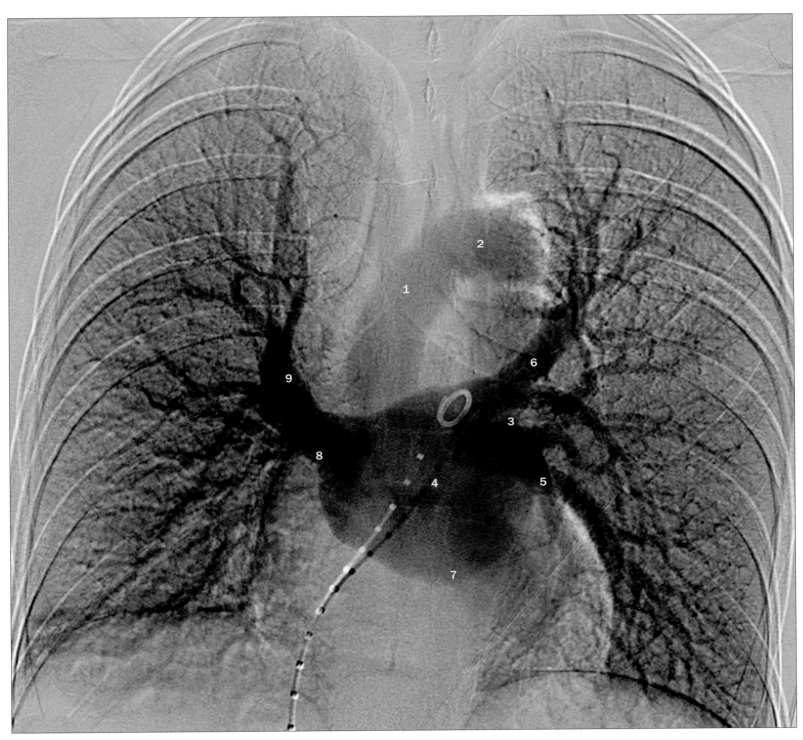

Pulmonary arteriogram, venous phase.

1 Aorta
2 Aortic arch
3 Left atrial appendage (auricle)
4 Left atrium
5 Left inferior pulmonary vein
6 Left superior pulmonary vein
7 Mitral valve
8 Right inferior pulmonary vein
9 Right superior pulmonary vein

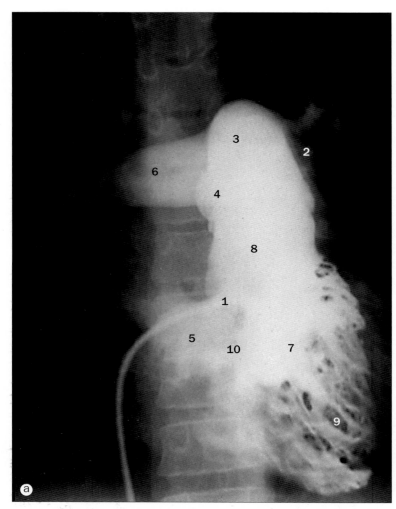 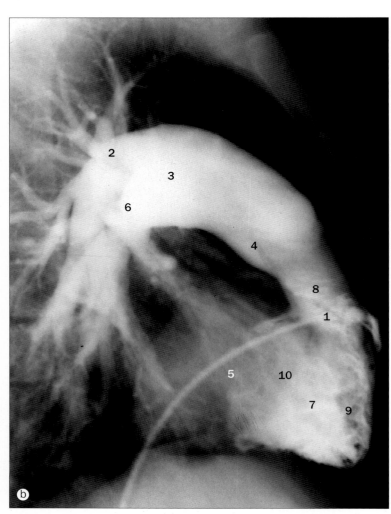

Right ventricular angiograms, (a) anteroposterior projection, (b) lateral projection.

 1 Catheter in right ventricle via inferior vena cava and right atrium
 2 Left main pulmonary artery
 3 Pulmonary artery
 4 Pulmonary valve
 5 Right atrium
 6 Right main pulmonary artery
 7 Right ventricle
 8 Right ventricular outflow tract
 9 Trabeculae of right ventricle
10 Tricuspid valve

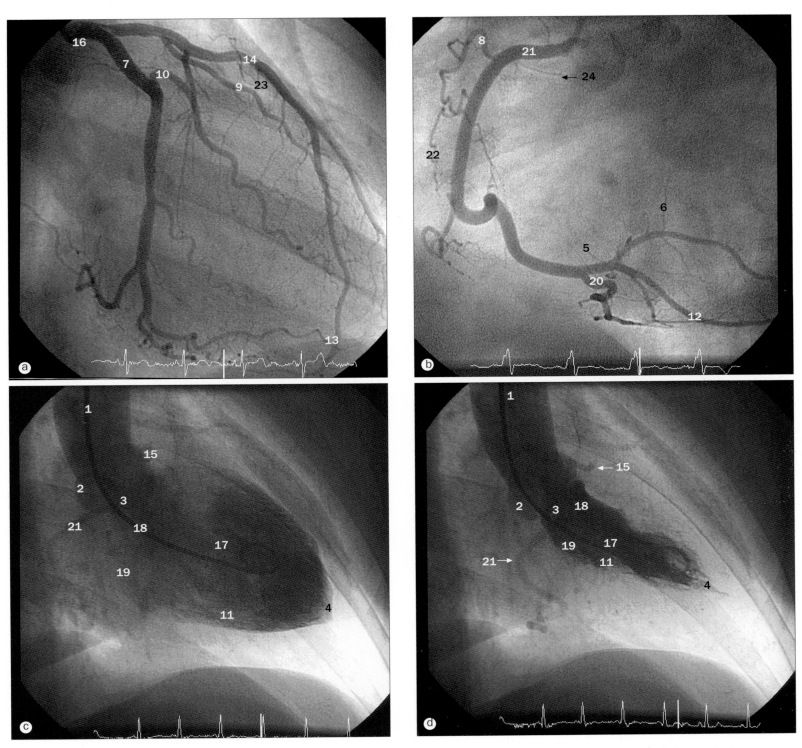

(a) Left coronary arteriogram, (b) right coronary arteriogram, (c) left ventricular angiogram, diastolic phase, (d) left ventricular angiogram, systolic phase.

1 Aorta
2 Aortic sinus
3 Aortic valve
4 Apex of the left ventricle
5 Atrioventricular nodal artery
6 Branch to left atrium
7 Circumflex artery
8 Conus artery
9 Diagonal arteries
10 First obtuse marginal branch of circumflex artery
11 Inferior wall of left ventricle
12 Lateral ventricular branch to left ventricle
13 Left anterior interventricular artery curving round apex of heart
14 Left anterior interventricular branch (left anterior descending)
15 Left coronary artery
16 Left main stem coronary artery
17 Left ventricular cavity
18 Left ventricular outflow tract
19 Mitral valve
20 Posterior interventricular septal artery (posterior descending artery)
21 Right coronary artery
22 Right marginal arteries
23 Septal arteries
24 Sinuatrial nodal artery

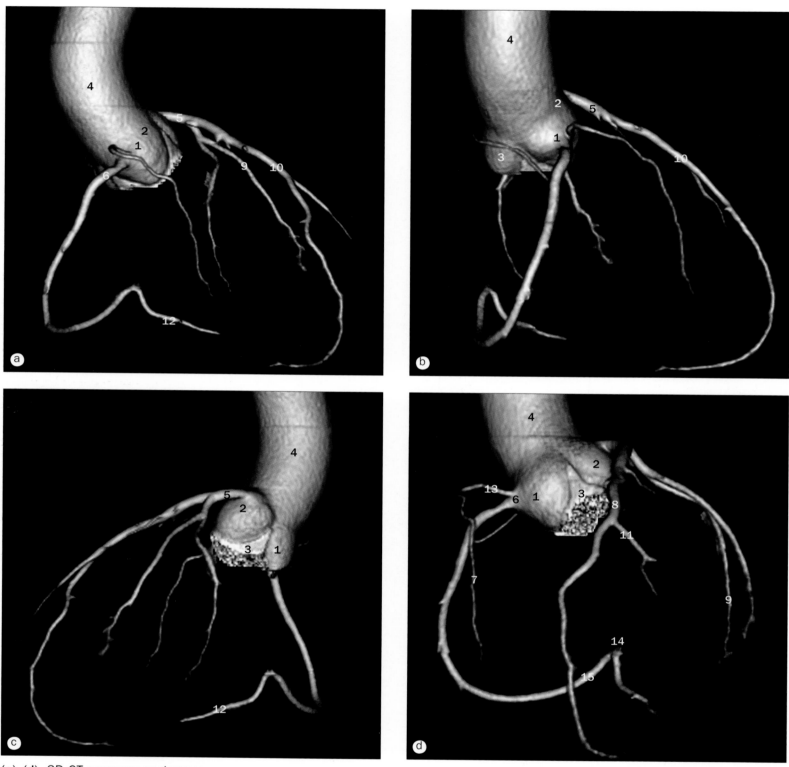

(a)–(d) 3D CT coronary angiograms.

1 Right coronary sinus
2 Left coronary sinus
3 Non coronary sinus
4 Ascending aorta
5 Left main coronary artery
6 Right main coronary artery
7 Right ventricular branch of right coronary artery
8 Circumflex artery
9 Diagonal artery
10 Left anterior descending artery
11 Obtuse marginal artery
12 Marginal artery
13 Right conal artery
14 Atrioventricular nodal artery
15 Posterior interventricular branch, right coronary artery

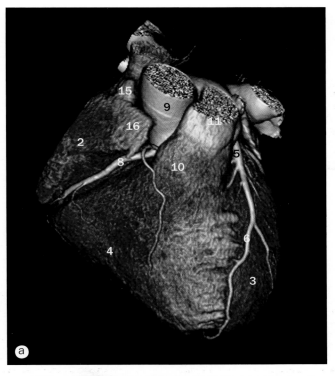

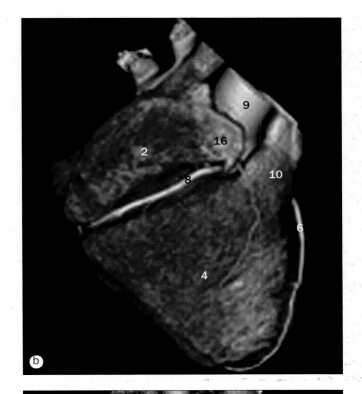

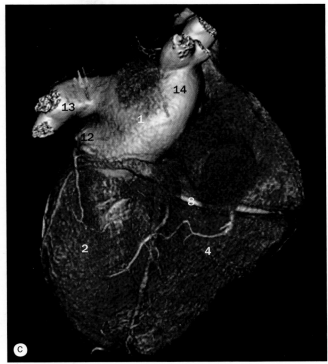

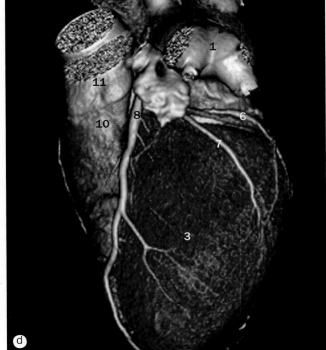

(a)–(d) 3D CT heart reconstructions.

1 Left atrium	**7** Circumflex artery	**12** Left atrial appendage
2 Right atrium	**8** Right coronary artery	**13** Right pulmonary veins
3 Left ventricle	**9** Aortic root	**14** Left pulmonary veins
4 Right ventricle	**10** Pulmonary outflow tract	**15** Superior vena cava
5 Left main coronary artery	**11** Pulmonary artery	**16** Right atrial appendage
6 Left anterior descending coronary artery		

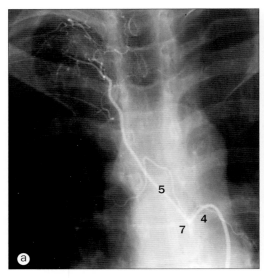 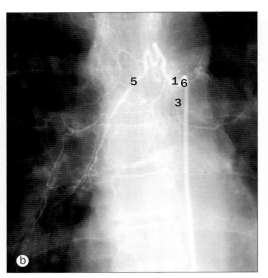 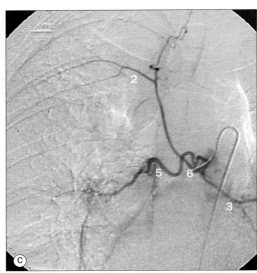

(a)–(c) Right bronchial arteriograms.

There is a great variability in the anatomy of the bronchial arteries, but the majority originate from the descending thoracic aorta, above the level of the left main stem bronchus between the upper border of the fifth thoracic vertebra and the lower border of the sixth thoracic vertebra. The number of bronchial arteries on each side may vary between one and four. Usually, there is one vessel to the right lung and two to the left. Accessory bronchial arteries may arise from the brachiocephalic artery and subclavian arteries, or from other branches such as the internal thoracic, pericardiophrenic and oesophageal arteries. In many cases the right bronchial artery arises from an intercostobronchial trunk, but in this example the trunk is very short and divides almost immediately into a right bronchial artery, which is directed towards the hilum, and the first right aortic intercostal artery. Reflux filling of the left bronchial artery is seen. A second larger bronchial artery which has been catheterised **(b)** has a common trunk arising from the front of the aorta, giving rise to a right and left bronchial artery.

1 Common bronchial trunk
2 Intercostal artery
3 Left bronchial branches
4 Reflux filling of left bronchial artery
5 Right bronchial artery
6 Tip of catheter in common bronchial arterial trunk
7 Tip of catheter in intercostobronchial trunk

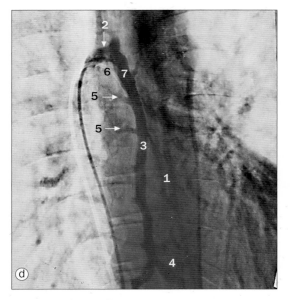

(d) Azygos venogram.

In the thorax the vertebral veins drain into intercostal veins, while in the lumbar region the lumbar veins drain into the ascending lumbar veins. The right ascending lumbar vein becomes the azygos vein on entering the thorax, and the left ascending lumbar vein becomes the hemi-azygos vein. At the level of the fourth thoracic vertebra, the azygos vein turns anteriorly (the arch of the azygos) to enter the superior vena cava. The hemi-azygos vein crosses to join the azygos vein at the level of the eighth or ninth thoracic vertebral body. The accessory hemi-azygos vein is continuous with the hemi-azygos vein inferiorly and the left superior intercostal vein superiorly.

1 Accessory hemi-azygos vein
2 Azygos arch
3 Azygos vein
4 Hemi-azygos vein
5 Intercostal veins
6 Subtraction artefact caused by cardiac and catheter movement
7 Tip of catheter introduced via femoral vein into superior vena cava and azygos vein

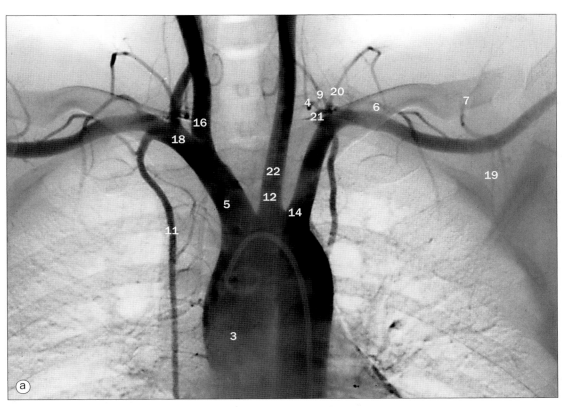

(a) Subtracted arch aortogram, anteroposterior image.
The vertebral artery (22) has a separate origin off the arch, projected over the left common carotid artery in this view. This is a normal variant.

(b) Subtracted arch aortogram, left anterior oblique image.
The origins of the supra-aortic branches are best shown by left anterior oblique projection, so that the origins of the vessels are not superimposed. There are many congenital variations in the way in which the major vessels arise from the aortic arch, but the most common is shown here.

(c) Left ventricular angiogram.

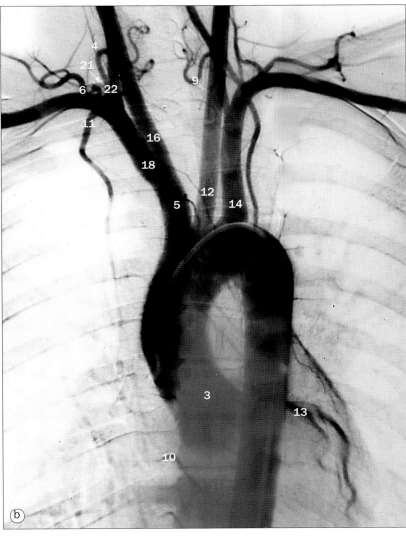

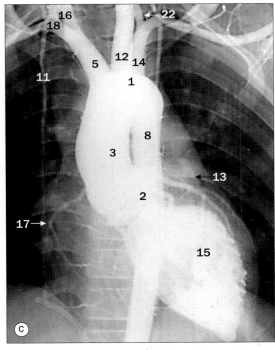

1 Aortic arch	**12** Left common carotid artery
2 Aortic valve	**13** Left coronary artery
3 Ascending aorta	**14** Left subclavian artery
4 Ascending cervical artery	**15** Left ventricle
5 Brachiocephalic trunk	**16** Right common carotid artery
6 Costocervical trunk	**17** Right coronary artery
7 Deltoid branch of thoraco-acromial artery	**18** Right subclavian artery
8 Descending aorta	**19** Superior thoracic artery
9 Inferior thyroid artery	**20** Suprascapular artery
10 Intercostal artery	**21** Thyrocervical trunk
11 Internal thoracic artery	**22** Vertebral artery

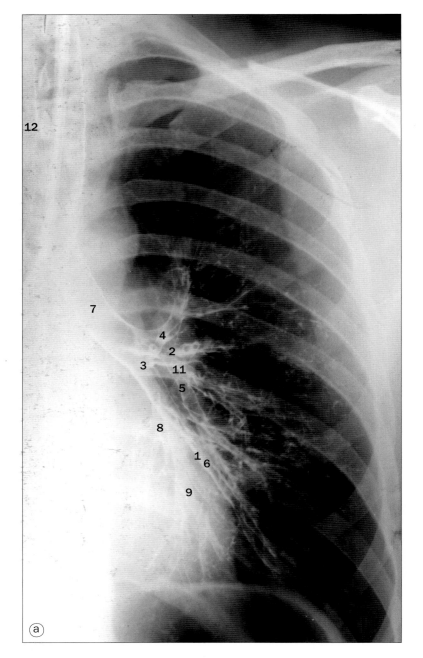

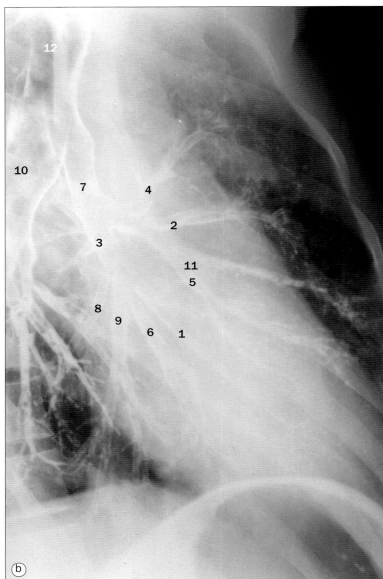

Left lung bronchogram, **(a)** postero-anterior image, **(b)** oblique projection.

 1 Anterior basal segmental bronchus
 2 Anterior segmental bronchus
 3 Apical (superior) segmental bronchus
 4 Apicoposterior segmental bronchus
 5 Inferior lingular segmental bronchus
 6 Lateral basal segmental bronchus
 7 Left main bronchus
 8 Medial basal segmental bronchus
 9 Posterior basal segmental bronchus
10 Right main bronchus
11 Superior lingular segmental bronchus
12 Trachea

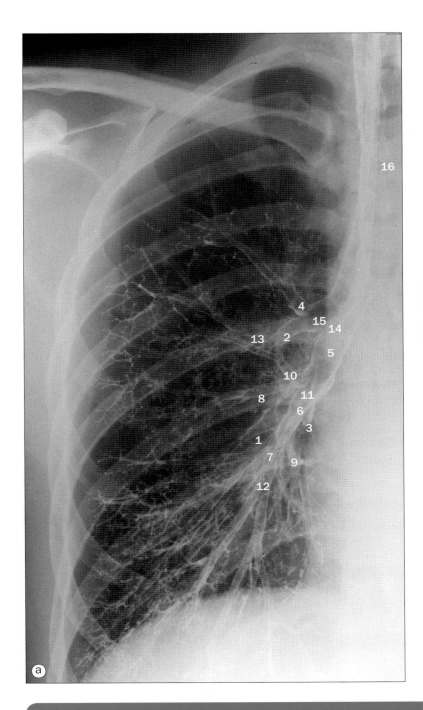

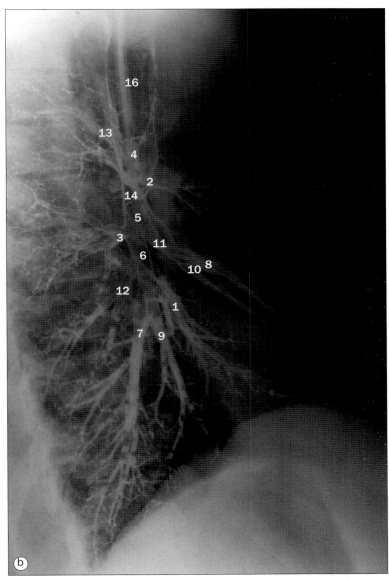

Right lung bronchogram, (a) postero-anterior projection, (b) lateral projection.

1 Anterior basal segmental bronchus	**9** Medial basal segmental bronchus
2 Anterior segmental bronchus	**10** Medial segmental bronchus of middle lobe
3 Apical (superior) segmental bronchus	**11** Middle lobe bronchus
4 Apical segmental bronchus	**12** Posterior basal segmental bronchus
5 Bronchus intermedius	**13** Posterior segmental bronchus
6 Inferior lobe bronchus	**14** Right main bronchus
7 Lateral basal segmental bronchus	**15** Right superior lobe bronchus
8 Lateral segmental bronchus of middle lobe	**16** Trachea

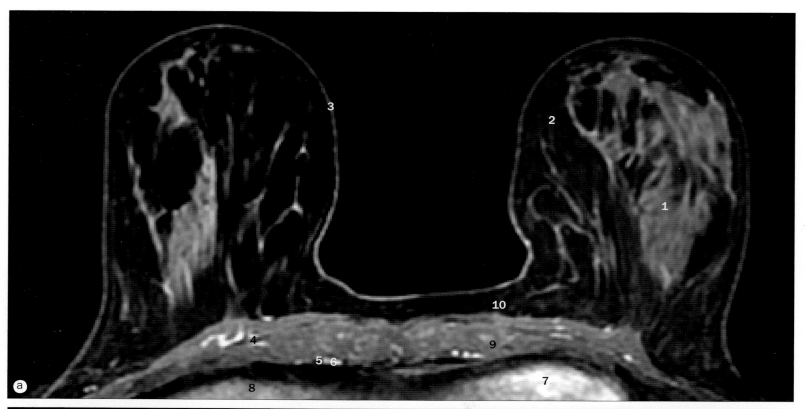

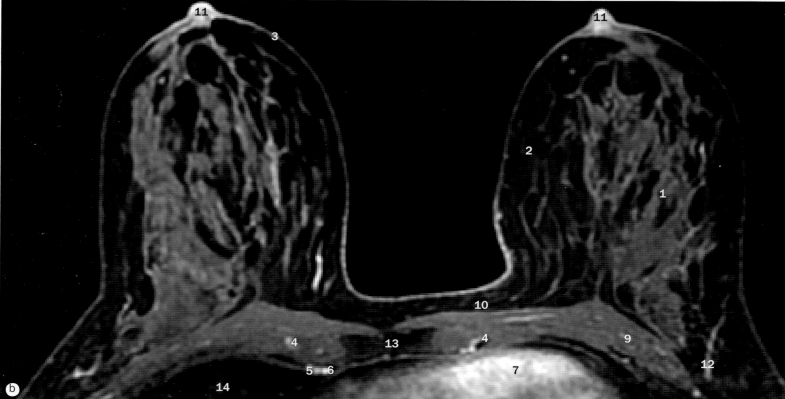

Mammograms, MR images.

1 Fibroglandular tissue (of the right breast)	6 Internal mammary artery	12 Intramammary branches of lateral thoracic artery
2 Adipose tissue of the breast	7 Heart	13 Sternum
3 Skin	8 Liver	14 Middle lobe of the right lung
4 Anterior perforating branch of the internal mammary artery	9 Pectoralis major muscle	
5 Internal mammary vein	10 Anterior pectoralis fascia	
	11 Nipple/areolar complex	

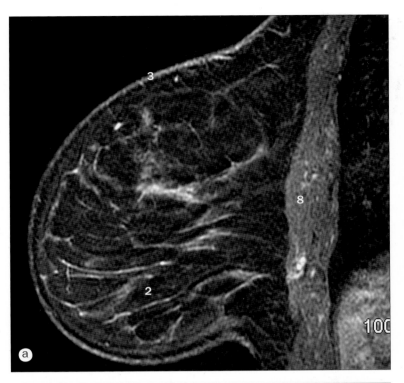

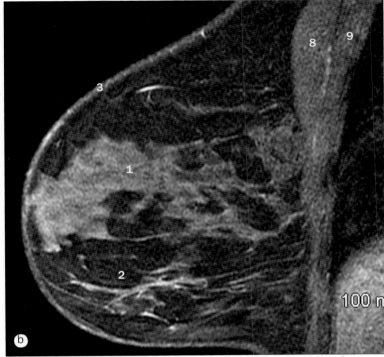

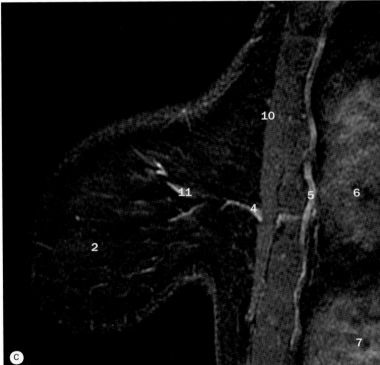

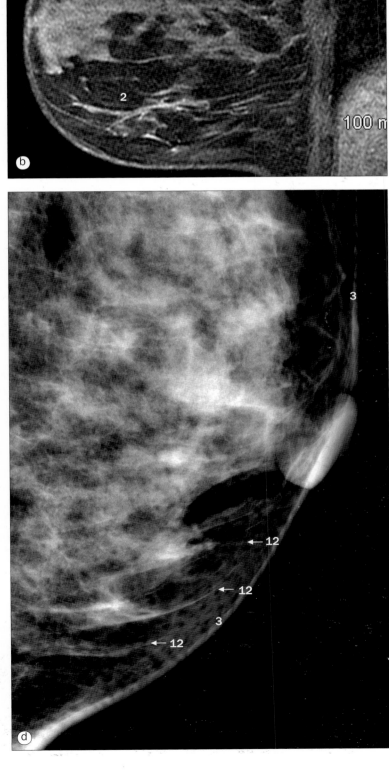

Mammograms, (a)–(c) MR images, (d) mammographic X-ray image.

1 Fibroglandular tissue (of the right breast)
2 Adipose tissue of the breast
3 Skin
4 Anterior perforating branch of the internal mammary artery
5 Internal mammary artery
6 Heart
7 Liver
8 Pectoralis major muscle
9 Pectoralis minor muscle
10 Anterior pectoralis fascia
11 Intramammary vessels
12 Cooper's ligaments

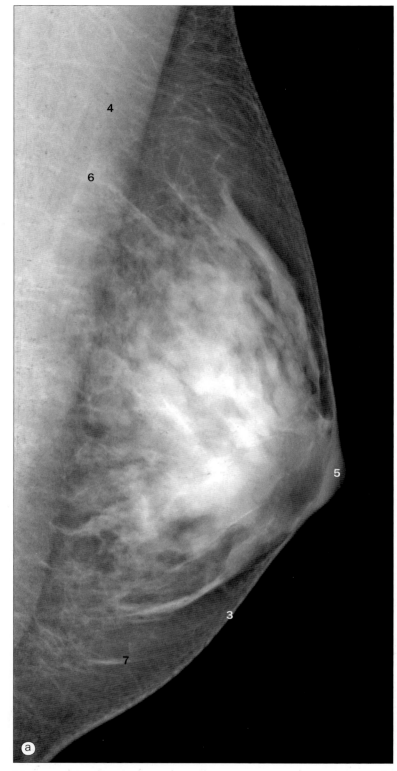
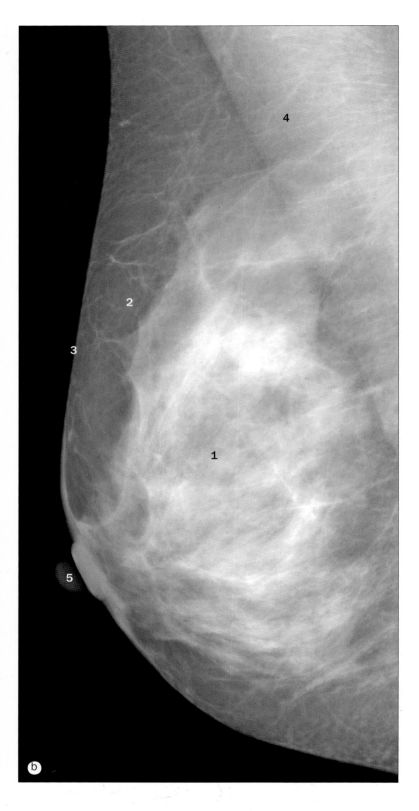

Mammograms.

1 Fibroglandular tissue (of the right breast)	**4** Pectoralis major muscle
	5 Nipple–areolar complex
2 Adipose tissue of the breast	**6** Vessel
3 Skin	**7** Cooper's ligament

5 Abdomen and pelvis – Cross-sectional

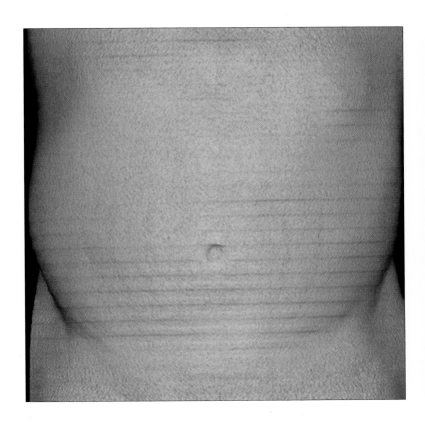

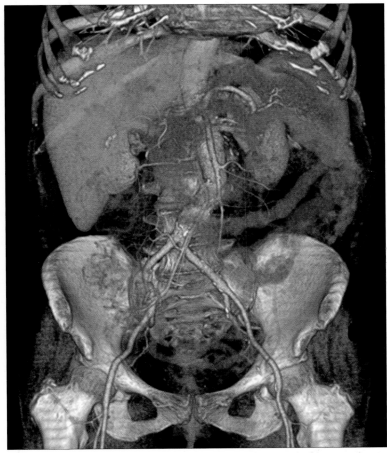

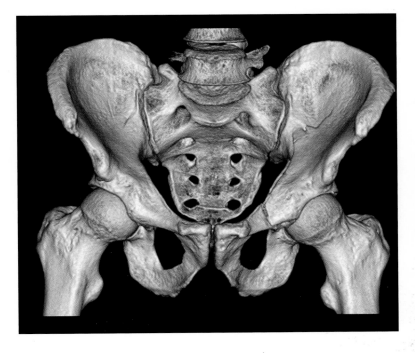

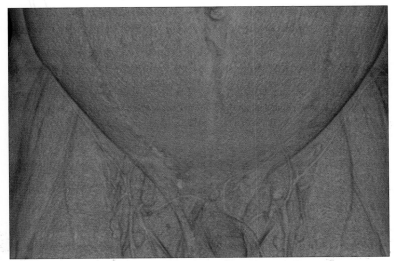

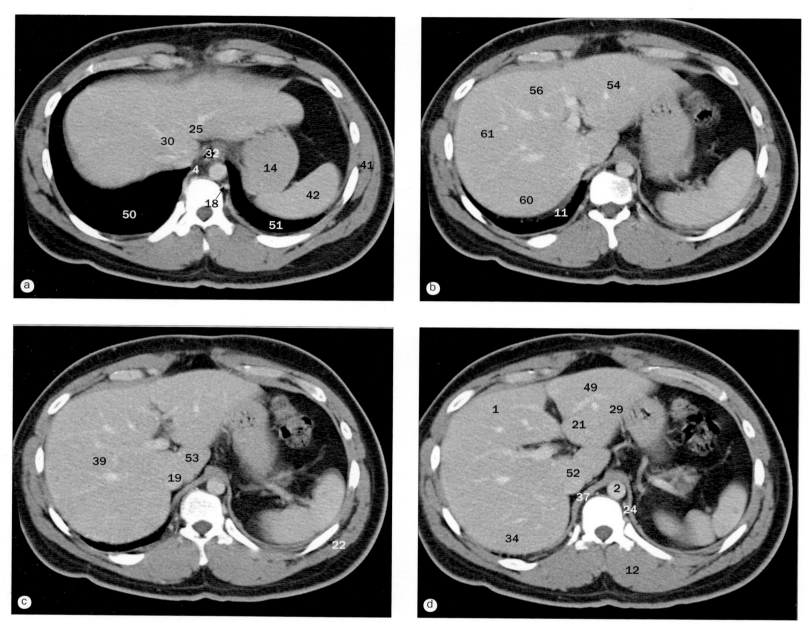

(a)–(h) Sequential axial CT images of abdomen and pelvis in a male, from superior to inferior.
Note: pages 124–135 show sequential images of the abdomen and pelvis of the same male patient.

1 Anterior segment of right lobe of liver	**14** Fundus of stomach	**27** Left suprarenal gland
2 Aorta	**15** Gall bladder	**28** Lesser curvature of stomach
3 Decending colon	**16** Greater curvature of stomach	**29** Medial segment of left lobe of liver
4 Azygos vein	**17** Head of pancreas	**30** Middle hepatic vein
5 Body of pancreas	**18** Hemi-azygos vein	**31** Neck of pancreas
6 Body of stomach	**19** Inferior vena cava	**32** Oesophagus
7 Body of vertebra	**20** Jejunum	**33** Portal vein
8 Coeliac trunk	**21** Lateral segment of left lobe of liver	**34** Posterior segment of right lobe of liver
9 Common hepatic artery	**22** Latissimus dorsi muscle	**35** Renal cortex
10 Descending (second) part of duodenum	**23** Left colic (splenic) flexure	**36** Renal fascia
11 Diaphragm	**24** Left crus of diaphragm	**37** Right crus of diaphragm
12 Erector spinae muscle	**25** Left hepatic vein	**38** Right kidney
13 Fissure for ligamentum venosum	**26** Left kidney	**39** Right lobe of liver

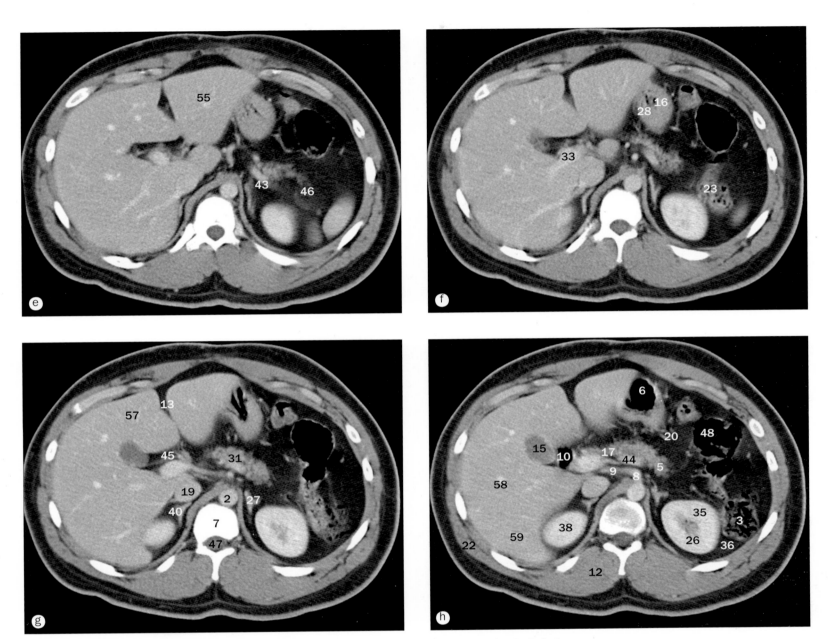

(a)–(h) Sequential axial CT images of abdomen and pelvis in a male, from superior to inferior.

40 Right suprarenal gland	**50** Right inferior lobe of lung
41 Serratus anterior muscle	**51** Left inferior lobe of lung
42 Spleen	**52** Caudate lobe of liver
43 Splenic artery	**53** Segment 1 of liver (caudate)
44 Splenic vein	**54** Segment 2 of liver (left lateral superior subsegment)
45 Superior (first) part of duodenum	**55** Segment 3 of liver (left lateral inferior subsegment)
46 Tail of pancreas	**56** Segment 4A of liver (left medial superior subsegment)
47 Thecal sac	
48 Transverse colon	
49 Left lobe of liver	

57 Segment 4B of liver (left medial m inferior subsegment)
58 Segment 5 of liver (right anterior inferior subsegment)
59 Segment 6 of liver (right posterior inferior subsegment)
60 Segment 7 of liver (right posterior superior subsegment)
61 Segment 8 of liver (right anterior superior subsegment)

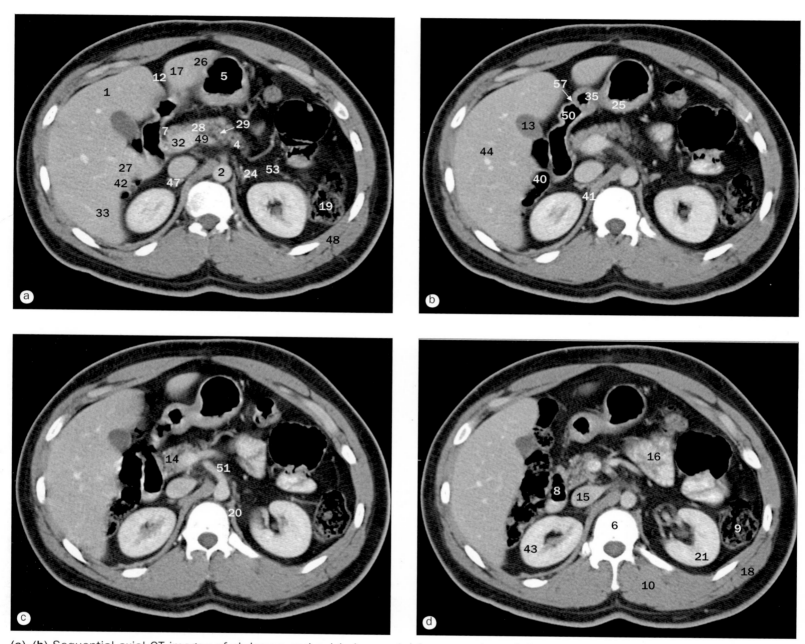

(a)–(h) Sequential axial CT images of abdomen and pelvis in a male, from superior to inferior.

1 Anterior segment of right lobe of liver	**11** External oblique muscle	**21** Left kidney
2 Aorta	**12** Fissure for ligamentum venosum	**22** Left renal artery
3 Ascending colon	**13** Gall bladder	**23** Left renal vein
4 Body of pancreas	**14** Head of pancreas	**24** Left suprarenal gland
5 Body of stomach	**15** Inferior vena cava	**25** Lesser curvature of stomach
6 Body of vertebra	**16** Jejunum	**26** Medial segment of left lobe of liver
7 Common bile duct	**17** Lateral segment of left lobe of liver	**27** Middle hepatic vein
8 Descending (second) part of duodenum	**18** Latissimus dorsi muscle	**28** Neck of pancreas
9 Descending colon	**19** Left colic (splenic) flexure	**29** Pancreatic duct
10 Erector spinae muscle	**20** Left crus of diaphragm	**30** Pararenal fat

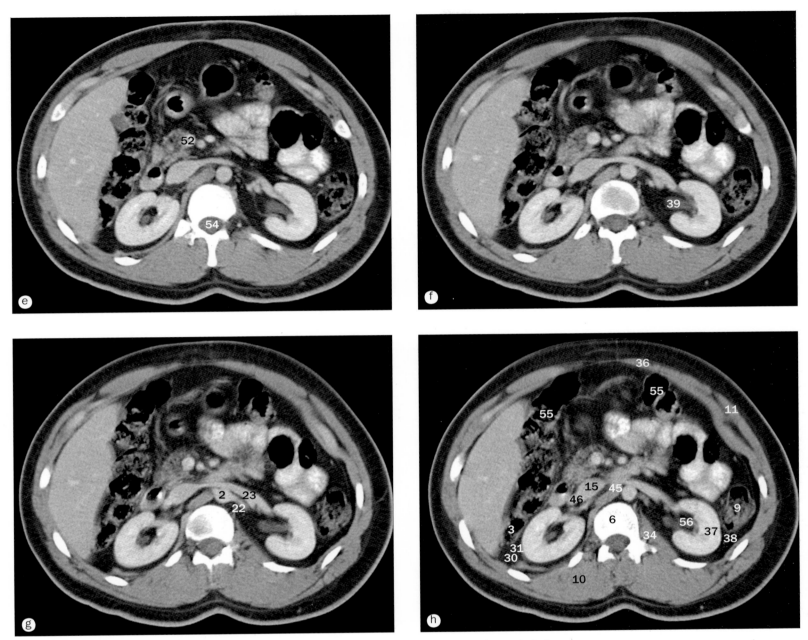

(a)–(h) Sequential axial CT images of abdomen and pelvis in a male, from superior to inferior.

31 Perirenal fat	40 Right colic (hepatic) flexure	49 Splenic vein
32 Portal vein	41 Right crus of diaphragm	50 Superior (first) part of duodenum
33 Posterior segment of right lobe of liver	42 Right hepatic vein	51 Superior mesenteric artery
34 Psoas major muscle	43 Right kidney	52 Superior mesenteric vein
35 Pyloric part of stomach	44 Right lobe of liver	53 Tail of pancreas
36 Rectus abdominis muscle	45 Right renal artery	54 Thecal sac
37 Renal cortex	46 Right renal vein	55 Transverse colon
38 Renal fascia	47 Right suprarenal gland	56 Renal sinus fat
39 Renal pelvis	48 Serratus anterior muscle	57 Pylorus

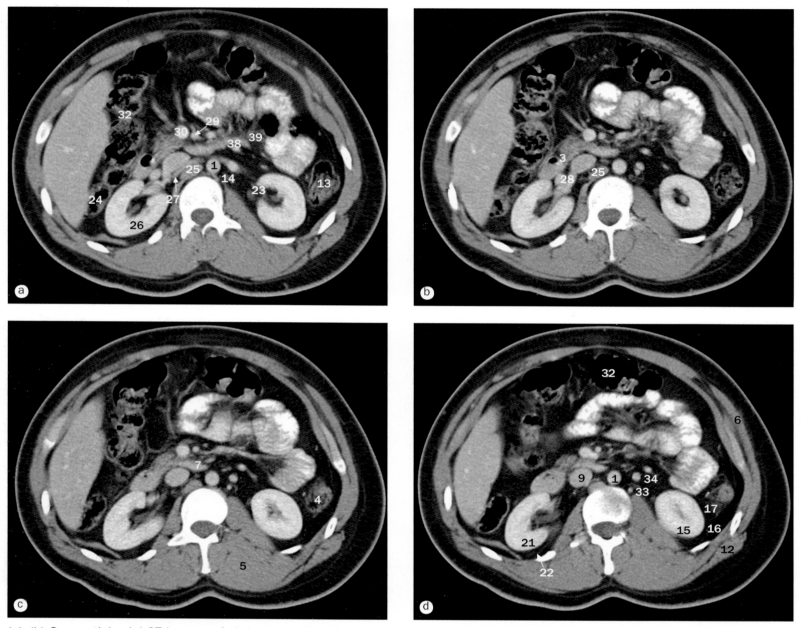

(a)–(h) Sequential axial CT images of abdomen and pelvis in a male, from superior to inferior.

1 Aorta	**8** Ileum	**15** Left kidney
2 Ascending colon	**9** Inferior vena cava	**16** Pararenal fat
3 Descending (second) part of duodenum	**10** Internal oblique muscle	**17** Perirenal fat
4 Descending colon	**11** Jejunum	**18** Psoas major muscle
5 Erector spinae muscle	**12** Latissimus dorsi muscle	**19** Quadratus lumborum muscle
6 External oblique muscle	**13** Left colic (splenic) flexure	**20** Rectus abdominis muscle
7 Horizontal (third) part of duodenum	**14** Left crus of diaphragm	**21** Renal cortex

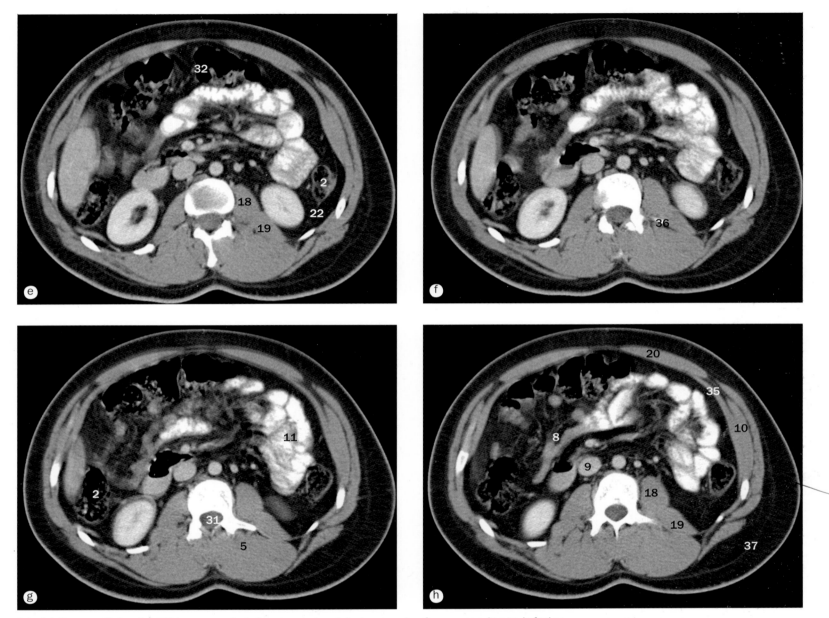

(a)–(h) Sequential axial CT images of abdomen and pelvis in a male, from superior to inferior.

22 Renal fascia
23 Renal pelvis
24 Right colic (hepatic) flexure
25 Right crus of diaphragm
26 Right kidney
27 Right renal artery

28 Right renal vein
29 Superior mesenteric artery
30 Superior mesenteric vein
31 Thecal sac
32 Transverse colon
33 Left testicular artery

34 Left testicular vein
35 Transversus abdominis muscle
36 Twelfth rib
37 Subcutaneous fascia
38 Fourth (ascending) part of duodenum
39 Duodenal–jejunal flexure

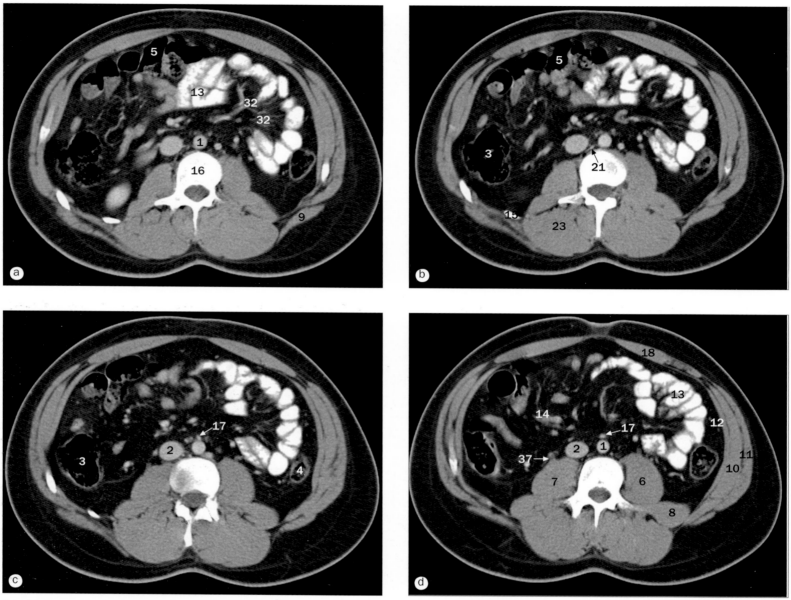

(a)–(h) Sequential axial CT images of abdomen and pelvis in a male, from superior to inferior.

1 Aorta	8 Quadratus lumborum muscle	15 Twelfth rib
2 Inferior vena cava	9 Latissimus dorsi muscle	16 Vertebral body
3 Ascending colon	10 Internal oblique muscle	17 Inferior mesenteric artery
4 Descending colon	11 External oblique muscle	18 Rectus abdominis muscle
5 Transverse colon	12 Transversus abdominis muscle	19 Appendicular artery
6 Left psoas muscle	13 Jejunum	20 Lumbar vein
7 Right psoas muscle	14 Ileum	21 Lumbar artery

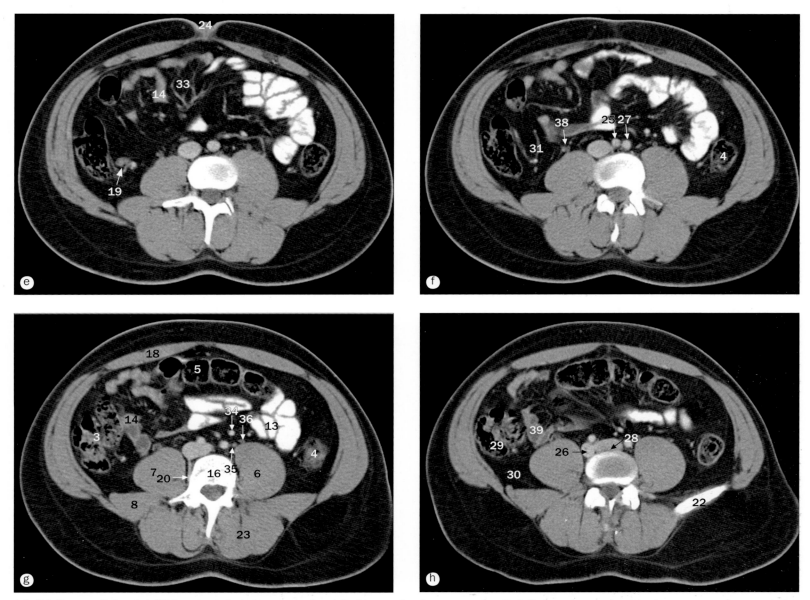

(a)–(h) Sequential axial CT images of abdomen and pelvis in a male, from superior to inferior.

22 Ilium	**29** Caecum	**34** Left testicular artery
23 Erector spinae muscles	**30** Appendix	**35** Left testicular vein
24 Umbilicus	**31** Ileocolic artery	**36** Left ureter
25 Right common iliac artery	**32** Jejunal branches of superior mesenteric	**37** Right ureter
26 Right common iliac vein	artery	**38** Right testicular vessels
27 Left common iliac artery	**33** Ileal branches of superior mesenteric	**39** Terminal ileum
28 Left common iliac vein	artery	

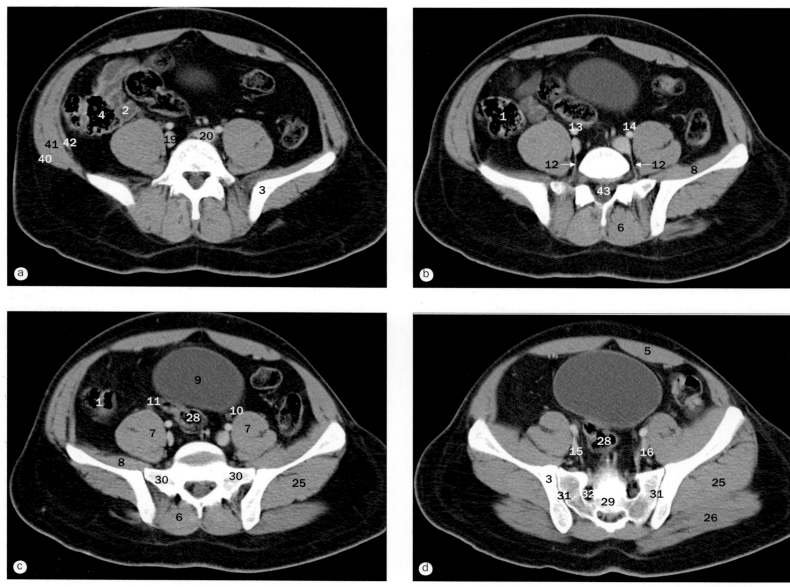

(a)–(h) Sequential axial CT images of abdomen and pelvis in a male, from superior to inferior.

1 Caecum	**9** Urinary bladder	**17** Right external iliac artery
2 Terminal ileum	**10** Left ureter	**18** Left external iliac artery
3 Ilium	**11** Right ureter	**19** Right common iliac vein
4 Ascending colon	**12** Lumbar veins	**20** Left common iliac vein
5 Rectus abdominis muscle	**13** Right common iliac artery	**21** Right internal iliac vein
6 Erector spinae muscles	**14** Left common iliac artery	**22** Left internal iliac vein
7 Psoas major muscle	**15** Right internal iliac artery	**23** Right external iliac vein
8 Iliacus muscle	**16** Left internal iliac artery	**24** Left external iliac vein

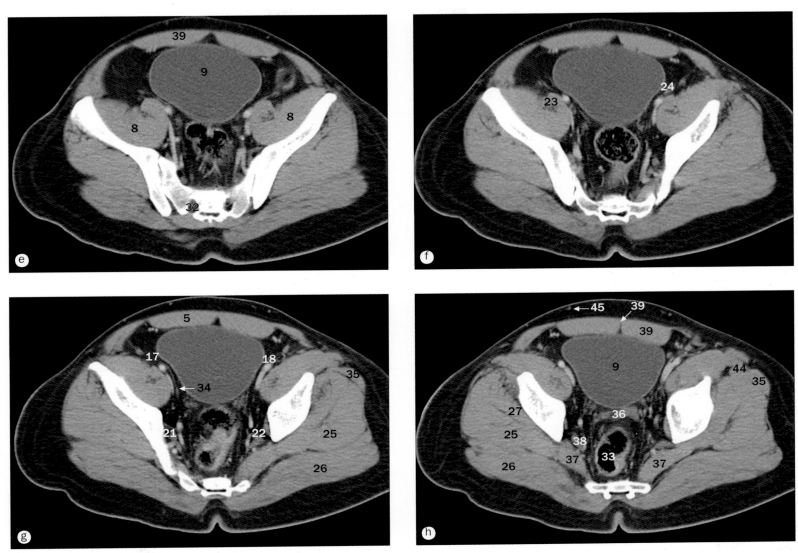

(a)–(h) Sequential axial CT images of abdomen and pelvis in a male, from superior to inferior.

25 Gluteus medius muscle	**32** Sacral foramen	**39** Linea alba
26 Gluteus maximus muscle	**33** Rectum	**40** External oblique muscle
27 Gluteus minimus muscle	**34** Vas deferens	**41** Internal oblique muscle
28 Sigmoid colon	**35** Tensor fasciae latae muscle	**42** Transversus abdominis muscle
29 Sacrum	**36** Seminal vesicle	**43** Thecal sac
30 Sacral alum	**37** Piriformis muscle	**44** Sartorius muscle
31 Sacroiliac joint	**38** Superior gluteal artery and vein	**45** Superficial inferior epigastric artery

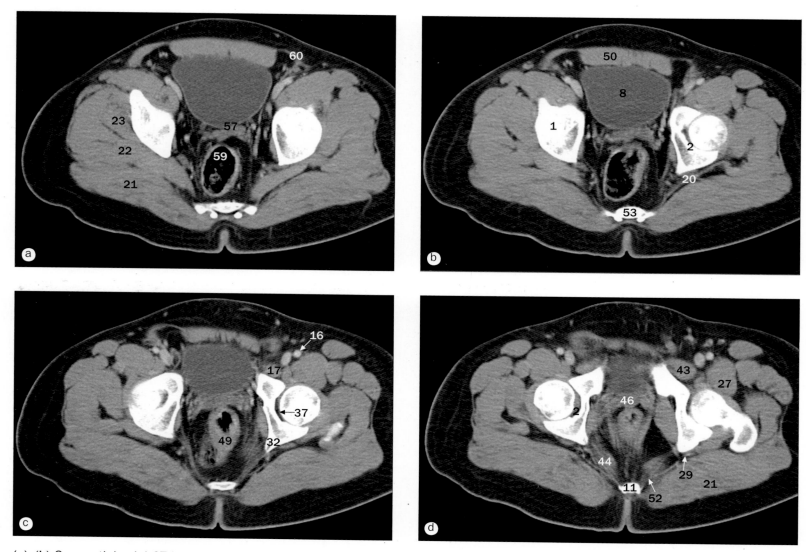

(a)–(h) Sequential axial CT images of abdomen and pelvis in a male, from superior to inferior.

1 Acetabular roof
2 Acetabulum
3 Adductor brevis muscle
4 Adductor longus muscle
5 Adductor magnus muscle
6 Anal canal
7 Biceps femoris muscle
8 Bladder
9 Body of pubis
10 Bulb of penis
11 Coccyx

12 Corpus cavernosum
13 Crus of corpus cavernosum
14 Epididymis
15 External anal sphincter
16 External iliac artery
17 External iliac vein
18 Femoral artery
19 Femoral vein
20 Gemellus muscle
21 Gluteus maximus muscle
22 Gluteus medius muscle

23 Gluteus minimus muscle
24 Gracilis muscle
25 Greater trochanter of femur
26 Head of femur
27 Iliopsoas muscle
28 Iliotibial tract
29 Inferior gluteal artery and vein
30 Inferior ramus of pubis
31 Internal pudendal artery and vein
32 Ischial spine
33 Ischio-anal fossa

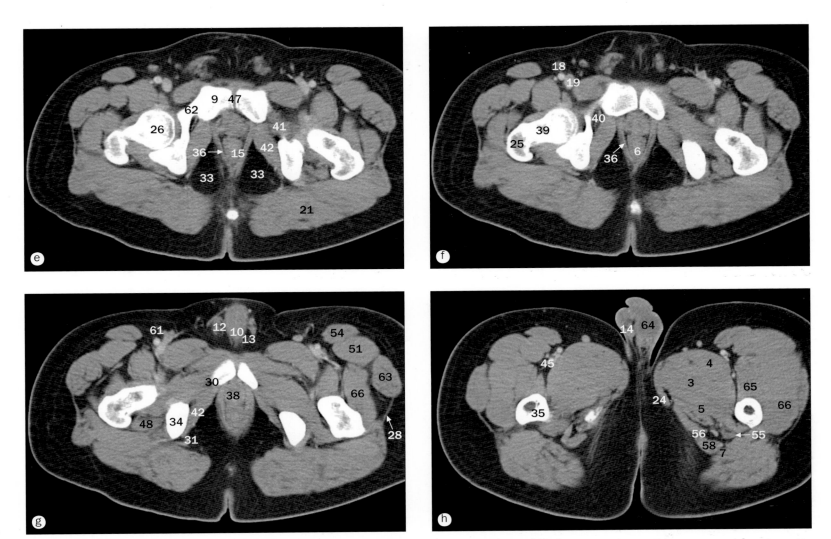

(a)–(h) Sequential axial CT images of abdomen and pelvis in a male, from superior to inferior.

34 Ischium	**45** Profunda femoris artery	**56** Semimembranosus muscle
35 Lesser trochanter of femur	**46** Prostate	**57** Seminal vesicle
36 Levator ani muscle	**47** Pubic symphysis	**58** Semitendinosus muscle
37 Ligament of head of femur	**48** Quadratus femoris muscle	**59** Sigmoid colon
38 Membranous urethra	**49** Rectum	**60** Spermatic cord
39 Neck of femur	**50** Rectus abdominis muscle	**61** Superficial femoral artery
40 Obturator artery and vein	**51** Rectus femoris muscle	**62** Superior ramus of pubis
41 Obturator externus muscle	**52** Sacrospinous ligament	**63** Tensor fasciae latae muscle
42 Obturator internus muscle	**53** Sacrum	**64** Testis
43 Pectineus muscle	**54** Sartorius muscle	**65** Vastus intermedius muscle
44 Piriformis muscle	**55** Sciatic nerve	**66** Vastus lateralis muscle

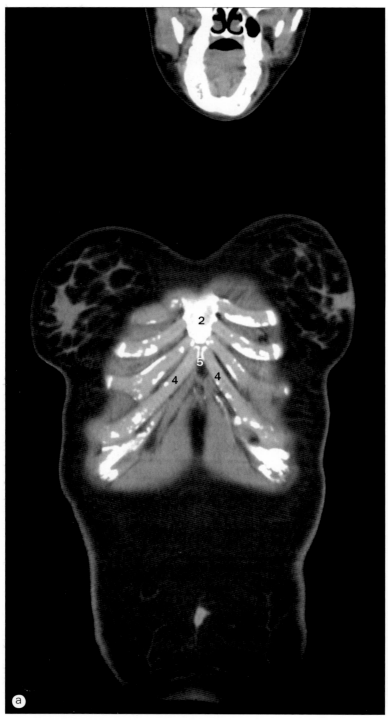

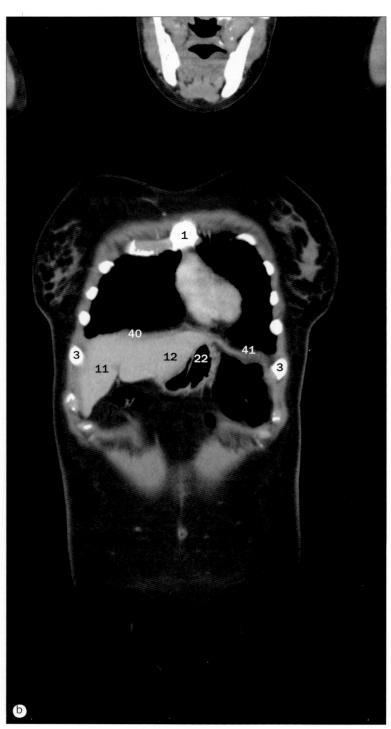

(a)–(d) Sequential coronal CT images of the chest, abdomen and pelvis in a female, from anterior to posterior.
Note: pages 136–145 show sequential images of the same female patient.

1 Manubrium	**8** Right ventricle	**15** Rectus abdominis muscle
2 Body of sternum	**9** Left ventricle	**16** Internal oblique muscle
3 Rib	**10** Pulmonary conus	**17** External oblique muscle
4 Costal cartilage	**11** Right lobe of liver	**18** Tranversus abdominis muscle
5 Xiphisternum	**12** Left lobe of liver	**19** Transverse colon
6 Breast	**13** Gall bladder	**20** Left colic flexure
7 Clavicle	**14** Fissure for ligamentum venosum	**21** Right colic flexure

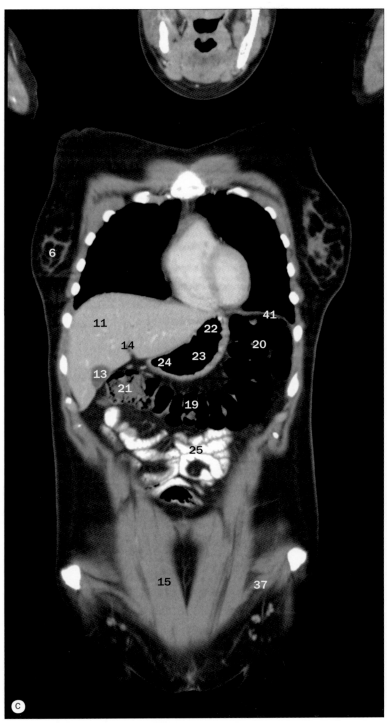

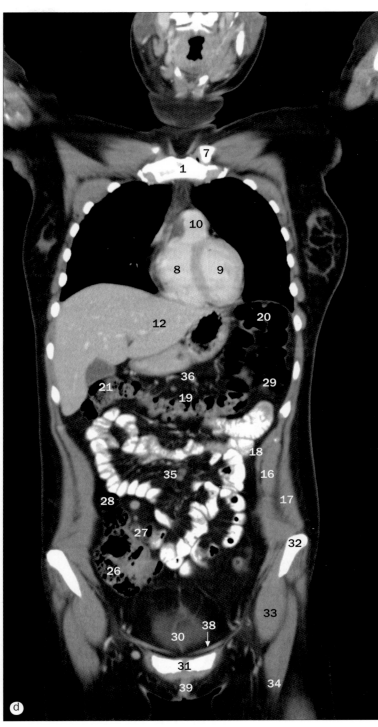

(a)–(d) Sequential coronal CT images of the chest, abdomen and pelvis in a female, from anterior to posterior.

22 Fundus of stomach	29 Descending colon	36 Transverse mesocolon
23 Body of stomach	30 Urinary bladder	37 Pectineus muscle
24 Antrum of stomach	31 Pubic symphysis	38 Levator ani muscle
25 Jejunum	32 Iliac crest	39 Labium majus
26 Caecum	33 Iliopsoas muscle	40 Right hemidiaphragm
27 Ileum	34 Sartorius muscle	41 Left hemidiaphragm
28 Ascending colon	35 Small bowel mesentery	

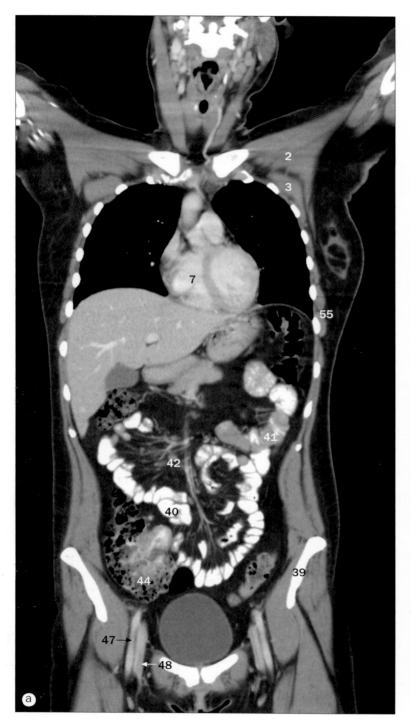
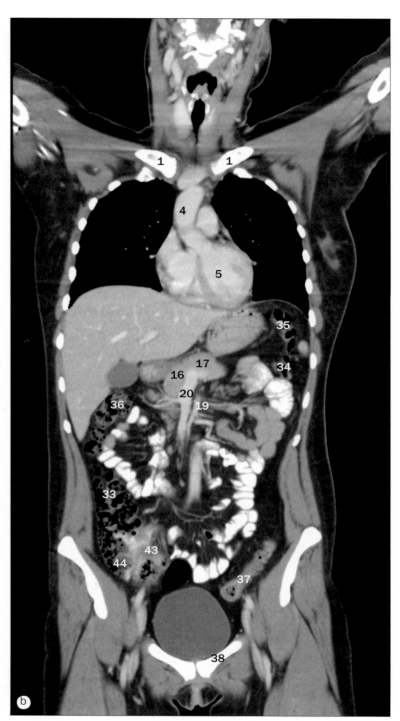

(a)–(d) Sequential coronal CT images of the chest, abdomen and pelvis in a female, from anterior to posterior.

1 Clavicle	**11** Brachiocephalic trunk	**21** Splenic vein
2 Pectoralis major muscle	**12** Right lung	**22** Portal vein
3 Pectoralis minor muscle	**13** Left lung	**23** Gall bladder
4 Ascending aorta	**14** Right lobe of liver	**24** Inferior vena cava
5 Left ventricle	**15** Left lobe of liver	**25** Aorta
6 Pulmonary artery	**16** Head of pancreas	**26** Right common iliac artery
7 Right ventricle	**17** Neck of pancreas	**27** Left common iliac artery
8 Right atrium	**18** Body of pancreas	**28** Psoas muscle
9 Superior vena cava	**19** Superior mesenteric artery (SMA)	**29** Iliacus muscle
10 Left brachiocephalic vein	**20** Superior mesenteric vein (SMV)	**30** Iliopsoas muscle

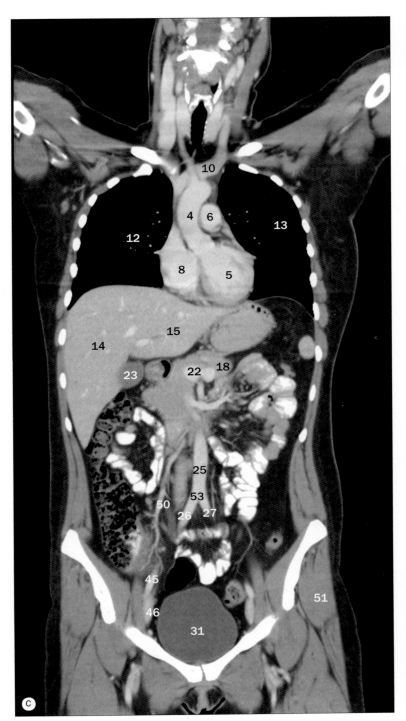
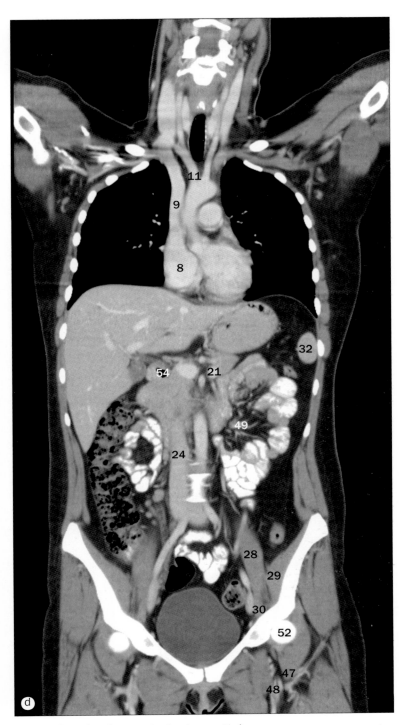

(a)–(d) Sequential coronal CT images of the chest, abdomen and pelvis in a female, from anterior to posterior.

31 Urinary bladder	**40** Ileum	**49** Jejunal branches of SMA
32 Spleen	**41** Jejunum	**50** Ileal branches of SMA
33 Ascending colon	**42** Small bowel mesentery	**51** Gluteus medius muscle
34 Descending colon	**43** Terminal ileum	**52** Head of femur
35 Left colic flexure	**44** Caecum	**53** Aortic bifurcation
36 Right colic flexure	**45** External iliac artery	**54** First part of duodenum
37 Sigmoid colon	**46** External iliac vein	**55** Serratus anterior muscle
38 Superior pubic ramus	**47** Femoral artery	
39 Ilium	**48** Femoral vein	

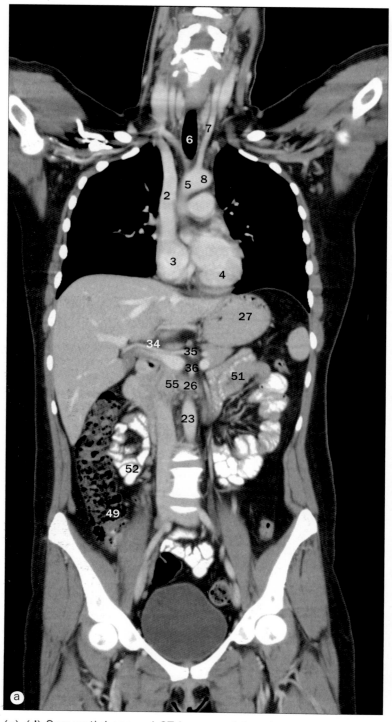

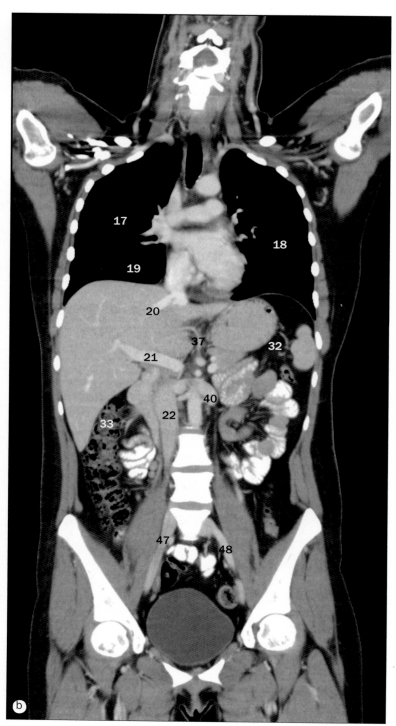

(a)–(d) Sequential coronal CT images of the chest, abdomen and pelvis in a female, from anterior to posterior.

1 Oesophagus	**12** Right upper lobe bronchus	**23** Aorta
2 Superior vena cava	**13** Bronchus intermedius	**24** Right kidney
3 Right atrium	**14** Left main bronchus	**25** Right renal artery
4 Left ventricle	**15** Left upper lobe bronchus	**26** Left renal vein
5 Ascending aorta	**16** Left atrium	**27** Fundus of stomach
6 Trachea	**17** Right lung	**28** Spleen
7 Left common carotid artery	**18** Left lung	**29** Ascending colon
8 Aortic arch	**19** Right lower lobe	**30** Descending colon
9 Right pulmonary artery	**20** Hepatic vein	**31** Sigmoid colon
10 Left pulmonary artery	**21** Portal vein	**32** Left colic flexure
11 Right main bronchus	**22** Inferior vena cava	**33** Right colic flexure

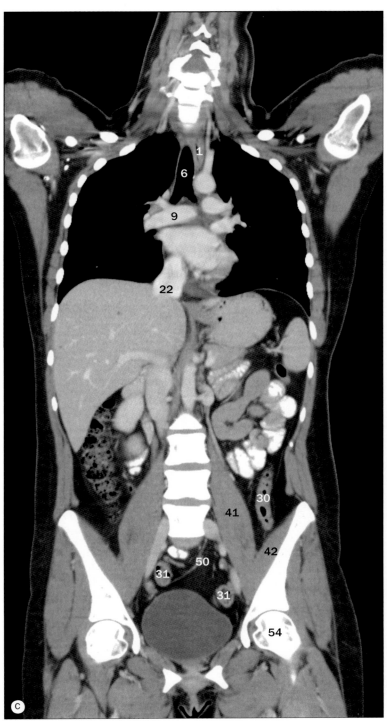 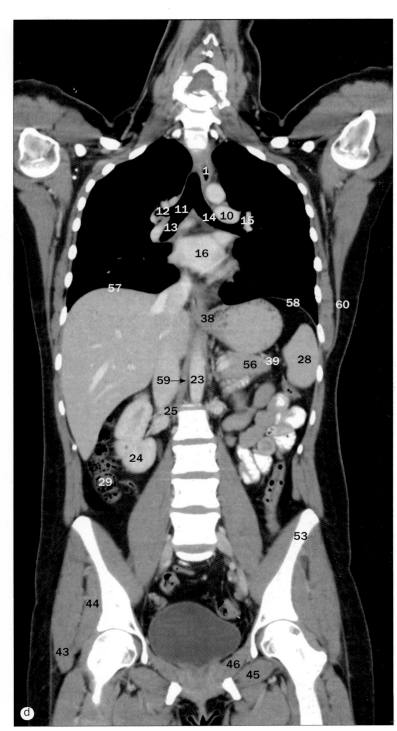

(a)–(d) Sequential coronal CT images of the chest, abdomen and pelvis in a female, from anterior to posterior.

34 Common hepatic artery	44 Gluteus medius muscle	53 Iliac bone
35 Coeliac axis	45 Obturator externus muscle	54 Head of femur
36 Superior mesenteric artery	46 Obturator internus muscle	55 Body of pancreas
37 Left gastric artery	47 Right common iliac vein	56 Tail of pancreas
38 Oesophagogastric junction	48 Left common iliac vein	57 Right hemidiaphragm
39 Splenic artery	49 Caecum	58 Left hemidiaphragm
40 Left renal artery	50 Sigmoid arteries (from inferior mesenteric	59 Right crus of diaphragm
41 Psoas muscle	artery)	60 Latissimus dorsi muscle
42 Iliacus muscle	51 Jejunum	
43 Gluteus maximus muscle	52 Ileum	

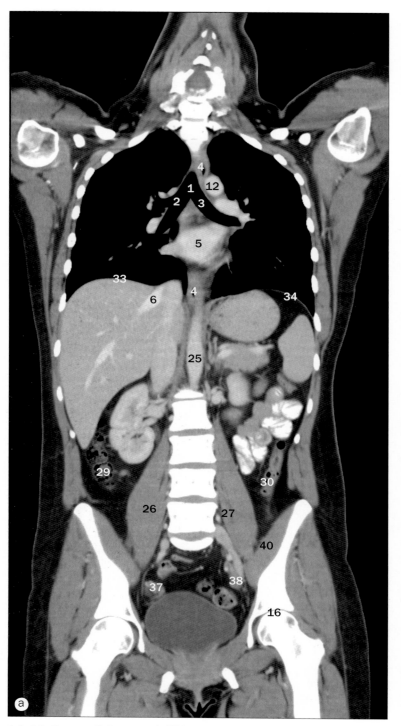

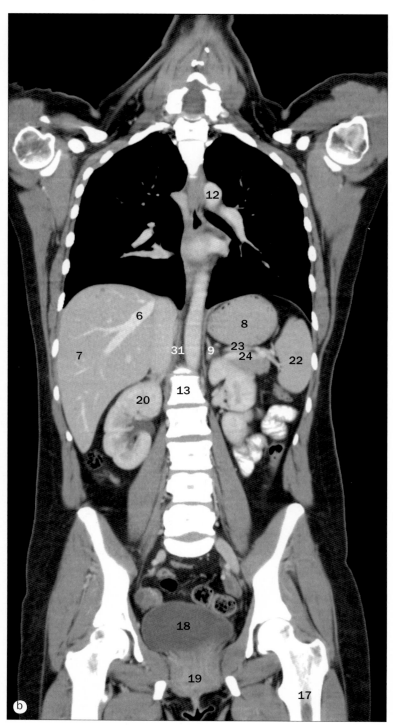

(a)–(d) Sequential coronal CT images of the chest, abdomen and pelvis in a female, from anterior to posterior.

1 Carina	**9** Left suprarenal gland	**17** Femur
2 Right main bronchus	**10** Right suprarenal gland	**18** Urinary bladder
3 Left main bronchus	**11** Descending thoracic aorta	**19** Vagina
4 Oesophagus	**12** Aortic arch (knuckle)	**20** Right kidney
5 Left atrium	**13** Vertebral body of L1	**21** Left kidney
6 Hepatic vein	**14** Sacrum	**22** Spleen
7 Right lobe of liver	**15** Sacroiliac joint	**23** Splenic artery
8 Fundus of stomach	**16** Acetabulum	**24** Splenic vein

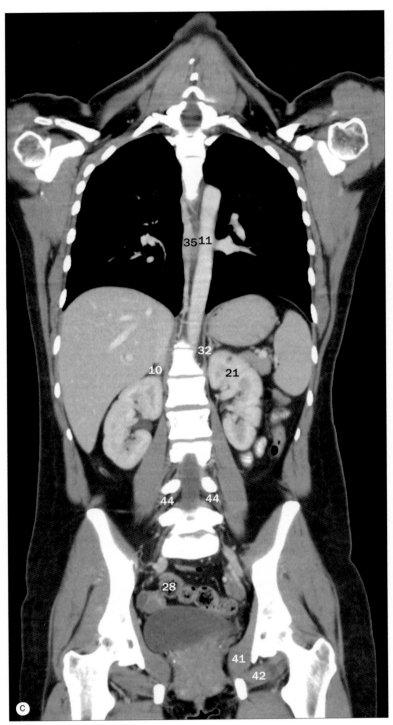
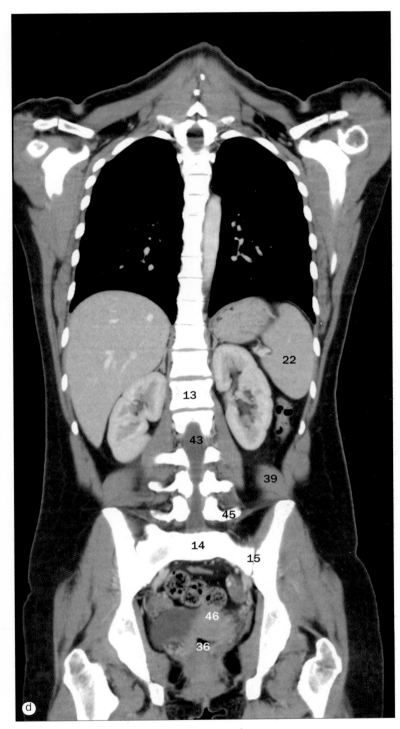

(a)–(d) Sequential coronal CT images of the chest, abdomen and pelvis in a female, from anterior to posterior.

25 Abdominal aorta	**33** Right hemidiaphragm	**41** Obturator internus muscle
26 Psoas major muscle	**34** Left hemidiaphragm	**42** Obturator externus muscle
27 Psoas minor muscle	**35** Azygos vein	**43** Spinal canal
28 Sigmoid colon	**36** Rectum	**44** Lumbar nerve roots
29 Ascending colon	**37** Right internal iliac vessels	**45** Transverse process of L5
30 Descending colon	**38** Left internal iliac vessels	**46** Uterus
31 Right crus of diaphragm	**39** Quadratus lumborum muscle	
32 Left crus of diaphragm	**40** Iliacus muscle	

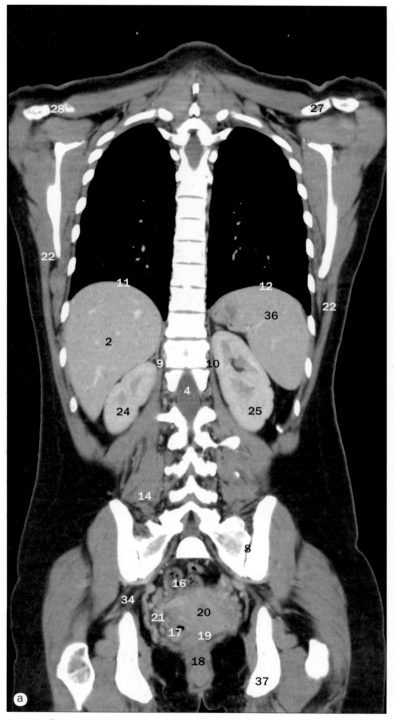

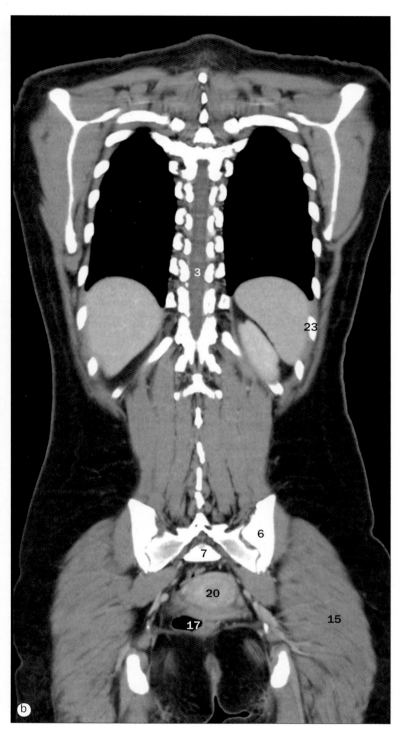

(a)–(d) Sequential coronal CT images of the chest, abdomen and pelvis in a female, from anterior to posterior.

1 Twelfth rib	**8** Sacroiliac joint	**15** Gluteus maximus muscle
2 Liver	**9** Right crus of diaphragm	**16** Sigmoid colon
3 Spinal cord	**10** Left crus of diaphragm	**17** Rectum
4 Spinal canal	**11** Right hemidiaphragm	**18** Vagina
5 Spinous process	**12** Left hemidiaphragm	**19** Cervix
6 Ilium	**13** Erector spinae muscles	**20** Uterus
7 Sacrum	**14** Quadratus lumborum muscle	**21** Uterine veins

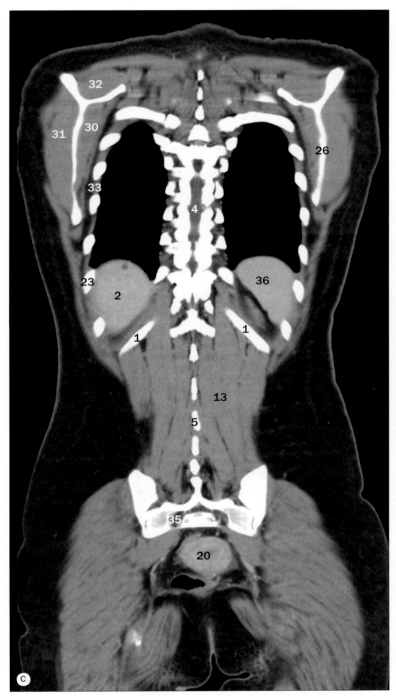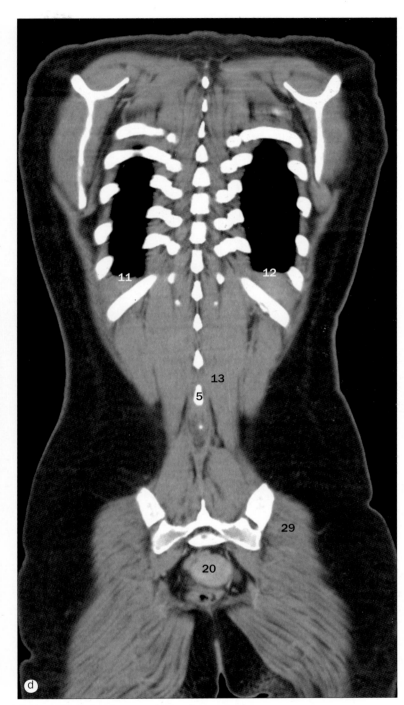

(a)–(d) Sequential coronal CT images of the chest, abdomen and pelvis in a female, from anterior to posterior.

22 Latissimus dorsi muscle	28 Acromioclavicular joint	34 Sciatic nerve
23 Tenth rib	29 Gluteus medius muscle	35 Sacral nerve foramen
24 Right kidney	30 Subscapularis muscle	36 Spleen
25 Left kidney	31 Infraspinatus muscle	37 Ischium
26 Scapula	32 Supraspinatus muscle	
27 Clavicle	33 Intercostal muscle	

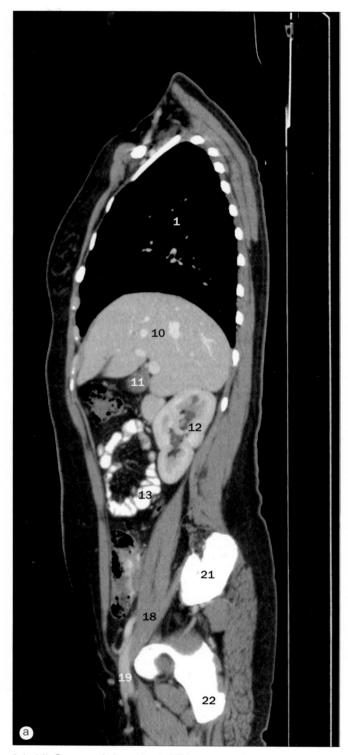
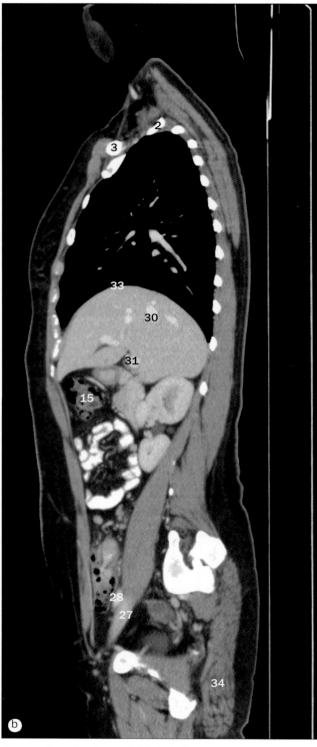

(a)–(d) Sequential sagittal CT images of the chest, abdomen and pelvis in a female, from right to left.
Note: pages 146–149 show sequential images of the same female patient.

1 Right lung	**7** Inferior vena cava	**13** Jejunum
2 Right first rib	**8** Superior vena cava	**14** Ileum
3 Right clavicle	**9** Right atrium	**15** Right colic flexure
4 Manubrium	**10** Right lobe of liver	**16** Pancreas
5 Right internal jugular vein	**11** Gall bladder	**17** Psoas major muscle
6 Aorta	**12** Right kidney	**18** Iliopsoas muscle

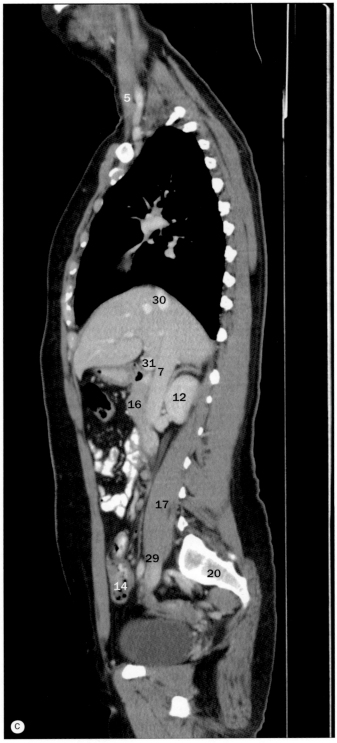

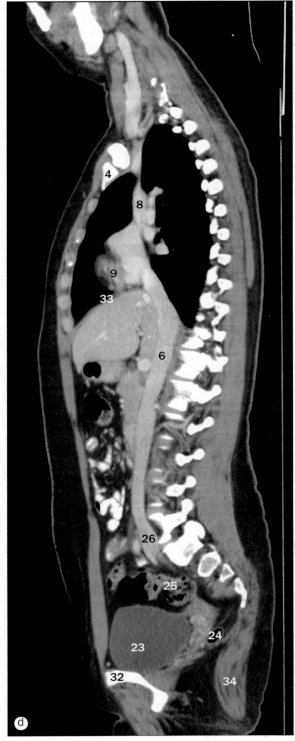

(a)–(d) Sequential sagittal CT images of the chest, abdomen and pelvis in a female, from right to left.

19 Common femoral vessels	25 Sigmoid colon	31 Portal vein
20 Sacrum	26 Right common iliac artery	32 Pubic bone
21 Ilium	27 Right external iliac vein	33 Right hemidiaphragm
22 Ischium	28 Right external iliac artery	34 Gluteus maximus muscle
23 Urinary bladder	29 Right common iliac vein	
24 Rectum	30 Hepatic vein	

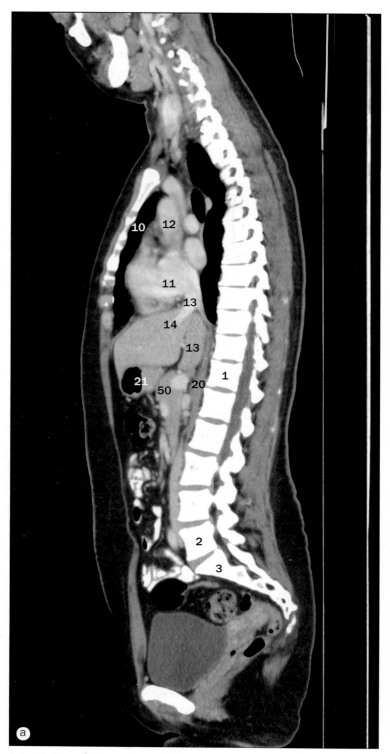

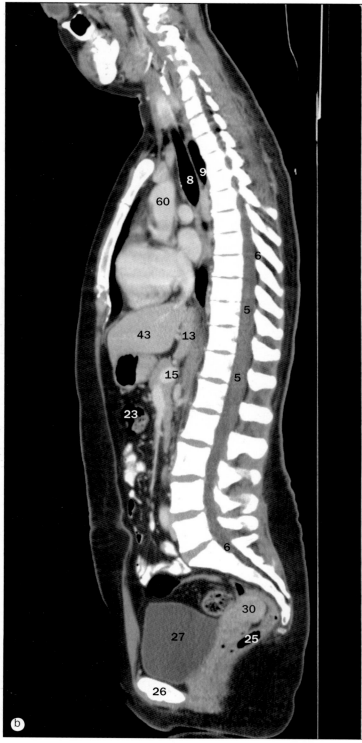

(a)–(d) Sequential sagittal CT images of the chest, abdomen and pelvis in a female, from right to left.

1	Body of T12 vertebra	11	Right atrium	21	Stomach
2	Body of L5 vertebra	12	Superior vena cava	22	Descending colon
3	Sacrum	13	Inferior vena cava	23	Transverse colon
4	Coccyx	14	Hepatic vein	24	Sigmoid colon
5	Spinal cord	15	Splenic vein	25	Rectum
6	Spinal canal	16	Superior mesenteric vein	26	Pubic bone
7	Filum terminale	17	Superior mesenteric artery	27	Urinary bladder
8	Trachea	18	Coeliac axis	28	Cervix
9	Oesophagus	19	Aorta	29	Vagina
10	Right lung	20	Right crus of diaphragm	30	Uterus

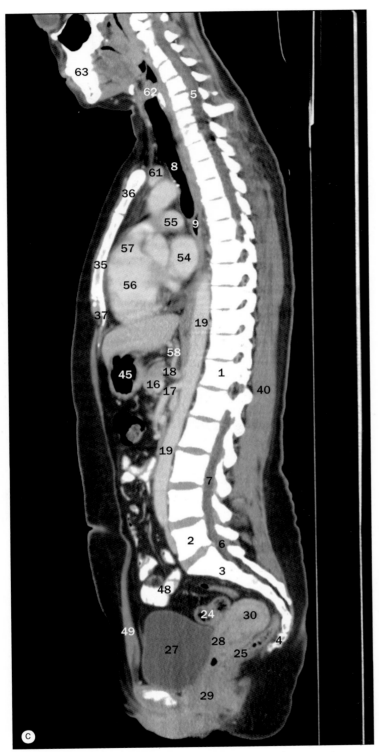

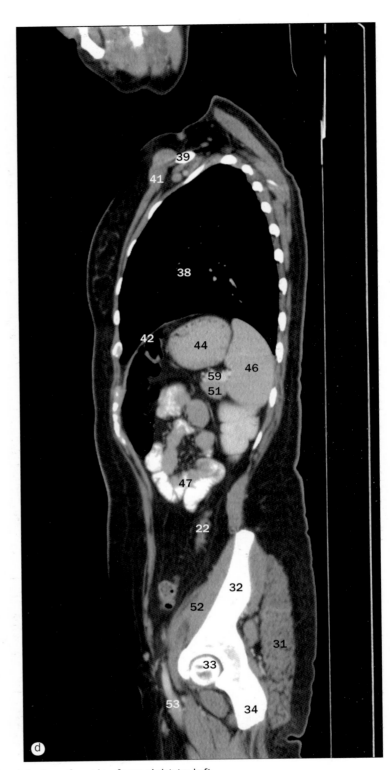

(a)–(d) Sequential sagittal CT images of the chest, abdomen and pelvis in a female, from right to left.

31 Gluteus maximus muscle	**42** Left hemidiaphragm	**53** Left femoral vessels
32 Ilium	**43** Liver	**54** Left atrium
33 Head of femur	**44** Fundus of stomach	**55** Right pulmonary artery
34 Ischium	**45** Body of stomach	**56** Right ventricle
35 Sternum	**46** Spleen	**57** Pulmonary outflow tract
36 Manubrium	**47** Jejunum	**58** Common hepatic artery
37 Xiphisternum	**48** Ileum	**59** Splenic artery
38 Left lung	**49** Rectus abdominis muscle	**60** Ascending thoracic aorta
39 Left clavicle	**50** Body of pancreas	**61** Left brachiocephalic vein
40 Erector spinae muscles	**51** Tail of pancreas	**62** Larynx
41 Left pectoralis major muscle	**52** Iliacus muscle	**63** Mandible

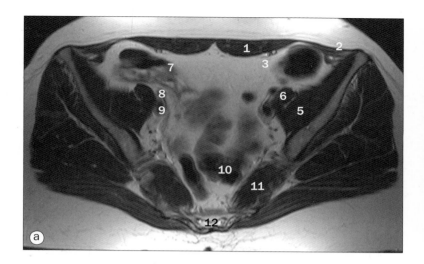

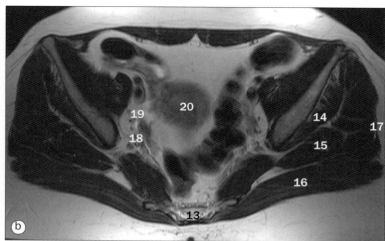

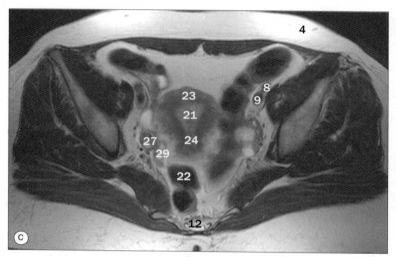

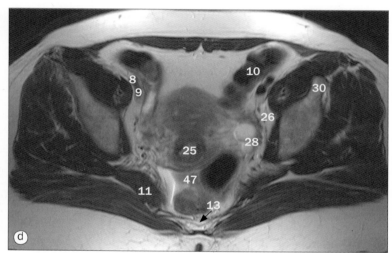

(a)–(p) Sequential axial T2w MR images of the female pelvis, from superior to inferior.

1 Rectus abdominis muscle	**11** Piriformis muscle	**21** Uterine cavity
2 External oblique aponeurosis	**12** Sacrum	**22** Rectosigmoid junction
3 Inferior epigastric vessels	**13** Central sacral canal	**23** Myometrium of uterus
4 Superficial epigastric vessels	**14** Gluteus minimis muscle	**24** Internal cervical os
5 Iliacus muscle	**15** Gluteus medius muscle	**25** External cervical os
6 Psoas muscle	**16** Gluteus maximus muscle	**26** Obturator vessels
7 Ileum	**17** Fascia lata	**27** Right ovary
8 External iliac artery	**18** Superior gluteal vessels	**28** Left ovary
9 External iliac vein	**19** Ovarian vessels	**29** Right uterine tube
10 Sigmoid colon	**20** Uterine fundus	**30** Antero-inferior iliac spine

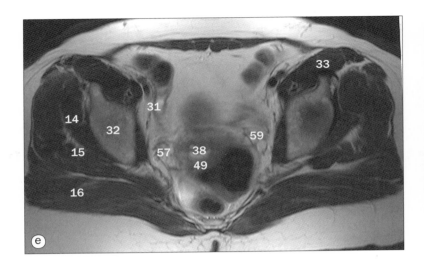

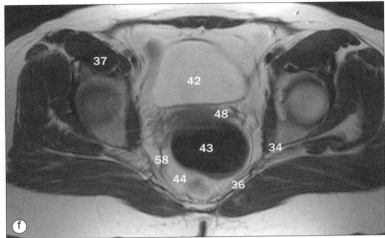

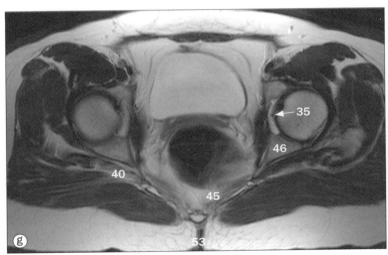

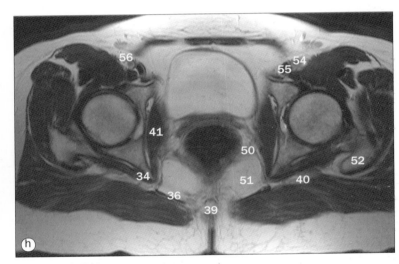

(a)–(p) Sequential axial T2w MR images of the female pelvis, from superior to inferior.

31 Round ligament of uterus	**41** Obturator internus muscle	**51** Ischio-anal fossa
32 Acetabular roof	**42** Bladder	**52** Greater trochanter of femur
33 Rectus femoris muscle	**43** Rectum	**53** Natal cleft
34 Ischial spine	**44** Mesorectum	**54** Common femoral artery
35 Ligamentum teres	**45** Waldeyer's fascia	**55** Common femoral vein
36 Sacrospinous ligament	**46** Ischium	**56** Femoral nerve branches
37 Iliopsoas muscle	**47** Recto-uterine pouch (of Douglas)	**57** Transverse cervical ligament
38 Cervical wall	**48** Posterior vaginal fornix	**58** Uterosacral ligament
39 Coccyx	**49** Cervical os	**59** Broad ligament
40 Sciatic nerve	**50** Levator ani muscle (puborectalis)	

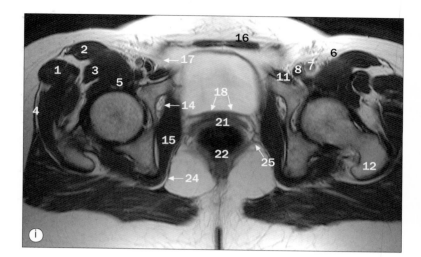

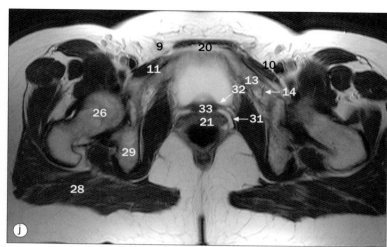

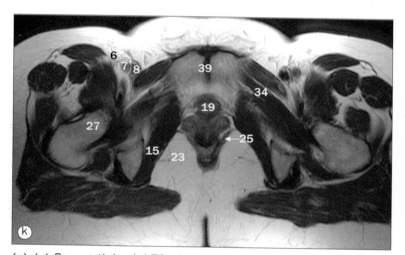

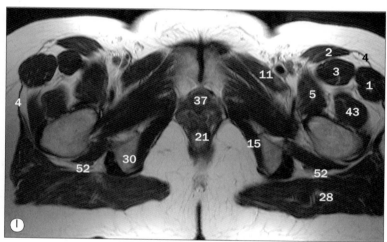

(a)–(p) Sequential axial T2w MR images of the female pelvis, from superior to inferior.

1 Tensor fasciae latae muscle	**11** Pectineus	**21** Vagina
2 Sartorius muscle	**12** Greater trochanter of femur	**22** Rectum
3 Rectus femoris muscle	**13** Superior pubic ramus	**23** Ischio-anal fossa
4 Fascia lata	**14** Obturator vessels	**24** Pudendal neurovascular bundle (Alcock's
5 Iliopsoas muscle	**15** Obturator internus muscle	canal)
6 Femoral nerve branches	**16** Rectus abdominis muscle	**25** Puborectalis muscle
7 Common femoral artery	**17** Inguinal ligament	**26** Femoral head
8 Common femoral vein	**18** Bladder base	**27** Femoral neck
9 Round ligament of the uterus	**19** Bladder neck	**28** Gluteus maximus muscle
10 Femoral canal	**20** Extraperitoneal fat (cave of Retzius)	**29** Ischium

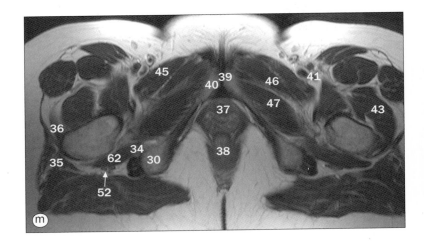

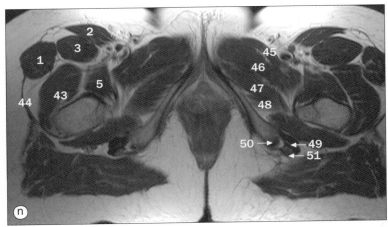

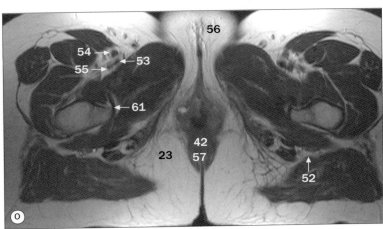

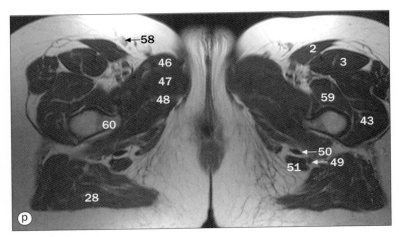

(a)–(p) Sequential axial T2w MR images of the female pelvis, from superior to inferior.

30 Ischial tuberosity	**41** Profunda femoris artery	**52** Sciatic nerve
31 Ureter	**42** Perineal body	**53** Superficial femoral vein
32 Vesico-ureteric junction	**43** Vastus lateralis muscle	**54** Superficial femoral artery
33 Trigone of bladder	**44** Iliotibial tract	**55** Profunda femoris vessels
34 Obturator externus muscle	**45** Pectineus muscle	**56** Labium majorum
35 Gluteus medius muscle	**46** Adductor longus muscle	**57** Anal canal
36 Gluteus minimis muscle (tendinous insertion)	**47** Adductor brevis muscle	**58** Long saphenous vein
	48 Adductor magnus muscle	**59** Vastus intermedius muscle
37 Urethra	**49** Semimembanosus muscle	**60** Lesser trochanter of femur
38 Anorectal junction	**50** Semitendinosus muscle	**61** Iliopsoas insertion
39 Symphysis pubis	**51** Biceps femoris muscle	**62** Quadratus femoris muscle
40 Pubic body		

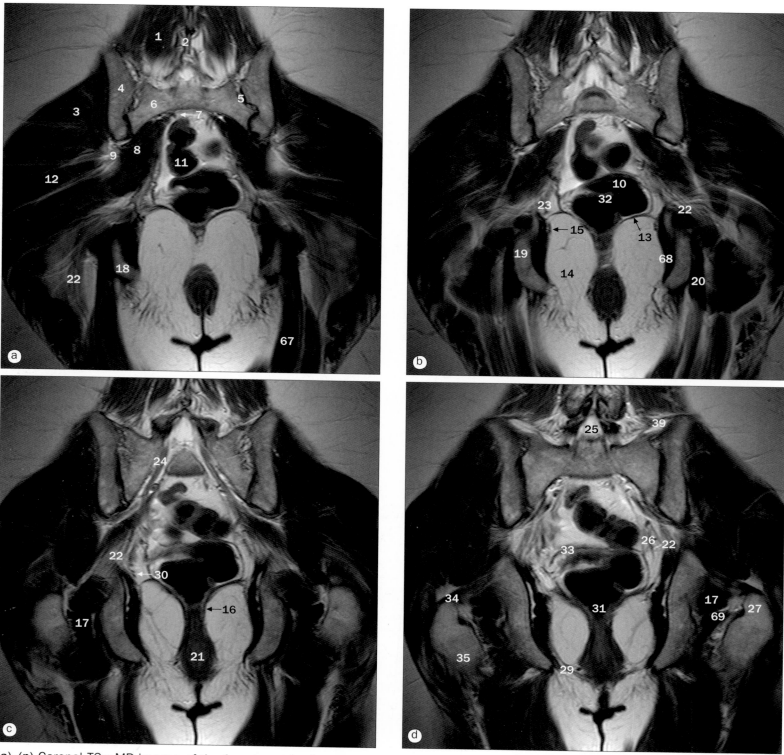

(a)–(p) Coronal T2w MR images of the female pelvis, from posterior to anterior.

1 Erector spinae muscle	**13** Levator ani muscle	**24** Sacral nerve (S1)
2 Spinous process L5	**14** Ischio-anal fossa	**25** Thecal sac
3 Gluteus maximus muscle	**15** Internal pudendal neurovascular bundle	**26** Superior rectal vessels
4 Ilium	(Alcock's canal)	**27** Greater trochanter of femur
5 Sacro-iliac joint	**16** External anal sphincter	**28** Acetabulum
6 Sacral ala	**17** Obturator externus muscle	**29** Urogenital diaphragm
7 Lumbosacral trunk	**18** Ischial tuberosity	**30** Obturator neurovascular bundle
8 Piriformis muscle	**19** Ischium	**31** Rectal ampulla
9 Superior gluteal vessels	**20** Common hamstring origin	**32** Transverse rectal fold (of Houston)
10 Rectum	**21** Anal canal	**33** Middle rectal vessels
11 Rectosigmoid junction	**22** Sciatic nerve	**34** Piriformis muscle (insertion)
12 Gluteus medius muscle	**23** Inferior gluteal vessels	**35** Intertrochanteric part of femur

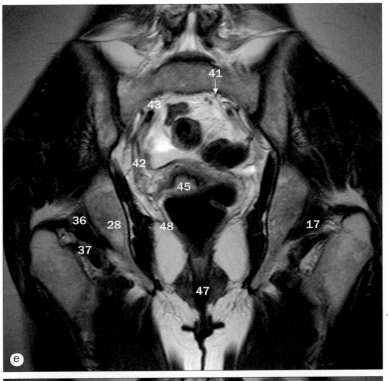

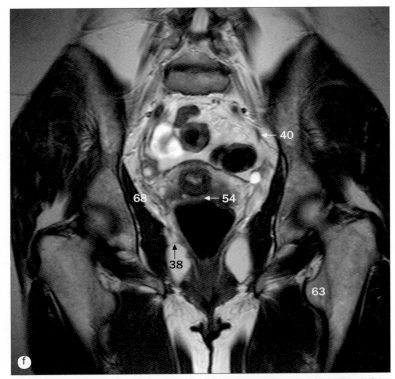

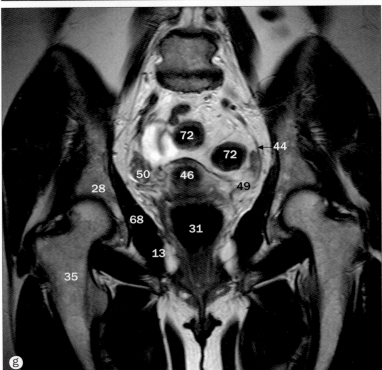

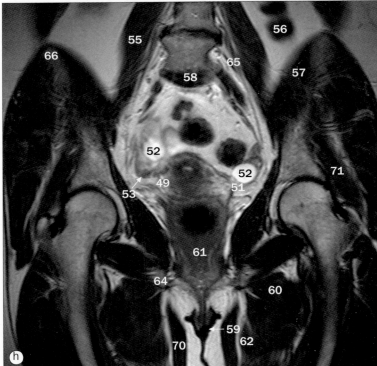

(a)–(p) Coronal T2w MR images of the female pelvis, from posterior to anterior.

36 Obturator externus muscle	49 Broad ligament of uterus	61 Vagina (posterior wall)
37 Gemelli muscle	50 Right ovary	62 Adductor longus muscle
38 Inferior rectal neurovascular bundle	51 Left ovary	63 Lesser trochanter of femur
39 Iliolumbar ligament	52 Physiological cyst of ovary (corpus luteum)	64 Inferior pubic ramus
40 Ureter	53 Uterine tube	65 Lumbar plexus
41 Sympathetic chain	54 Recto-uterine pouch (of Douglas)	66 Iliac crest
42 Internal iliac vessel branches	55 Psoas major muscle	67 Biceps femoris muscle
43 Common iliac vessel bifurcation	56 Descending colon	68 Obturator internus muscle
44 Gonadal vessels	57 Iliacus muscle	69 Quadratus femoris muscle
45 Cervix of uterus	58 Intervertebral disc at L5/S1	70 Gracilis muscle
46 Uterine cavity	59 Labium minorum	71 Gluteus minimis muscle
47 Perineal body	60 Adductor brevis muscle	72 Sigmoid colon
48 Puborectalis muscle		

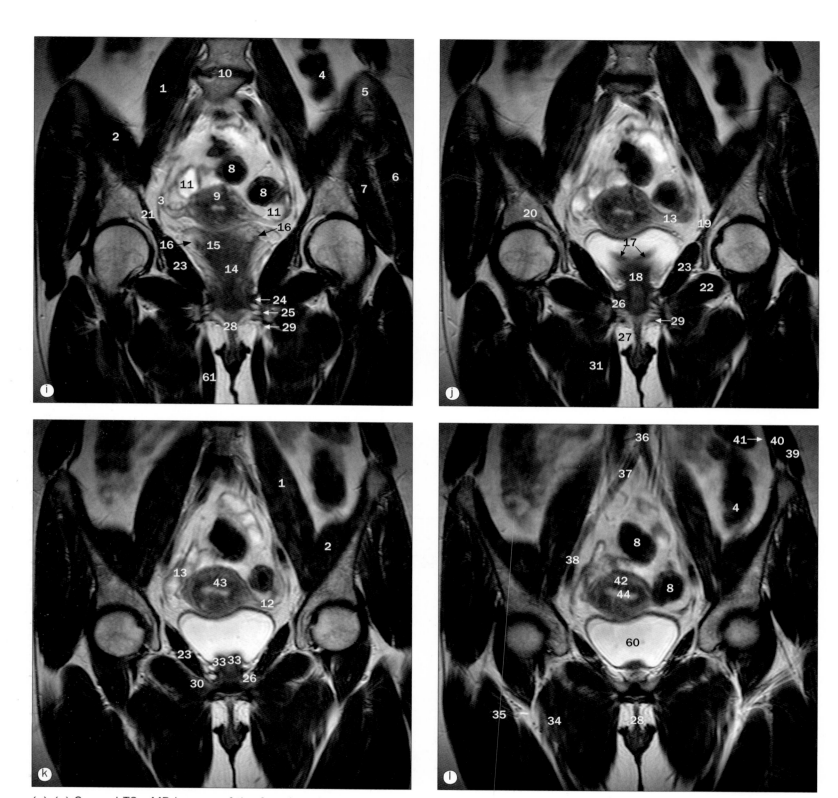

(a)–(p) Coronal T2w MR images of the female pelvis, from posterior to anterior.

1 Psoas major muscle	**11** Ovaries (corpora luteal cysts)	**21** Obturator internus muscle
2 Iliacus muscle	**12** Broad ligament of uterus	**22** Obturator externus muscle
3 Internal iliac artery branches	**13** Uterine tubes	**23** Levator ani muscle
4 Descending colon	**14** Vagina	**24** Pubovaginalis muscle
5 Iliac crest	**15** Posterior fornix of vagina	**25** Transverse perineii (urogenital diaphragm)
6 Gluteus medius muscle	**16** Ureter	**26** Deep perineal pouch
7 Gluteus minimis muscle	**17** Ureteric orifice	**27** Superficial perineal pouch
8 Sigmoid colon	**18** Trigone of bladder	**28** Urethra
9 Uterine myometrium	**19** Obturator neurovascular bundle	**29** Sphincter urethralis
10 Intervertebral disc at L4/5	**20** Acetabular roof	**30** Inferior pubic ramus

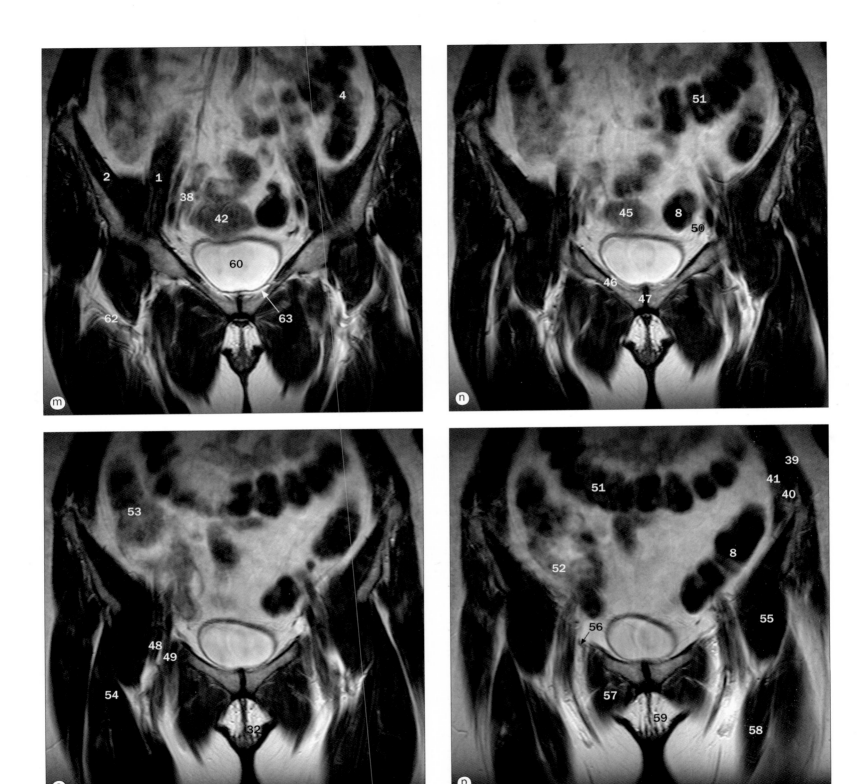

(a)–(p) Coronal T2w MR images of the female pelvis, from posterior to anterior.

31 Adductor longus muscle	42 Uterine myometrium	53 Caecum
32 Labia minora	43 Uterine endometrium	54 Rectus femoris muscle
33 Internal sphincter of bladder	44 Uterine cavity	55 Iliopsoas muscle
34 Vastus medialis muscle	45 Uterine fundus	56 Femoral canal
35 Vastus lateralis muscle	46 Superior pubic ramus	57 Adductor brevis muscle
36 Aorta	47 Symphysis pubis	58 Sartorius muscle
37 Common iliac artery	48 Common femoral artery	59 Labius majorum
38 External iliac artery	49 Common femoral vein	60 Bladder
39 External oblique muscle	50 Superior vesical vessels	61 Gracilis muscle
40 Internal oblique muscle	51 Transverse colon	62 Circumflex femoral vessels
41 Transversus abdominis muscle	52 Small bowel	63 Retropubic cave (of Retzius)

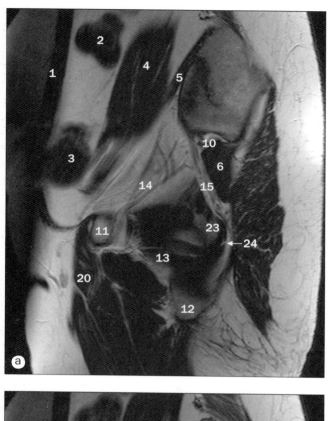

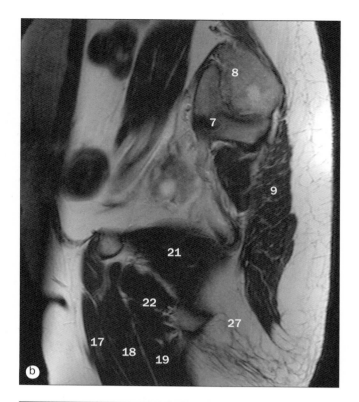

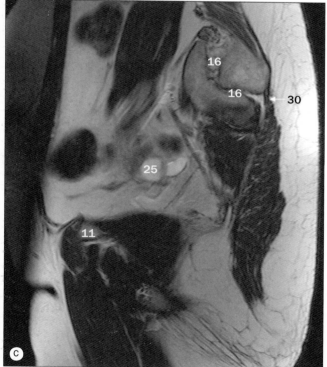

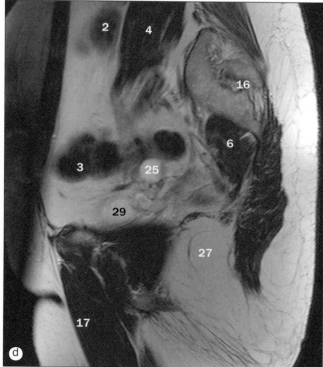

(a)–(p) Sequential sagittal T2w MR images of a female pelvis, from right to left through the midline.

1 Rectus abdominis muscle	10 Superior gluteal vessels	19 Adductor magnus muscle
2 Transverse colon	11 Superior pubic ramus	20 Iliopsoas muscle
3 Sigmoid colon	12 Inferior pubic ramus	21 Obturator internus muscle
4 Psoas major muscle	13 Obturator externus muscle	22 Pectineus muscle
5 Iliacus muscle	14 Obturator neurovascular bundle	23 Ischial tuberosity
6 Piriformis muscle	15 Sciatic nerve	24 Hamstring origin
7 Sacral ala	16 Sacro-iliac joint	25 Right ovary (corpus luteal cyst)
8 Ilium	17 Adductor longus muscle	26 Levator ani muscle
9 Gluteus maximus muscle	18 Adductor brevis muscle	27 Ischio-anal fossa

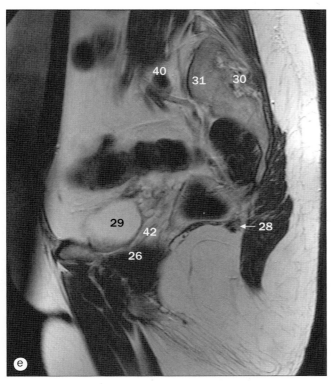

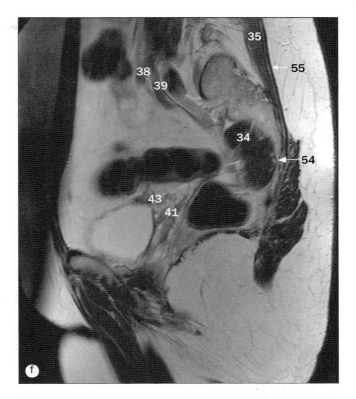

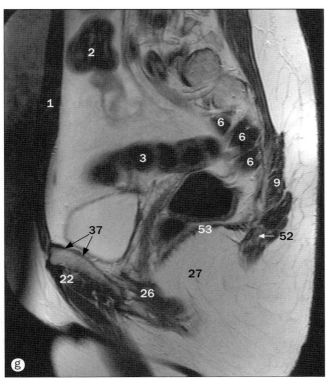

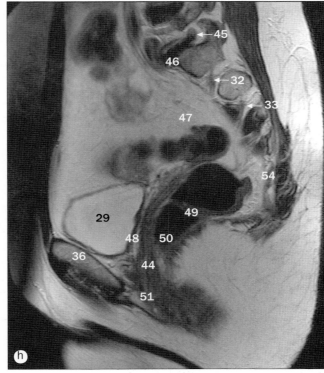

(a)–(p) Sequential sagittal T2w MR images of a female pelvis, from right to left through the midline.

28 Internal pudendal neurovascular bundle (Alcock's canal)
29 Bladder
30 Dorsal sacro-iliac ligaments
31 Sacral body
32 First sacral root
33 Second sacral root
34 Rectosigmoid junction
35 Erector spinae muscle
36 Pubic body

37 Retropubic space (cave of Retzius, extraperitoneal fat)
38 External iliac artery
39 Internal iliac artery
40 Internal iliac vein
41 Broad ligament of uterus
42 Transverse (cardinal) cervical ligament
43 Uterine tube
44 Vagina
45 Fifth lumbar root
46 Intervertebral disc at L5/S1

47 Mesosigmoid
48 Trigone of bladder
49 Tranverse rectal fold (valve of Houston)
50 Rectal ampulla
51 Tranverse perineii muscle (urogenital diaphragm)
52 Coccyx
53 Coccygeus muscle
54 Waldeyer's fascia
55 Thoracolumbar fascia

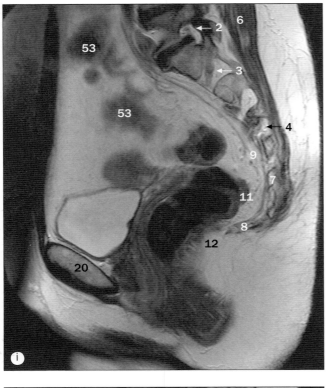

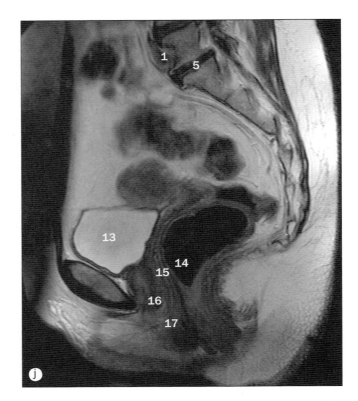

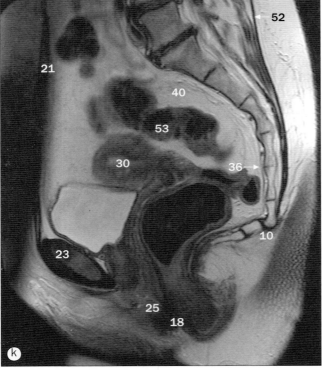

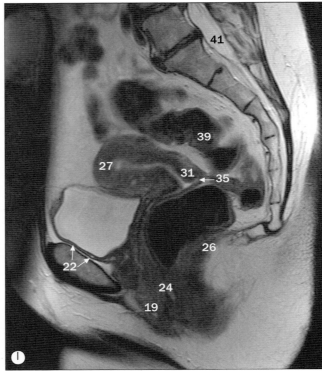

(a)–(p) Sequential sagittal T2w MR images of a female pelvis, from right to left through the midline.

1 Left common iliac vein	10 Sacro-coccygeal junction	19 External anal sphincter
2 L5 root (intervertebral foramen)	11 Levator ani muscle	20 Pubic body
3 S1 root	12 Puborectalis muscle	21 Rectus abdominis muscle
4 S3 root	13 Bladder	22 Retropubic space (extraperitoneal fat,
5 Intervertebral disc at L5/S1	14 Rectal ampulla	cave of Retzius)
6 Erector spinae muscle	15 Vagina	23 Symphysis pubis
7 Fifth sacral segment	16 Urethra	24 Anal canal
8 Coccyx	17 Vaginal introitus	25 Perineal body
9 Sacral plexus	18 Anus	26 Anococcygeal raphe

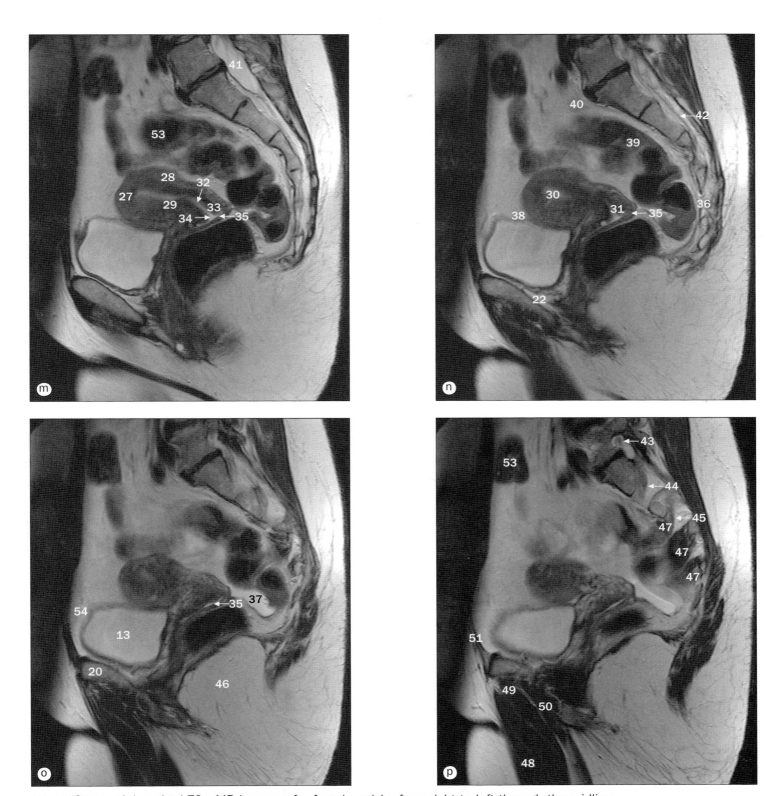

(a)–(p) Sequential sagittal T2w MR images of a female pelvis, from right to left through the midline.

27 Uterine fundus	**37** Recto-uterine pouch (of Douglas)	**46** Ischio-anal fossa
28 Uterine myometrium	**38** Uterovesical pouch	**47** Piriformis (slips of origin)
29 Uterine endometrium	**39** Rectosigmoid junction	**48** Adductor longus muscle
30 Uterine cavity	**40** Mesosigmoid	**49** Adductor brevis muscle
31 Cervix	**41** Thecal sac	**50** Adductor magnus muscle
32 Internal cervical os	**42** Filum terminale	**51** Rectus sheath
33 Cervical wall	**43** Left L5 root	**52** Thoracolumbar fascia
34 External os of cervix	**44** Left S1 root	**53** Sigmoid colon
35 Posterior fornix of vagina	**45** Left S2 root	**54** Extraperitoneal fat
36 Waldeyer's fascia		

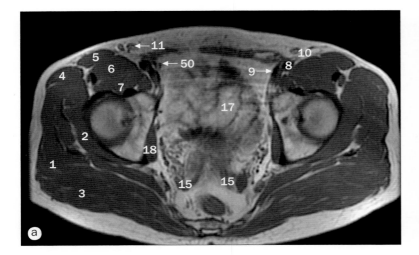

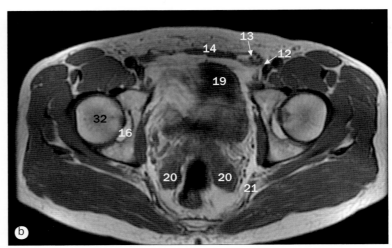

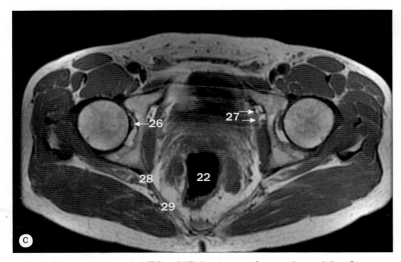

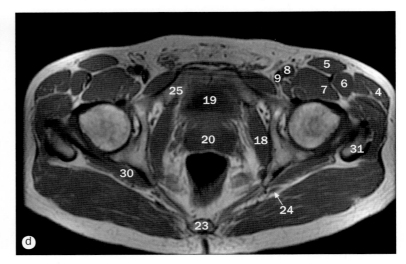

(a)–(l) Sequential axial T2w MR images of a male pelvis, from superior to inferior.

1 Gluteus medius muscle	9 Common femoral vein	17 Small bowel
2 Gluteus minimis muscle	10 Femoral nerve branches	18 Obturator internus muscle
3 Gluteus maximus muscle	11 Long saphenous vein	19 Bladder
4 Tensor fasciae latae muscle	12 Femoral canal	20 Seminal vesicle
5 Sartorius muscle	13 Spermatic cord	21 Inferior gluteal vessels
6 Rectus femoris muscle	14 Rectus abdominis muscle	22 Rectum
7 Iliopsoas muscle	15 Ductus (vas) deferens	23 Sacrum
8 Common femoral artery	16 Acetabulum	24 Sciatic nerve

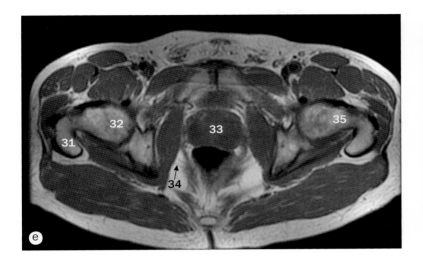

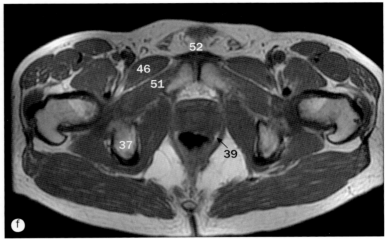

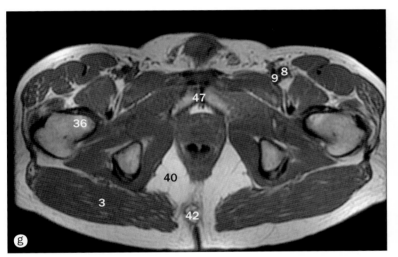

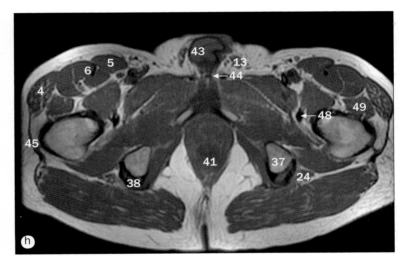

(a)–(l) Sequential axial T2w MR images of a male pelvis, from superior to inferior.

25 Superior pubic ramus
26 Ligamentum teres
27 Obturator vessels and nerve
28 Ischial spine
29 Sacrospinous ligament
30 Obturator externus muscle
31 Greater trochanter of femur
32 Femoral head
33 Prostate
34 Inferior rectal vessels and nerve

35 Femoral neck
36 Lesser trochanter of femur
37 Ischial tuberosity
38 Hamstrings (common tendinous origin)
39 Levator ani muscle (puborectalis)
40 Ischio-anal fossa
41 Anorectal junction
42 Coccyx
43 Corpus cavernosum

44 Dorsal penile vessels
45 Fascia lata
46 Pectineus muscle
47 Symphysis pubis
48 Iliopsoas tendon
49 Vastus lateralis muscle
50 Inferior epigastric vessels
51 Adductor longus muscle
52 Transverse pubic ligament

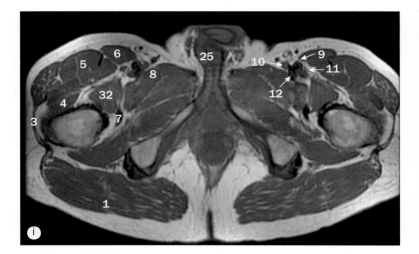

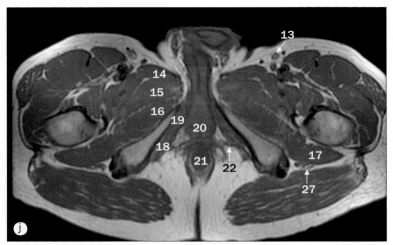

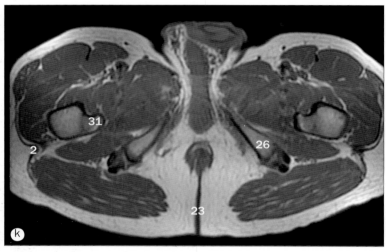

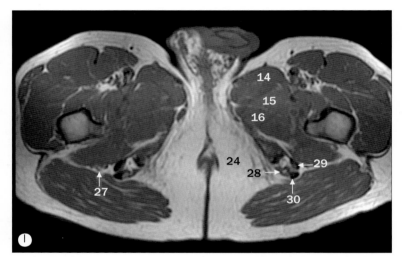

(a)–(l) Sequential axial T2w MR images of a male pelvis, from superior to inferior.

1 Gluteus maximus muscle	**12** Profunda femoris vein	**23** Natal cleft
2 Fascia lata	**13** Long saphenous vein	**24** Ischio-anal fossa
3 Iliotibial tract	**14** Adductor longus muscle	**25** Corpus cavernosum
4 Vastus lateralis muscle	**15** Adductor brevis muscle	**26** Ischial tuberosity
5 Rectus femoris muscle	**16** Adductor magnus muscle	**27** Sciatic nerve
6 Sartorius muscle	**17** Quadratus femoris muscle	**28** Semitendinosus tendinous origin
7 Iliopsoas tendon	**18** Ischiocavernosus muscle	**29** Semimembranosus tendinous origin
8 Pectineus muscle	**19** Crus of penis	**30** Biceps femoris tendinous origin
9 Superficial femoral artery	**20** Bulb of penis	**31** Lesser trochanter of femur
10 Superficial femoral vein	**21** Anus	**32** Iliopsoas muscle
11 Profunda femoris artery	**22** Inferior rectal neurovascular bundle	

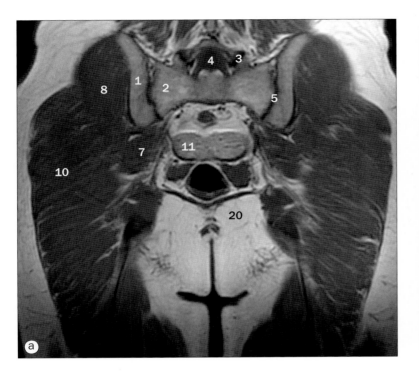

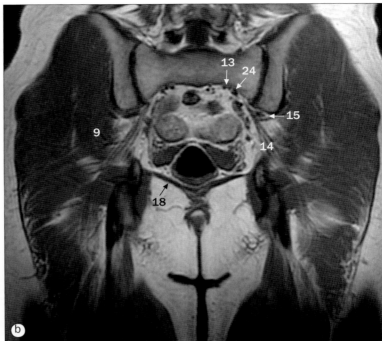

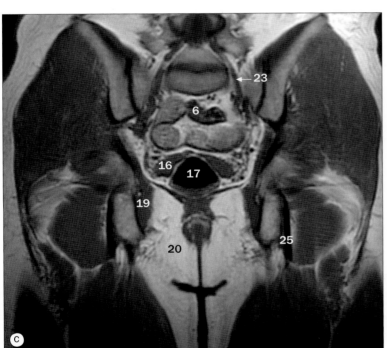

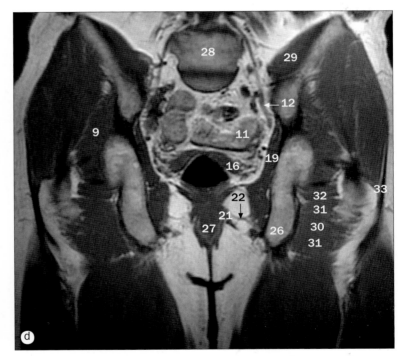

(a)–(p) Sequential coronal T2w MR images of a male pelvis, from posterior to anterior.

1 Ilium	12 Ureter	23 Fifth lumbar root
2 Sacral ala	13 Gonadal vessels	24 Lumbosacral trunk
3 Facet joint (L5/S1)	14 Sciatic nerve	25 Common hamstring origin
4 Thecal sac	15 Superior gluteal vessels	26 Ischial tuberosity
5 Sacro-iliac joint	16 Seminal vesicle	27 Anal canal
6 Rectosigmoid junction	17 Rectal ampulla	28 L5 vertebral body
7 Piriformis muscle	18 Levator ani muscle	29 Iliacus muscle
8 Gluteus medius muscle	19 Obturator internus muscle	30 Quadratus femoris muscle
9 Gluteus minimis muscle	20 Ischio-anal fossa	31 Gemelli muscles (superior and inferior)
10 Gluteus maximus muscle	21 External anal sphincter	32 Obturator externus muscle
11 Small bowel	22 Inferior rectal neurovascular bundle	33 Fascia lata

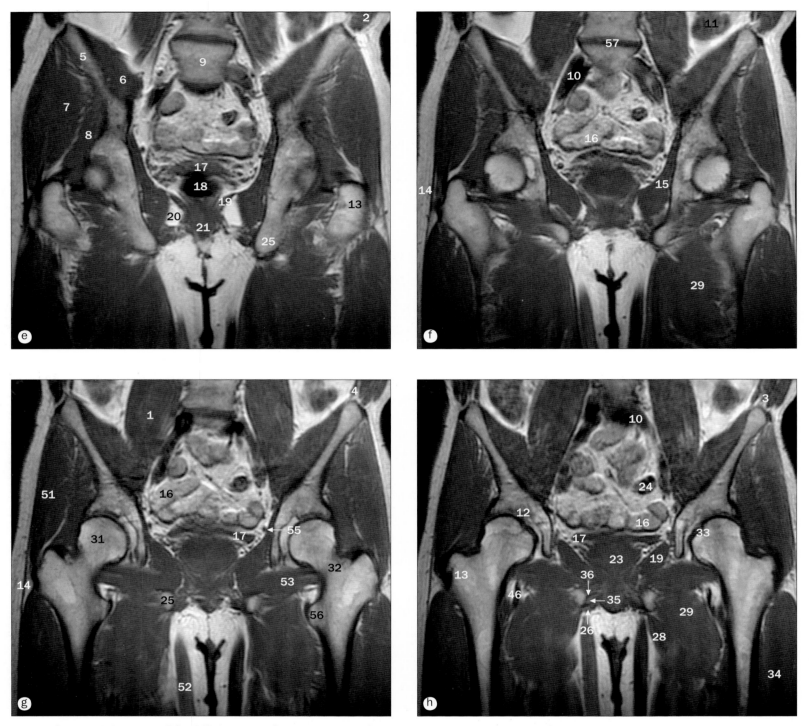

(a)–(p) Sequential coronal T2w MR images of a male pelvis, from posterior to anterior.

1 Psoas major muscle	**9** Fifth lumbar vertebral body	**17** Seminal vesicle
2 External oblique muscle	**10** Common iliac vessels	**18** Rectum
3 Internal oblique muscle	**11** Descending colon	**19** Levator ani muscle
4 Transversus abdominis muscle	**12** Acetabulum	**20** Ischio-anal fossa
5 Ilium	**13** Greater trochanter of femur	**21** Anal canal
6 Iliacus muscle	**14** Fascia lata	**22** Bladder
7 Gluteus medius muscle	**15** Obturator internus muscle	**23** Prostate
8 Gluteus minimis muscle	**16** Small bowel	**24** Sigmoid colon

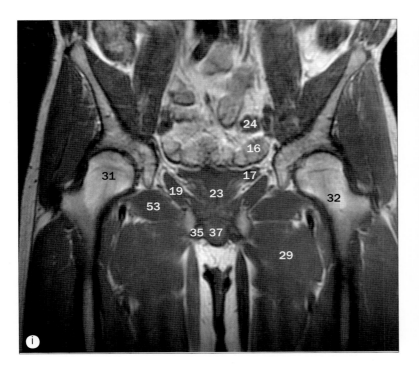

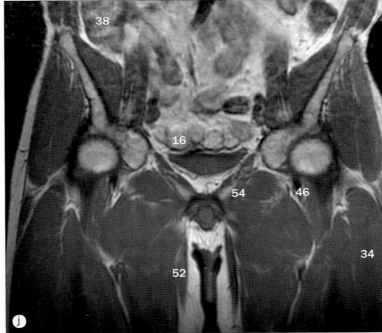

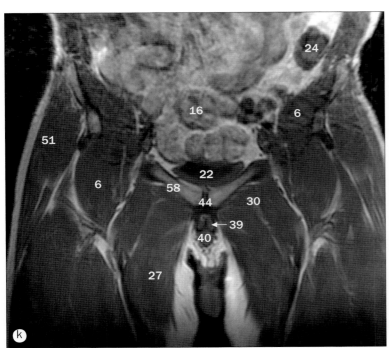

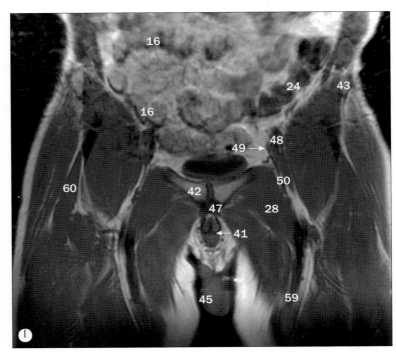

(a)–(p) Sequential coronal T2w MR images of a male pelvis, from posterior to anterior.

25 Ischium	37 Bulb of penis	49 External iliac vein
26 Transverse perineii muscle	38 Caecum	50 Common femoral vessels
27 Adductor longus muscle	39 Corpus cavernosus	51 Gluteus maximus muscle
28 Adductor brevis muscle	40 Corpus spongiosus	52 Gracilis muscle
29 Adductor magnus muscle	41 Penile (spongy) urethra	53 Obturator externus muscle
30 Pectineus muscle	42 Pubic body	54 Inferior pubic ramus
31 Femoral head	43 Anterior superior iliac spine	55 Obturator neurovascular bundle
32 Femoral neck	44 Symphysis pubis	56 Lesser trochanter of femur
33 Fovea capitalis of femur	45 Testicle	57 Intervertebral disc at L4/5
34 Vastus lateralis muscle	46 Profunda femoris vessels	58 Superior pubic ramus
35 Crus of penis	47 Suspensory ligament of penis	59 Superficial femoral vessels
36 Ischiocavernosus	48 External iliac artery	60 Tensor fasciae latae muscle

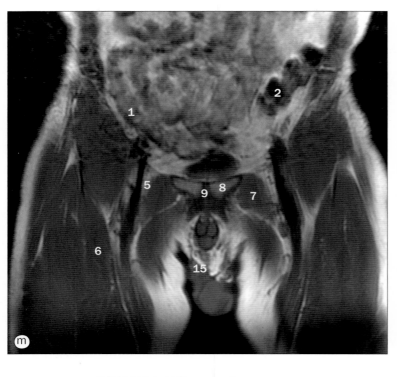

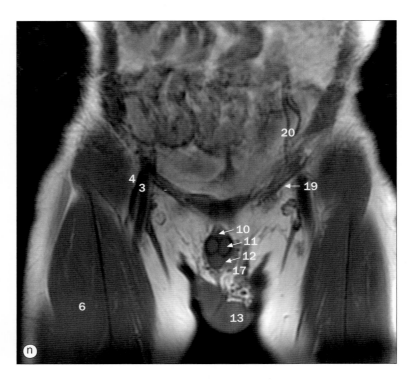

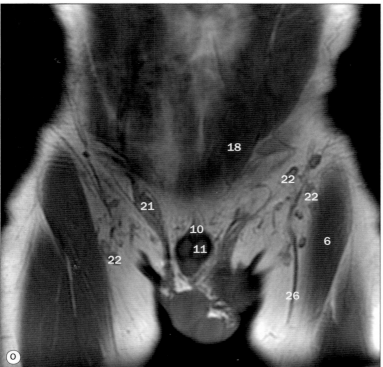

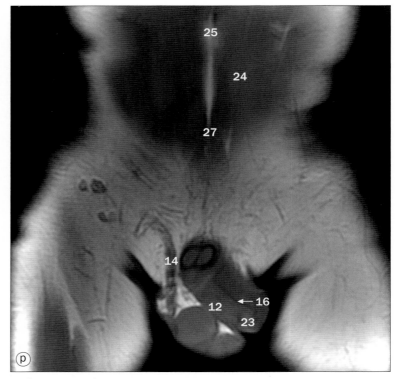

(a)–(p) Sequential coronal T2w MR images of a male pelvis, from posterior to anterior.

1 Small bowel	10 Suspensory ligament of penis	19 Inguinal ligament
2 Sigmoid colon	11 Corpus cavernosum of penis	20 Inferior epigastric vessels
3 Common femoral vein	12 Corpus spongiosum of penis	21 Inguinal canal (external ring)
4 Common femoral artery	13 Testicle	22 Superficial inguinal lymph nodes
5 Femoral canal	14 Spermatic cord	23 Glans penis
6 Rectus femoris muscle	15 Epididymal head	24 Rectus abdominis muscle
7 Pectineus muscle	16 Penile (spongy) urethra	25 Umbilicus
8 Pubic body	17 Pampiniform plexus	26 Long saphenous vein
9 Symphysis pubis	18 External oblique muscle	27 Linea alba

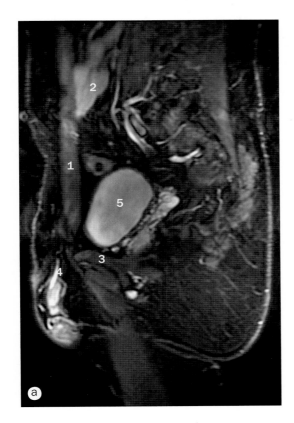

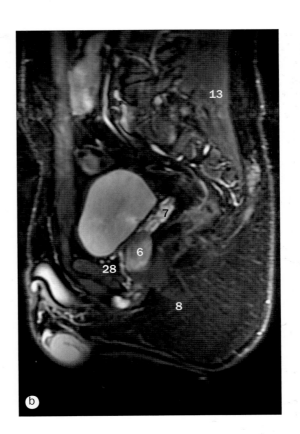

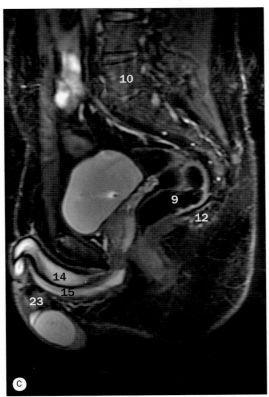

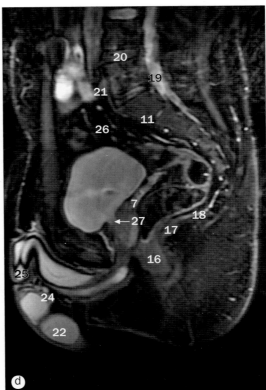

(a)–(h) Sequential sagittal MR images of a male pelvis, from right to left, through the midline (T2 Fat Sat images).

1 Rectus abdominis muscle
2 Small bowel
3 Pubic body
4 Spermatic cord
5 Bladder
6 Prostate
7 Seminal vesicle
8 Ischio-anal fossa

9 Rectum
10 Fifth lumbar vertebra
11 Sacrum
12 Coccyx
13 Erector spinae muscle
14 Corpus cavernosum
15 Corpus spongiosum

16 Anal canal
17 Puborectalis muscle
18 Anococcygeal raphe
19 Thecal sac
20 Intervertebral disc (L4/5)
21 Common iliac vein
22 Testicle

23 Epididymal head
24 Epididymal body
25 Glans penis
26 Sigmoid colon
27 Prostatic urethra
28 Retropubic space (cave of
   Retzius)

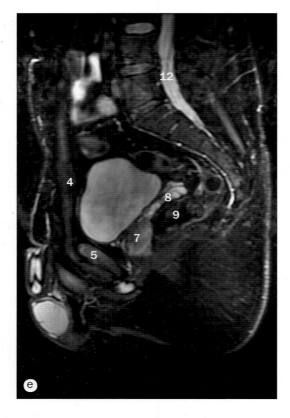

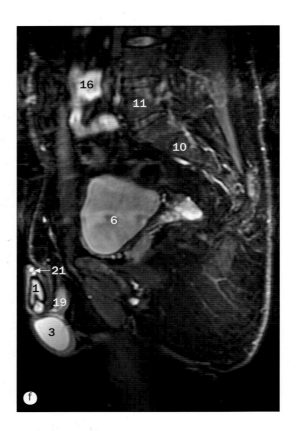

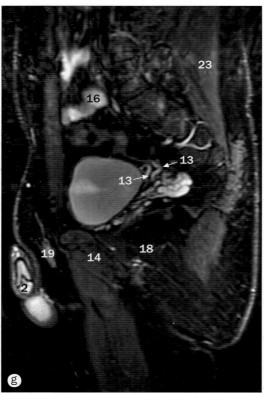

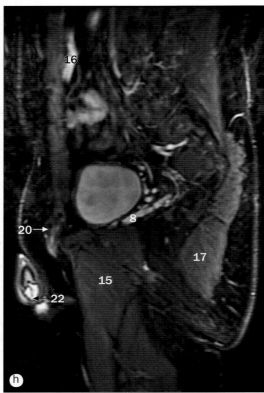

(a)–(h) Sequential sagittal MR images of a male pelvis, from right to left, through the midline (T2 Fat Sat images).

1 Corpus cavernosum	**7** Prostate	**13** Ductus (vas) deferens	**19** Spermatic cord
2 Glans penis	**8** Seminal vesicle	**14** Pectineus muscle	**20** Inguinal canal (external ring)
3 Testicle	**9** Rectum	**15** Adductor brevis muscle	**21** Dorsal vessels of penis
4 Rectus abdominis muscle	**10** Sacrum	**16** Small bowel	**22** External meatus of urethra
5 Pubic body	**11** Fifth lumbar vertebra	**17** Gluteus maximus muscle	**23** Erector spinae muscle
6 Bladder	**12** Thecal sac	**18** Ischio-anal fossa	

6 Abdomen and pelvis – Non cross-sectional

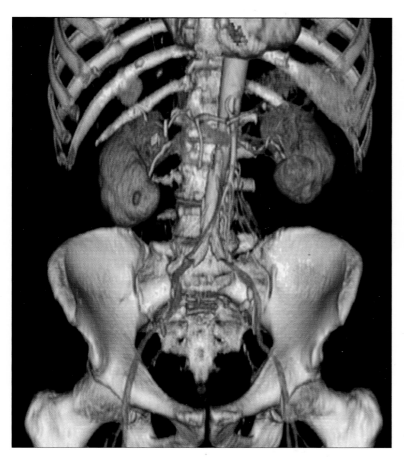

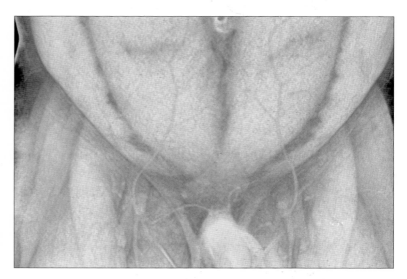

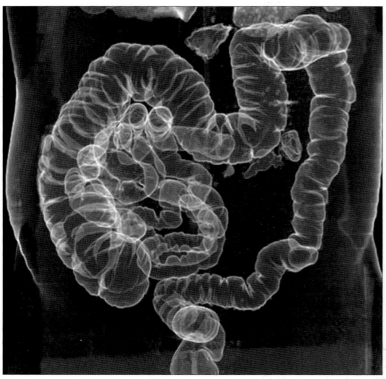

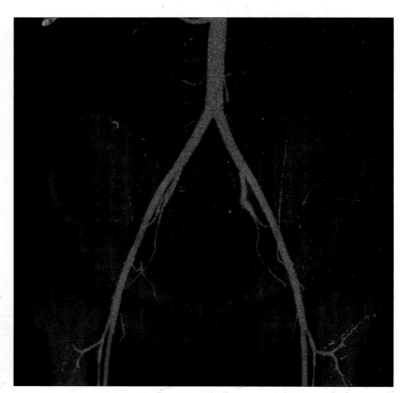

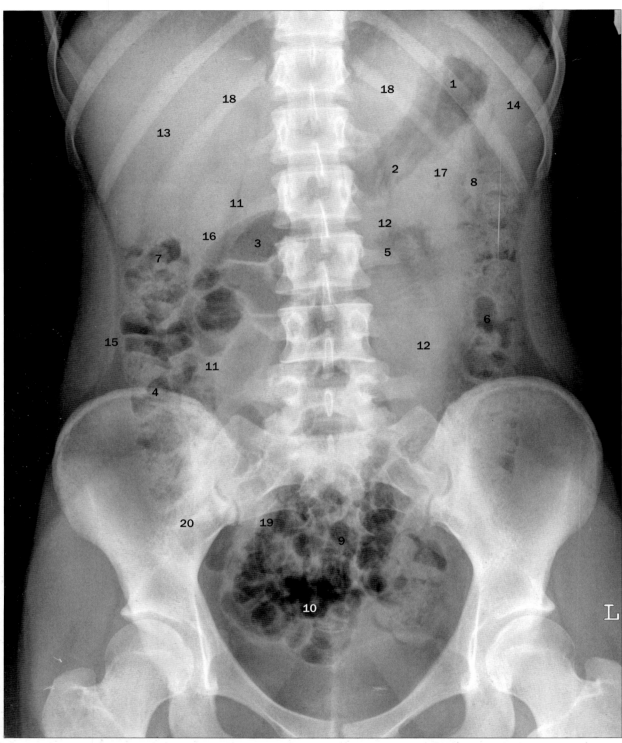

Supine abdominal radiograph.

1 Gas in fundus of stomach	7 Hepatic flexure of colon	14 Spleen
2 Gas in body of stomach	8 Splenic flexure of colon	15 Properitoneal fat line
3 Gas in first part of duodenum (duodenal cap)	9 Sigmoid colon	16 Right kidney
4 Ascending colon	10 Rectum	17 Left kidney
5 Transverse colon	11 Right psoas margin	18 Twelfth rib
6 Descending colon	12 Left psoas margin	19 Gas in ileum
	13 Liver	20 Gas in caecum

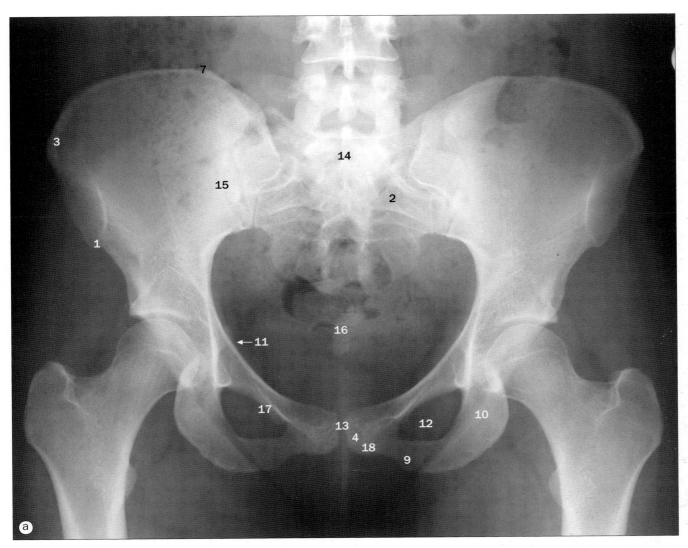

(a) Pelvis and hips of an adult female, anteroposterior projection.
(b) and (c) Pelvis of a 17-year-old male, anteroposterior projections.

1 Anterior inferior iliac spine	**7** Iliac crest	**13** Pubic symphysis
2 Anterior sacral foramen	**8** Ilium	**14** Sacral crest
3 Anterior superior iliac spine	**9** Inferior ramus of pubis	**15** Sacro-iliac joint
4 Body of pubis	**10** Ischial ramus	**16** Segment of coccyx
5 Centre for iliac crest	**11** Ischial spine	**17** Superior ramus of pubis
6 Centre for ischial tuberosity	**12** Obturator foramen	**18** Tubercle of pubis

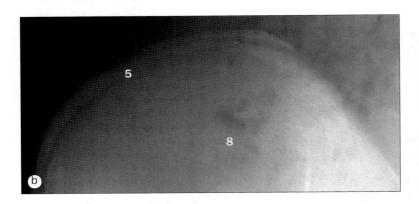

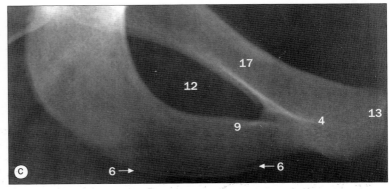

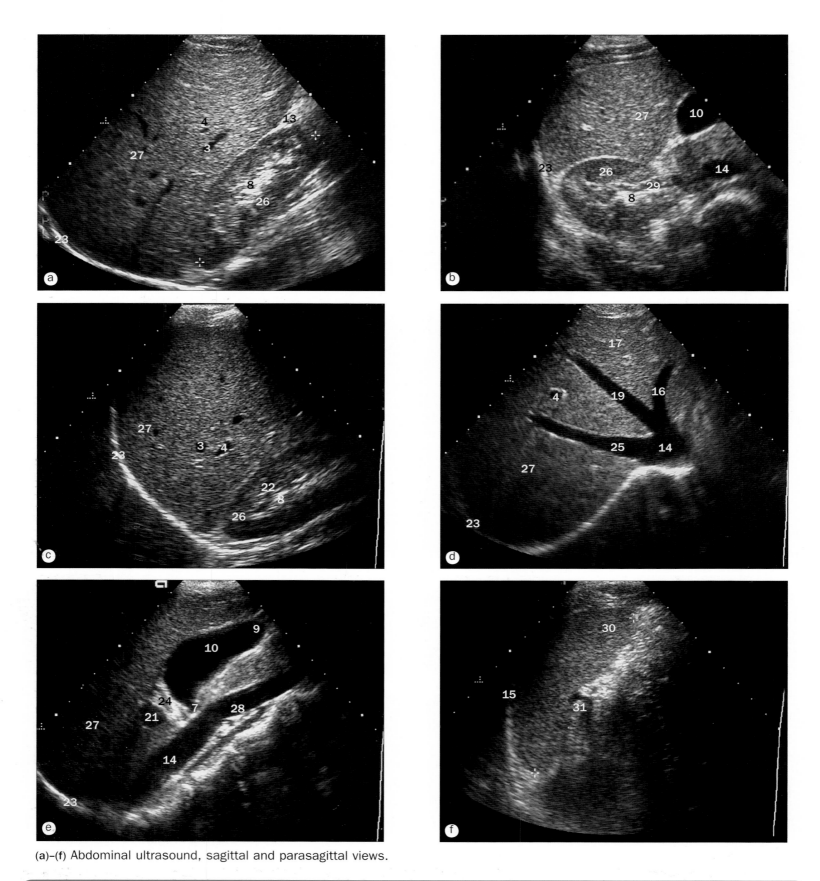

(a)–(f) Abdominal ultrasound, sagittal and parasagittal views.

1 Abdominal aorta	6 Common bile duct	11 Head of pancreas
2 Body of pancreas	7 Cystic duct	12 Hepatic artery
3 Branch of hepatic vein	8 Fat in renal sinus	13 Hepatorenal recess
4 Branch of portal vein	9 Fundus of gall bladder	14 Inferior vena cava
5 Coeliac trunk	10 Gall bladder	15 Left dome of diaphragm

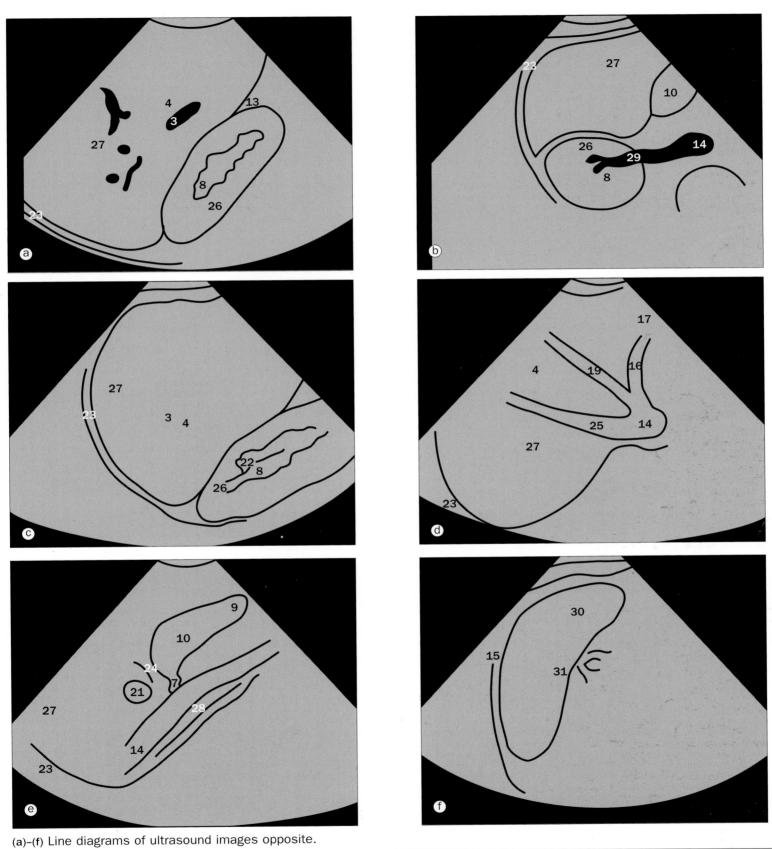

(a)–(f) Line diagrams of ultrasound images opposite.

16 Left hepatic vein	**23** Right dome of diaphragm	**30** Spleen
17 Left lobe of liver	**24** Right hepatic artery	**31** Splenic vein
18 Left renal vein	**25** Right hepatic vein	**32** Superior mesenteric artery
19 Middle hepatic vein	**26** Right kidney	**33** Superior mesenteric vein
20 Neck of pancreas	**27** Right lobe of liver	**34** Tail of pancreas
21 Portal vein	**28** Right renal artery	**35** Vertebral body
22 Renal papilla	**29** Right renal vein	

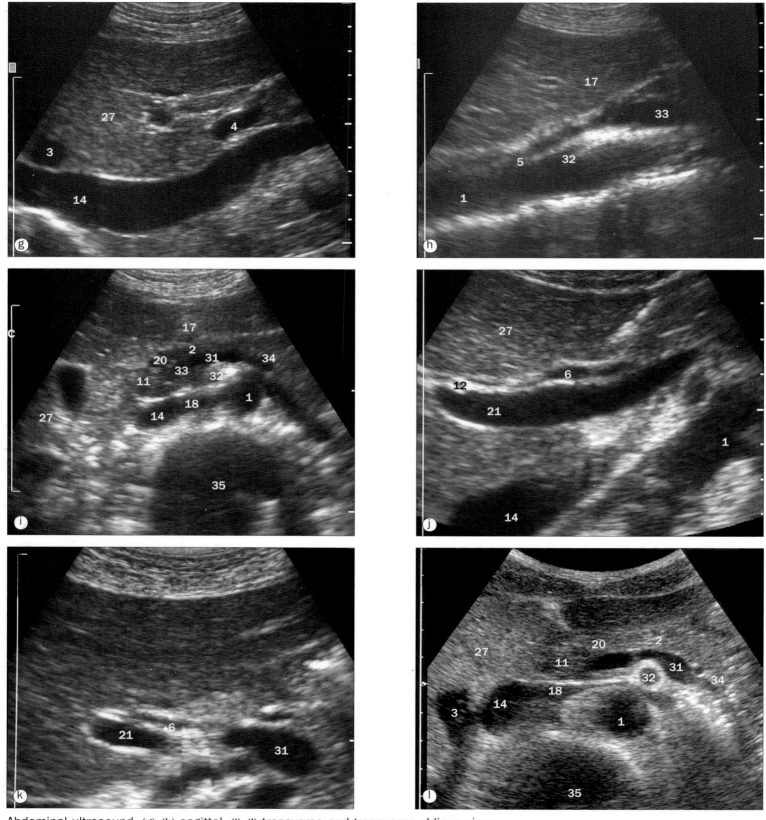

Abdominal ultrasound, (g)–(h) sagittal, (i)–(l) transverse and transverse oblique views.

1 Abdominal aorta	6 Common bile duct	11 Head of pancreas
2 Body of pancreas	7 Cystic duct	12 Hepatic artery
3 Branch of hepatic vein	8 Fat in renal sinus	13 Hepatorenal recess
4 Branch of portal vein	9 Fundus of gall bladder	14 Inferior vena cava
5 Coeliac trunk	10 Gall bladder	15 Left dome of diaphragm

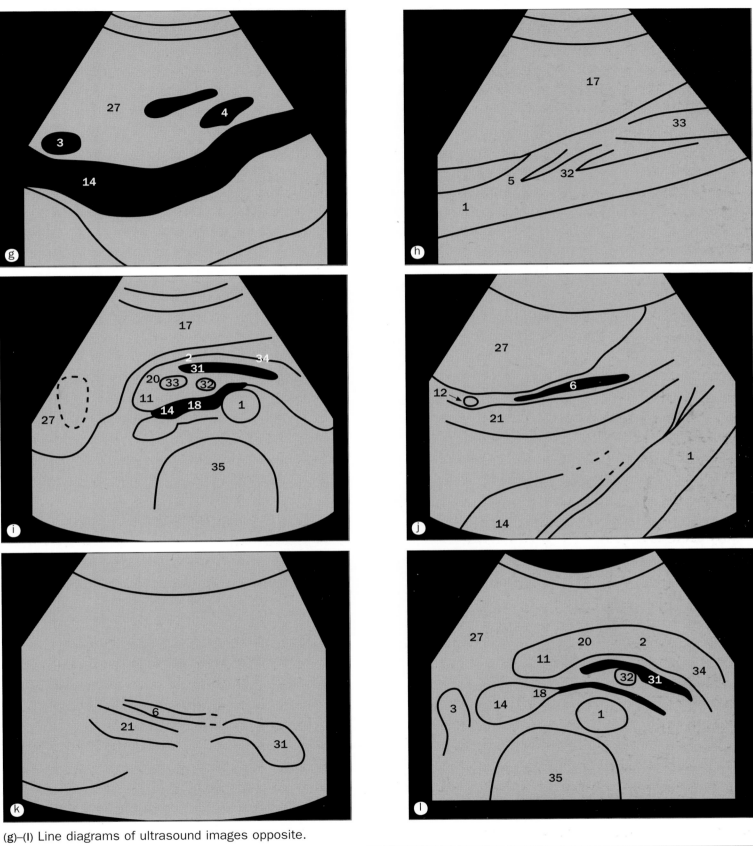

(g)–(l) Line diagrams of ultrasound images opposite.

16 Left hepatic vein	**23** Right dome of diaphragm	**30** Spleen
17 Left lobe of liver	**24** Right hepatic artery	**31** Splenic vein
18 Left renal vein	**25** Right hepatic vein	**32** Superior mesenteric artery
19 Middle hepatic vein	**26** Right kidney	**33** Superior mesenteric vein
20 Neck of pancreas	**27** Right lobe of liver	**34** Tail of pancreas
21 Portal vein	**28** Right renal artery	**35** Vertebral body
22 Renal papilla	**29** Right renal vein	

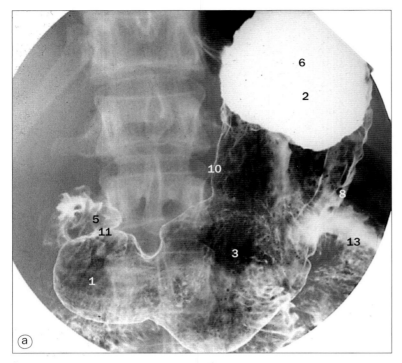

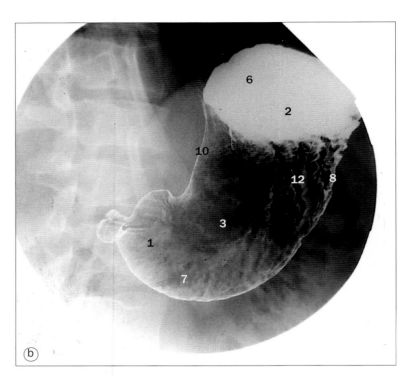

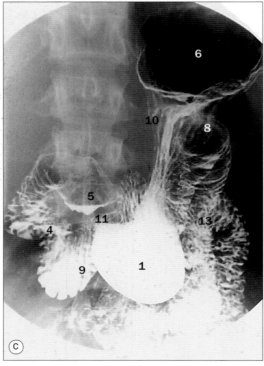

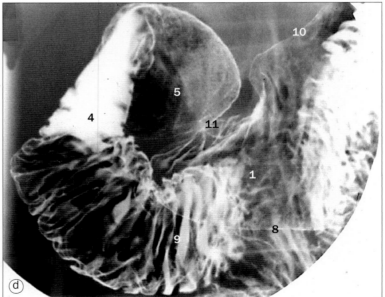

Abdomen. Double-contrast barium meals of stomach and duodenum, (**a**) and (**b**) with the patient supine (to show the mucosa of the stomach), (**c**) with the patient erect, (**d**) with the patient in a supine oblique position (to show the duodenum).

1	Antrum of stomach	**7**	Gas bubbles
2	Barium pooling in fundus of stomach	**8**	Greater curvature of stomach
3	Body of stomach	**9**	Horizontal (third) part of duodenum
4	Descending (second) part of duodenum	**10**	Lesser curvature of stomach
5	Duodenal cap (superior or first part of duodenum)	**11**	Region of pyloric canal
		12	Rugae of stomach
6	Fundus of stomach	**13**	Small bowel

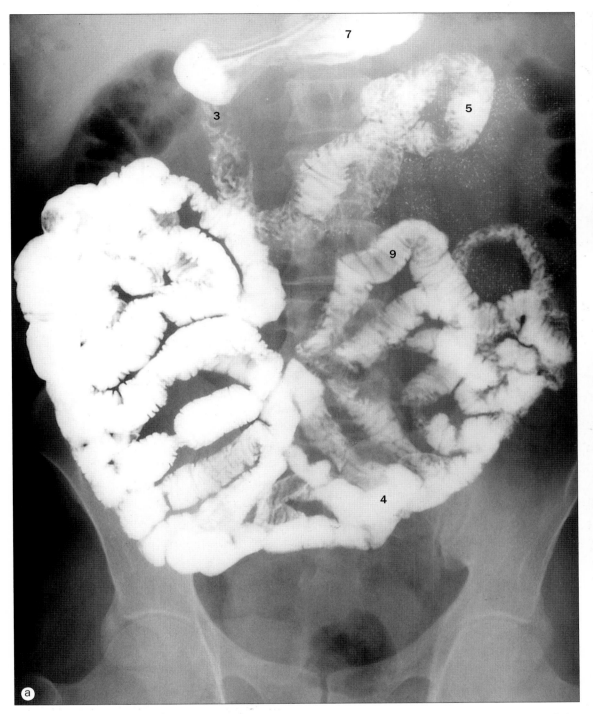

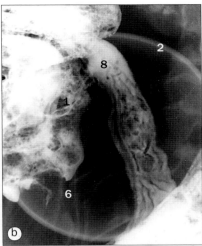

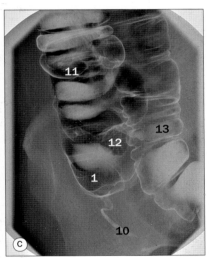

Abdomen, barium follow-throughs, **(a)** with the patient supine, **(b)** showing a localised view of the terminal ileum and **(c)** ileocaecal valve. Anteroposterior radiographs.

1 Caecum	**8** Terminal ileum
2 Compression device	**9** Valvulae conniventes (plicae circulares) of
3 Descending (second) part of duodenum	jejunum
4 Proximal ileum	**10** Appendix
5 Proximal jejunum	**11** Ascending colon
6 Right sacro-iliac joint	**12** Ileocaecal valve
7 Stomach	**13** Transverse colon

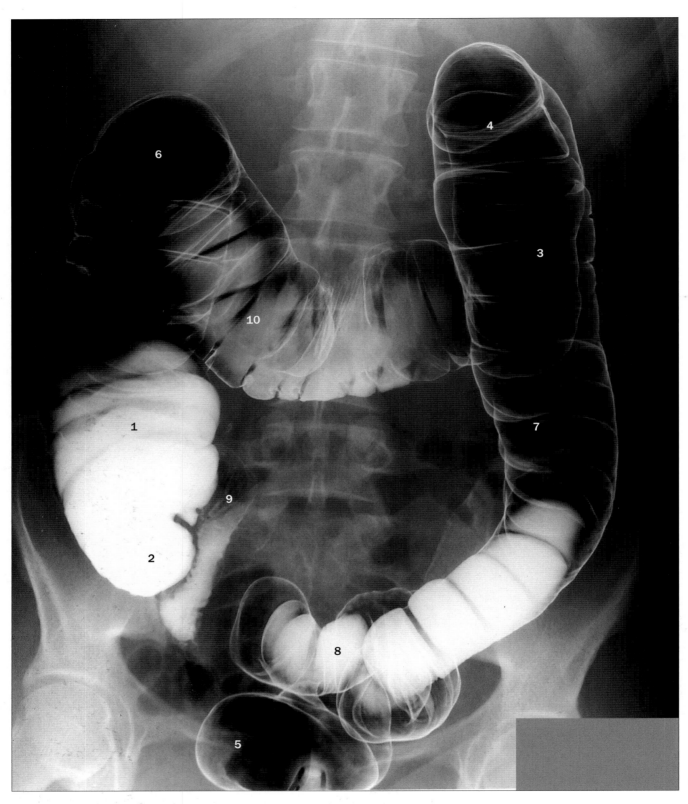

Abdomen, double-contrast barium enema of the large bowel (colon).

1 Ascending portion of colon	6 Right colic (hepatic) flexure of colon
2 Caecum	7 Sacculations (haustrations) of colon
3 Descending portion of colon	8 Sigmoid colon
4 Left colic (splenic) flexure of colon	9 Terminal ileum
5 Rectum	10 Transverse portion of colon

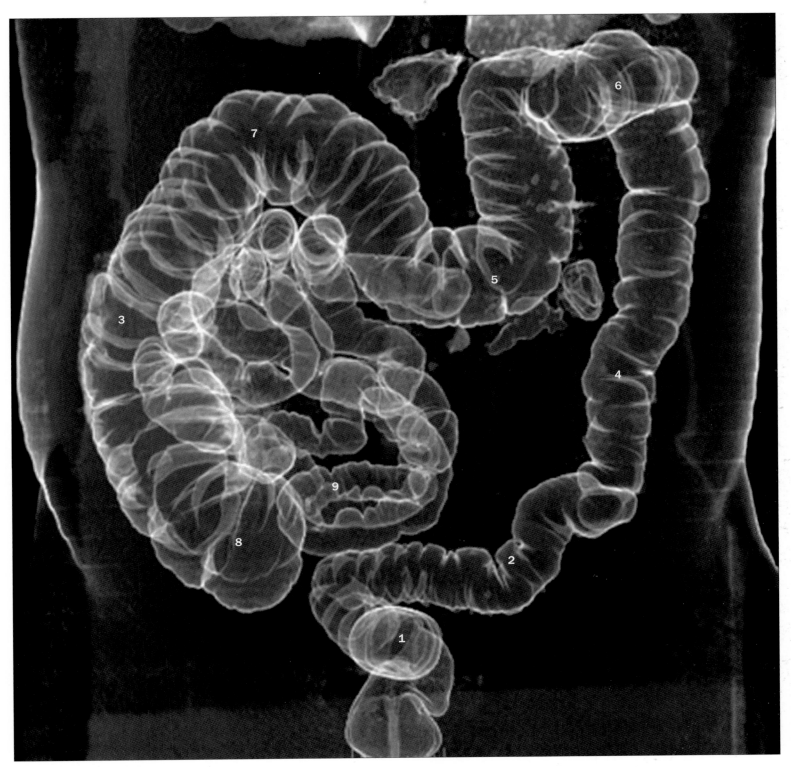

CT colonography.

1 Rectum
2 Sigmoid colon
3 Ascending colon
4 Descending colon
5 Transverse colon
6 Splenic flexure (left colic)
7 Hepatic flexure (right colic)
8 Caecum
9 Terminal ileum

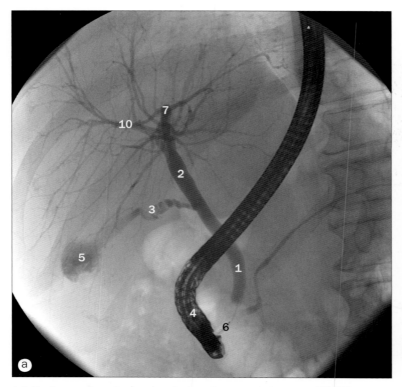

(a) Endoscopic retrograde cholangiopancreatogram (ERCP).

(b) Magnetic cholangiopancreatogram (MRCP).

1 Common bile duct	5 Gall bladder	8 Neck of gall bladder
2 Common hepatic duct	6 Hepatopancreatic (Vater's) ampulla	9 Pancreatic duct
3 Cystic duct	7 Left hepatic duct	10 Right hepatic duct
4 Endoscope in duodenum		

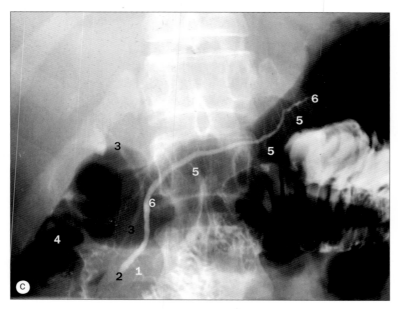

1 Accessory pancreatic duct (Santonni's)
2 Ampullary part of pancreatic duct
3 Common bile duct
4 Contrast and gas in descending (second) part of duodenum
5 Intralobular ducts
6 Main pancreatic duct

(c) ERCP.

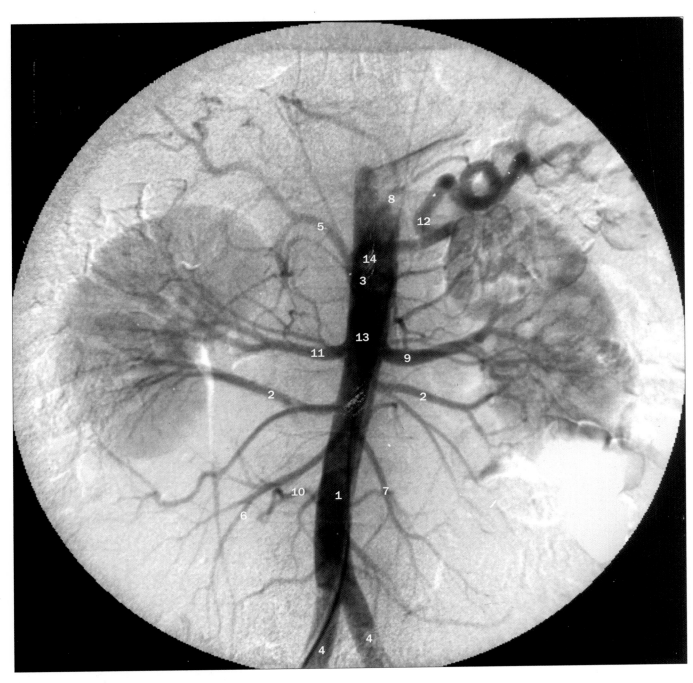

Abdominal aortogram.

1 Abdominal aorta
2 Accessory renal arteries
3 Coeliac trunk
4 Common iliac arteries
5 Hepatic artery
6 Ileocolic artery
7 Jejunal branches of superior mesenteric artery
8 Left gastric artery
9 Left renal artery
10 Lumbar arteries
11 Right renal artery
12 Splenic artery
13 Superior mesenteric artery
14 Tip of pigtail catheter in abdominal aorta

(a) and (b) Subtracted coeliac trunk arteriograms.

1 Dorsal pancreatic artery
2 Gastroduodenal artery
3 Hepatic artery
4 Left gastric artery
5 Left gastro-epiploic artery
6 Left hepatic artery
7 Pancreatica magna artery
8 Phrenic artery
9 Right gastro-epiploic artery
10 Right hepatic artery
11 Splenic artery
12 Superior pancreatico-duodenal artery
13 Tip of catheter in coeliac trunk
14 Transverse pancreatic artery

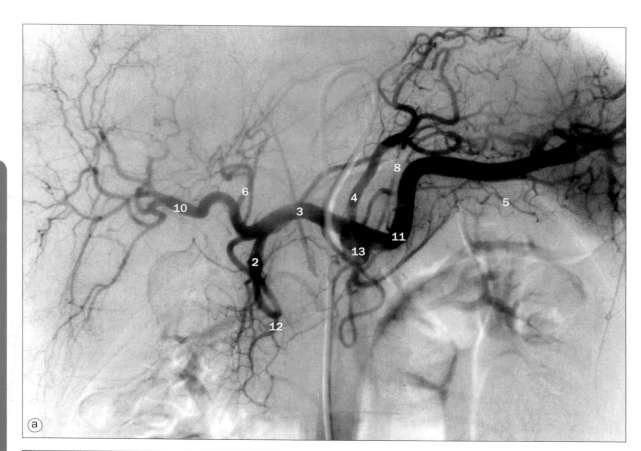

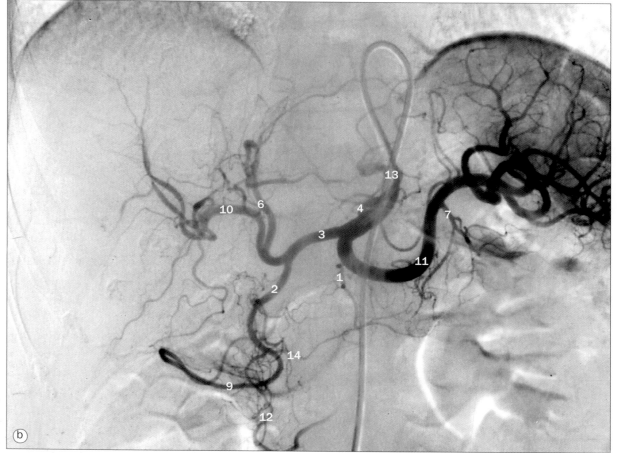

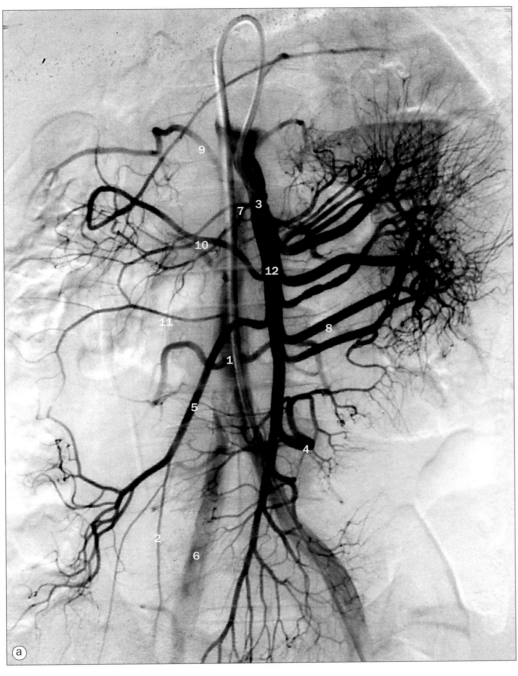

(a) Subtracted superior mesenteric arteriogram.

1 Aorta
2 Appendicular artery
3 Catheter with tip selectively in superior mesenteric artery
4 Ileal branches of superior mesenteric artery
5 Ileocolic artery
6 Iliac artery
7 Inferior pancreaticoduodenal artery
8 Jejunal branches of superior mesenteric artery
9 Lumbar arteries arising from abdominal aorta
10 Middle colic artery
11 Right colic artery
12 Superior mesenteric artery

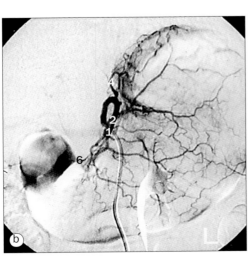

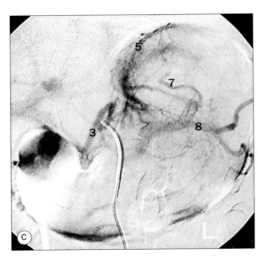

(b) Gastric arteries, (c) gastric veins.

1 Catheter in origin of left gastric artery
2 Left gastric artery
3 Left gastric vein
4 Oesophageal branch of left gastric artery
5 Oesophageal branches of left gastric vein
6 Right gastric artery
7 Short gastric veins
8 Splenic vein

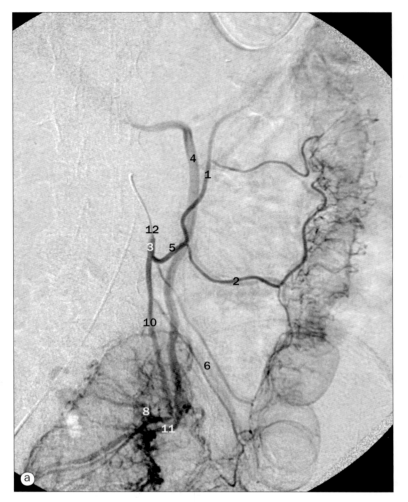

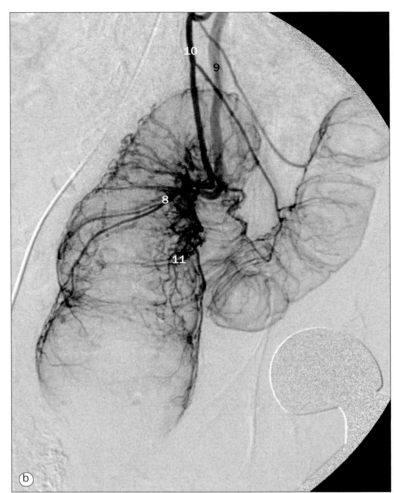

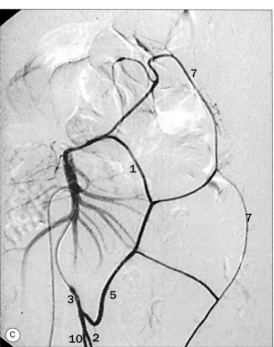

1 Ascending branch of left colic artery
2 Descending branch of left colic artery
3 Inferior mesenteric artery
4 Inferior mesenteric vein
5 Left colic artery
6 Left colic vein
7 Marginal artery of Drummond
8 Sigmoid arteries
9 Sigmoid vein
10 Superior rectal artery
11 Superior rectal vein
12 Tip of catheter in inferior mesenteric
   artery

(a)–(c) Inferior mesenteric arteriograms.

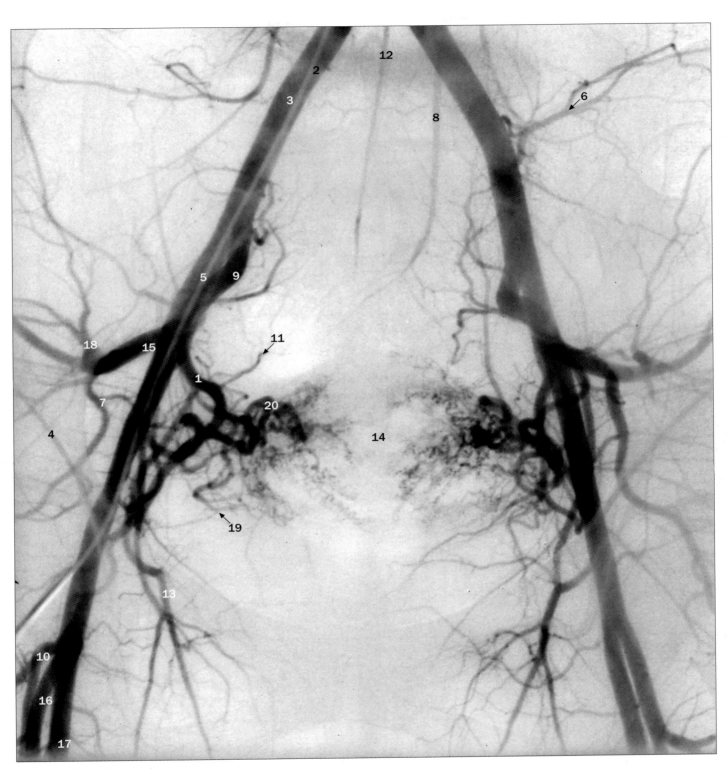

Subtracted pelvic arteriogram.

This anteroposterior film of the pelvis demonstrates both the internal and the external iliac arteries and their branches. Many of the vessels are superimposed: to see them more clearly oblique projections could be obtained. The contrast medium injected into the arteries is excreted by the kidneys, and a full bladder may obscure the branches. Selective catheterisation of the internal and external iliac arteries using a preshaped catheter gives better detail without superimposition of the vessels.

1 Anterior trunk of internal iliac artery
2 Catheter introduced into distal
    abdominal aorta via right
    femoral artery
3 Common iliac artery
4 Deep circumflex iliac artery
5 External iliac artery
6 Iliolumbar artery
7 Inferior gluteal artery
8 Inferior mesenteric artery
9 Internal iliac artery
10 Lateral circumflex femoral artery
11 Lateral sacral artery
12 Median sacral artery
13 Obturator artery
14 Position of uterus
15 Posterior trunk of internal iliac artery
16 Profunda femoris artery
17 Superficial femoral artery
18 Superior gluteal artery
19 Superior vesical artery
20 Uterine artery

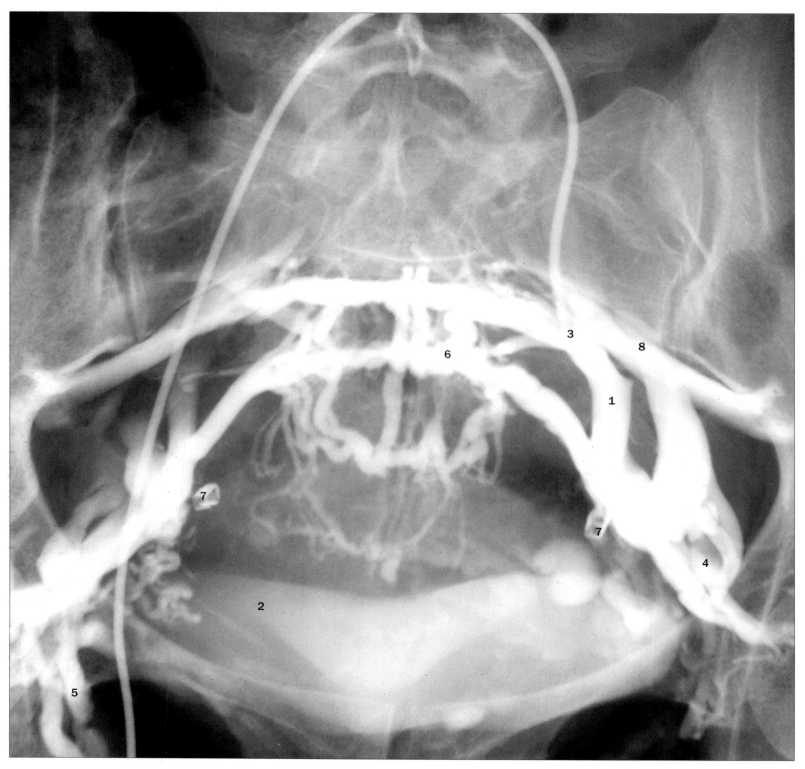

Female pelvic venogram.

1 Anterior division of internal iliac vein
2 Bladder containing contrast medium
3 Catheter introduced via right femoral vein, with tip in left internal
   iliac vein
4 Inferior gluteal veins
5 Obturator veins
6 Sacral plexus of veins
7 Sterilisation clips
8 Superior gluteal veins

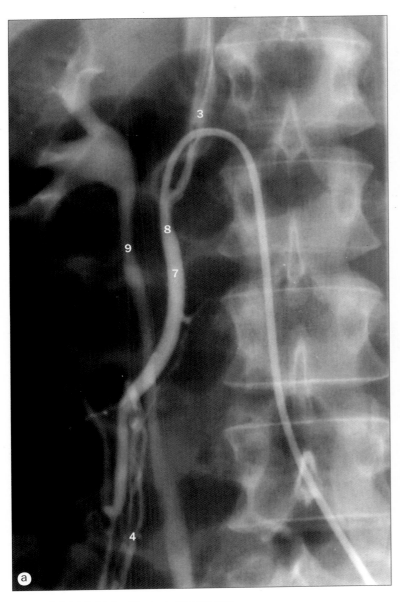

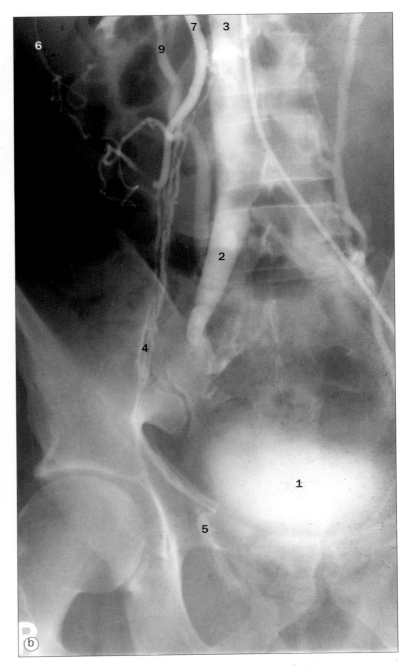

(a) and (b) Right testicular venograms.

The gonadal veins drain into one or two main veins via a venous plexus. On the left, the main vein drains into the left renal vein. It may occasionally communicate with the inferior mesenteric vein and drain into the portal venous system. On the right, the main vein usually drains into the inferior vena cava directly (as in the case illustrated), but it can drain into the right renal vein.

1 Bladder
2 Common iliac veins
3 Inferior vena cava
4 Pampiniform plexus of veins
5 Pampiniform plexus of veins (undescended testis in inguinal canal)
6 Renal capsular veins
7 Right testicular vein
8 Tip of catheter in right testicular vein, introduced via left femoral vein
9 Ureter

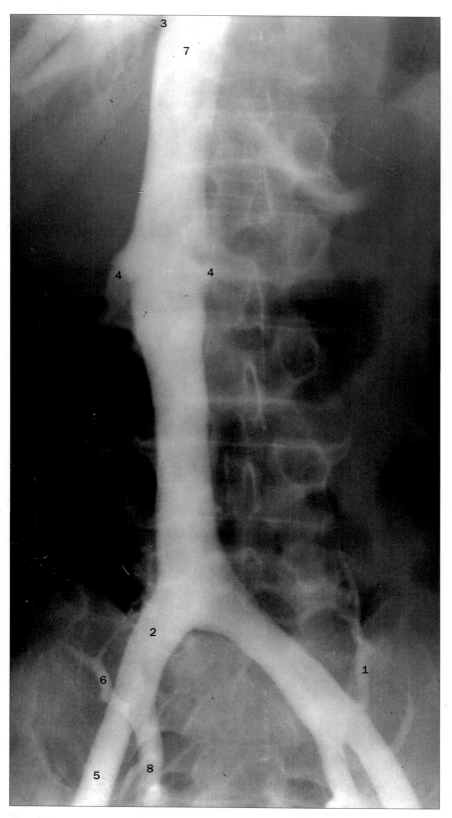

Inferior vena cavogram.

1	Ascending lumbar vein
2	Common iliac vein
3	Entrance of hepatic veins
4	Entrance of renal veins
5	External iliac vein
6	Iliolumbar vein
7	Inferior vena cava
8	Internal iliac vein

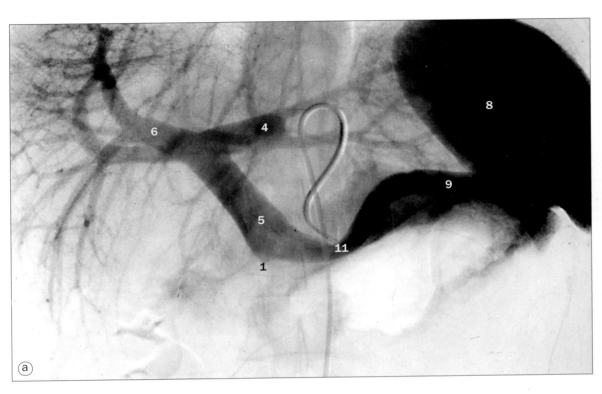

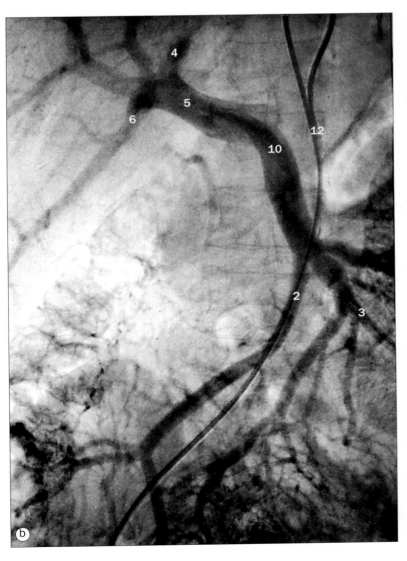

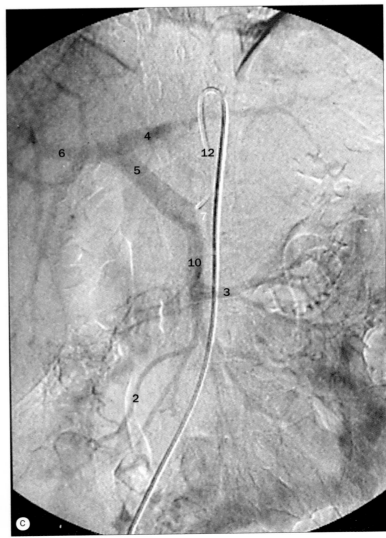

(a) Indirect splenoportogram.

(b) and (c) Venous phase of superior mesenteric arteriogram.

1 Entry of superior mesenteric vein
2 Ileocolic vein
3 Jejunal vein
4 Left branch of portal vein
5 Portal vein
6 Right branch of portal vein
7 Site of entry of splenic vein
8 Spleen
9 Splenic vein
10 Superior mesenteric vein
11 Tip of catheter in splenic artery
12 Tip of catheter in superior mesenteric artery

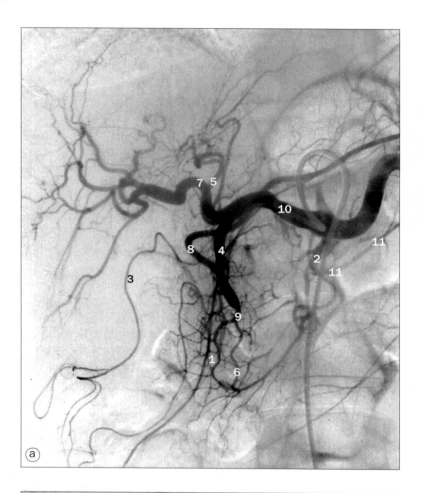

(a) Subtracted hepatic arteriogram.

1 Anterior branch of inferior pancreaticoduodenal artery
2 Dorsal pancreatic artery
3 Epiploic artery
4 Gastroduodenal artery
5 Left branch of hepatic artery
6 Posterior branch of superior pancreaticoduodenal artery
7 Right branch of hepatic artery
8 Right gastro-epiploic artery
9 Superior pancreaticoduodenal artery
10 Tip of catheter in hepatic artery
11 Transverse pancreatic artery

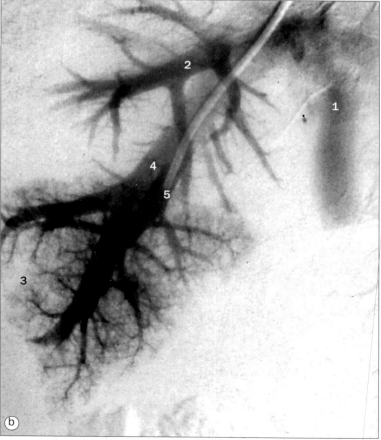

(b) Subtracted hepatic venogram.

1 Inferior vena cava
2 Middle hepatic vein
3 Parenchyma of liver
4 Right hepatic vein
5 Tip of catheter in hepatic vein

(a) Selective gastroduodenal arteriogram.

(b) Subtracted pancreatic arteriogram.

1 Anterior branch of inferior pancreatico-
   duodenal artery
2 Anterior branch of superior pancreatico-
   duodenal artery
3 Gastroduodenal artery
4 Left gastro-epiploic artery
5 Posterior branch of inferior pancreatico-
   duodenal artery
6 Posterior branch of superior
   pancreatico-duodenal artery
7 Right gastro-epiploic artery
8 Superior mesenteric artery
9 Tip of catheter in dorsal pancreatic
   artery
10 Transverse pancreatic artery

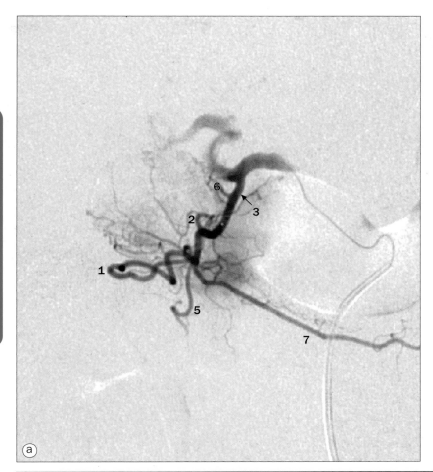

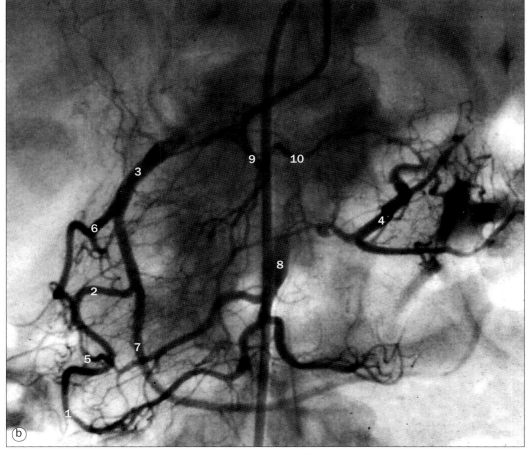

(a) Renal arteriogram.

1 Arcuate arteries
2 Interlobar arteries
3 Lobar arteries
4 Main renal artery
5 Tip of catheter in renal artery

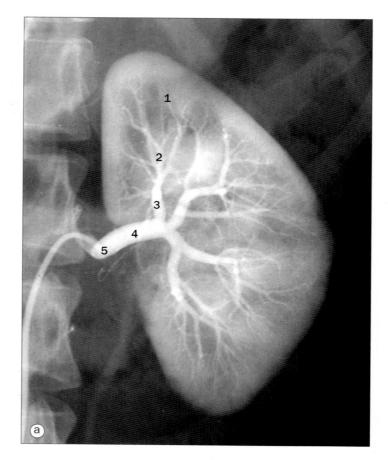

(b) Left suprarenal arteriogram.

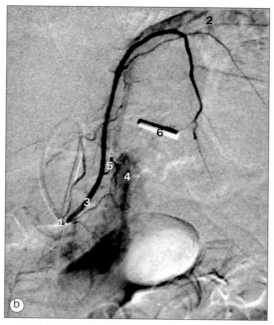

1 Catheter in origin of inferior
   phrenic artery
2 Diaphragm
3 Inferior phrenic artery
4 Left suprarenal gland
5 Superior suprarenal arteries
6 Tip of nasogastric tube

(c) Left suprarenal venogram.

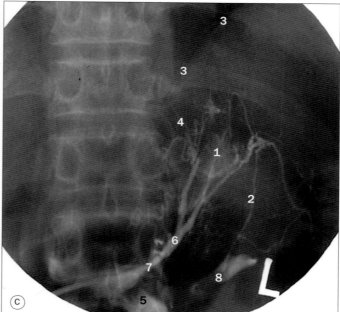

1 Adenoma in suprarenal
   gland
2 Capsular veins
3 Diaphragm
4 Inferior phrenic vein

5 Left renal vein
6 Left suprarenal vein
7 Tip of catheter in left
   suprarenal vein
8 Upper pole calyx

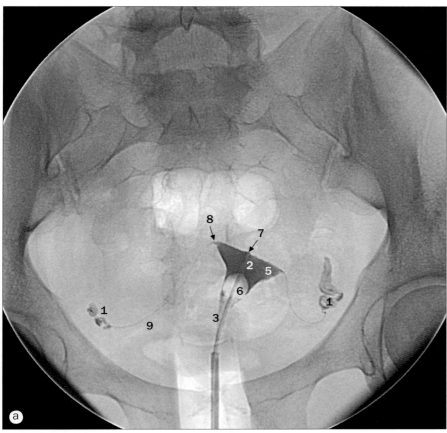

(a) Early phase of uterine filling.

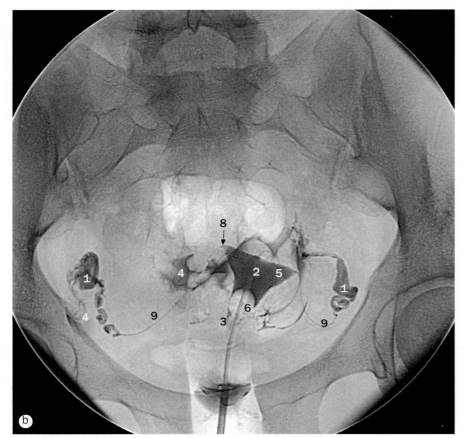

(b) Late phase with peritoneal spill.

1 Ampulla of uterine tube
2 Body of uterus
3 Cervix of uterus
4 Contrast spillage into peritoneal cavity
5 Cornu of uterus
6 Foley balloon catheter in uterus
7 Fundus of uterus
8 Isthmus of uterine tube
9 Uterine tube (fallopian tube)

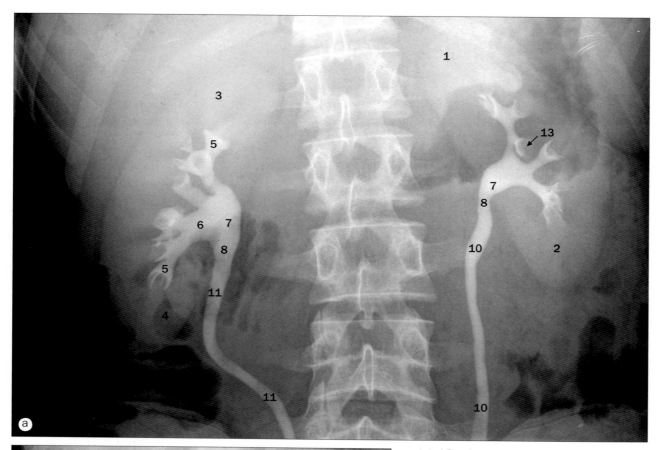

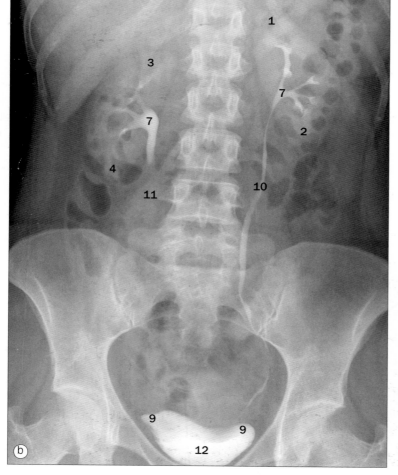

(a) 10 minutes IVU (intravenous urogram) with abdominal compression.

(b) Full length 15 minutes IVU after release of compression.

1 Upper pole of left kidney
2 Lower pole of left kidney
3 Upper pole of right kidney
4 Lower pole of right kidney
5 Minor calyx
6 Major calyx
7 Renal pelvis
8 Pelvi-ureteric junction
9 Vesico-ureteric junction
10 Left ureter
11 Right ureter
12 Urinary bladder
13 Renal papilla

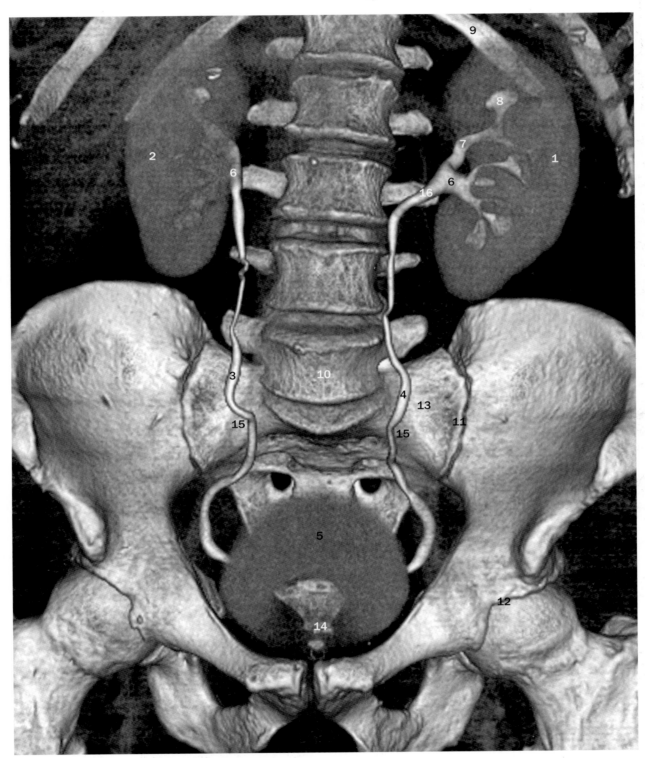

3D CT urogram at 10 minutes post intravenous injection.

1 Left kidney	**9** Twelfth rib
2 Right kidney	**10** Body of L5 vertebra
3 Right ureter	**11** Sacro-iliac joint
4 Left ureter	**12** Hip joint
5 Urinary bladder	**13** Sacral alum
6 Renal pelvis	**14** Coccyx
7 Major calyx	**15** Point of ureteric crossover of common iliac vessels
8 Minor calyx	**16** Pelvi-ureteric junction (PUJ)

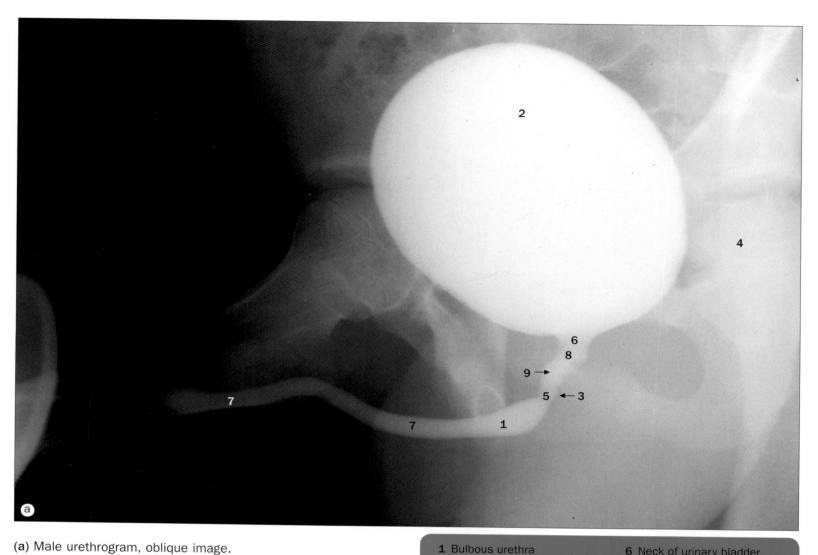

(a) Male urethrogram, oblique image.

(b) Penile arteriogram.

(c) Cavernosogram.

1 Bulbous urethra	6 Neck of urinary bladder
2 Contrast in urinary bladder	7 Penile urethra
3 External sphincter (sphincter urethrae)	8 Prostatic urethra
	9 Seminal colliculus (verumontanum)
4 Head of femur	
5 Membranous urethra	

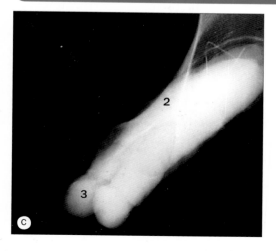

1 Artery of the penis	5 Dorsal artery of the penis
2 Corpus cavernosum	6 Internal pudendal artery
3 Crus of corpus cavernosum	7 Perineal artery
4 Deep artery of the penis	

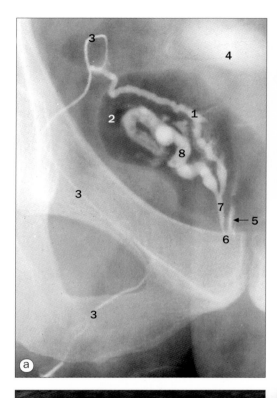

(a) Seminal vesiculogram.

1 Ampulla of ductus deferens
2 Colonic gas
3 Ductus deferens (vas deferens)
4 Full urinary bladder
5 Left ejaculatory duct
6 Position of seminal colliculus (verumontanum)
7 Right ejaculatory duct
8 Seminal vesicle

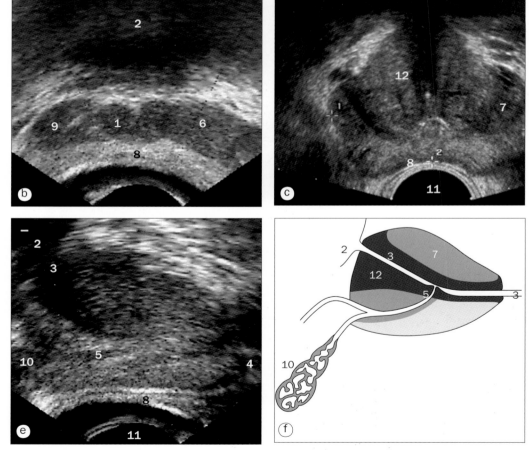

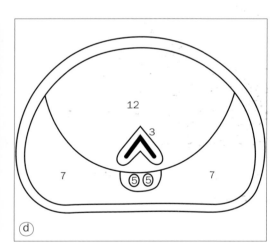

1 Ampulla of ductus deferens
2 Bladder
3 Course of urethra
4 Distal urethra
5 Ejaculatory duct
6 Left seminal vesicle
7 Peripheral zone of prostate
8 Rectal wall
9 Right seminal vesicle
10 Seminal vesicle
11 Transducer
12 Transitional zone of prostate

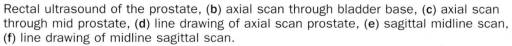

Rectal ultrasound of the prostate, (b) axial scan through bladder base, (c) axial scan through mid prostate, (d) line drawing of axial scan prostate, (e) sagittal midline scan, (f) line drawing of midline sagittal scan.

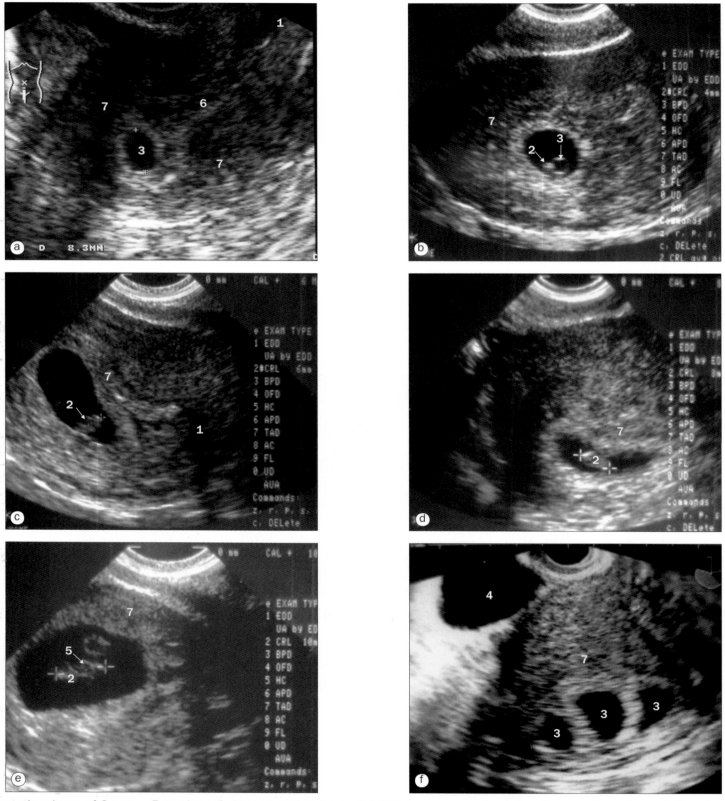

(a) Gestational sac of 8 mm = 5 weeks + 3 days gestational age, (b) CRL (crown rump length) = 4 mm = 6 weeks gestational age, (c) CRL = 6 mm = 6 weeks + 3 days gestational age, (d) CRL = 8 mm = 6 weeks + 5 days gestational age, (e) CRL = 10 mm = 7 weeks + 2 days gestational age, (f) triplets – three separate gestational sacs.

1 Cervix	3 Gestation sac	5 Position of fetal heart	7 Uterus
2 Fetus	4 Maternal bladder	6 Uterine cavity	

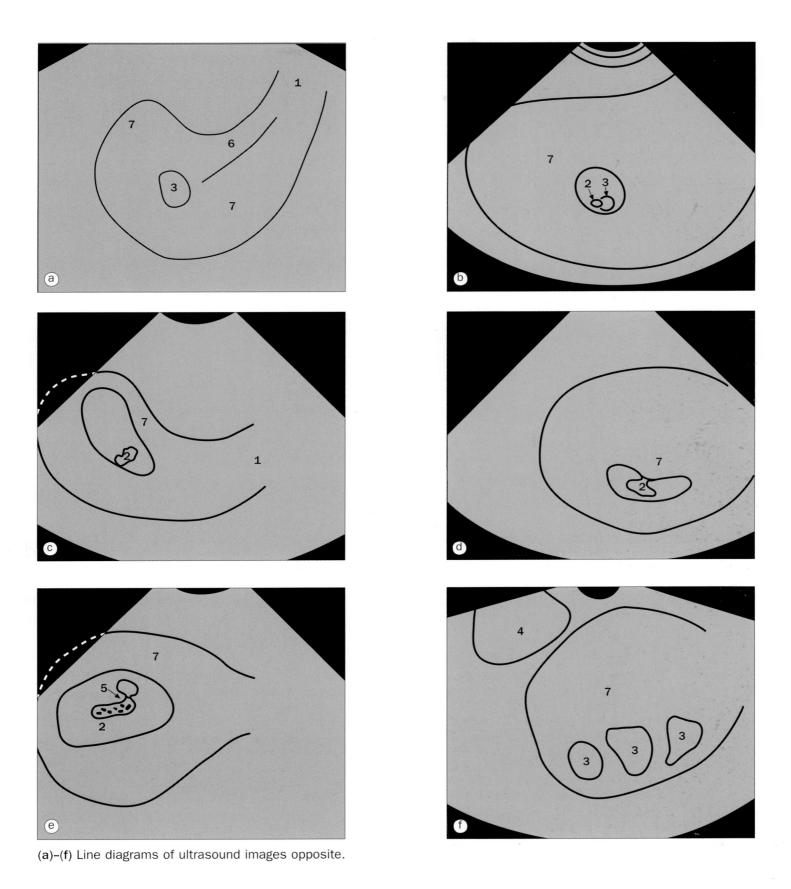

(a)–(f) Line diagrams of ultrasound images opposite.

1 Cervix
2 Fetus
3 Gestation sac
4 Maternal bladder
5 Position of fetal heart
6 Uterine cavity
7 Uterus

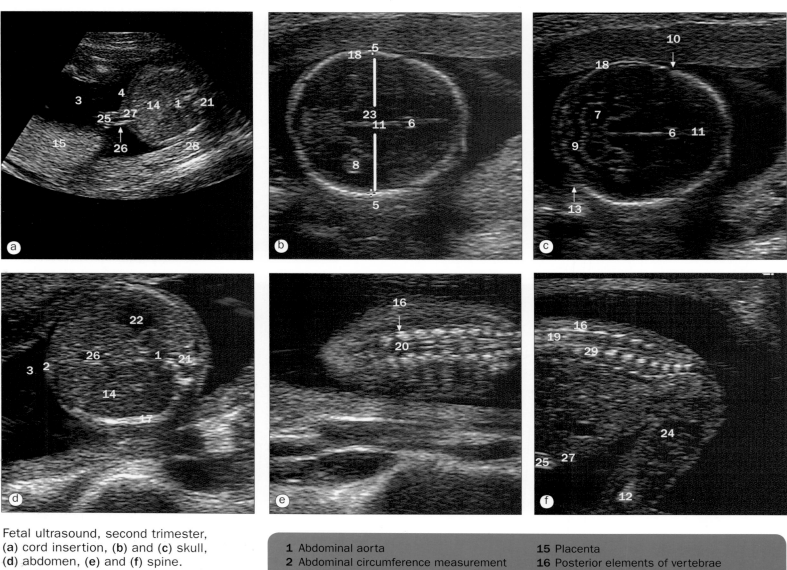

Fetal ultrasound, second trimester,
(a) cord insertion, (b) and (c) skull,
(d) abdomen, (e) and (f) spine.

1 Abdominal aorta	**15** Placenta
2 Abdominal circumference measurement	**16** Posterior elements of vertebrae
3 Amniotic fluid	**17** Ribs
4 Anterior abdominal wall	**18** Skull
5 Biparietal diameter measurement	**19** Spinal canal
6 Cavum septum pellucidum	**20** Spinal cord
7 Cerebellum	**21** Spine
8 Choroid plexus	**22** Stomach
9 Cisterna magna (cerebellomedullary cistern)	**23** Thalamus
	24 Thigh
10 Coronal suture	**25** Umbilical cord
11 Falx cerebri	**26** Umbilical vein
12 Femur	**27** Umbilicus
13 Lambdoid suture	**28** Uterine wall
14 Liver	**29** Vertebral body

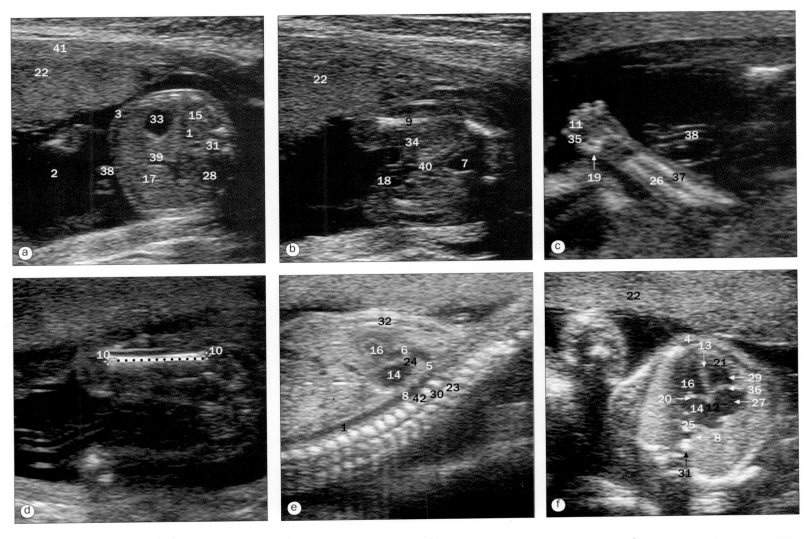

Fetal ultrasound, second trimester,
(a) abdomen, (b) pelvis, (c) forearm,
(d) femur, (e) heart and aorta,
(f) four chamber view of the heart.

1 Abdominal aorta	22 Placenta
2 Amniotic fluid	23 Posterior elements of vertebrae
3 Anterior abdominal wall	24 Pulmonary artery
4 Anterior chest wall	25 Pulmonary vein
5 Aortic arch	26 Radius
6 Ascending aorta	27 Right atrium
7 Bladder	28 Right kidney
8 Descending aorta	29 Right ventricle
9 Femur	30 Spinal canal
10 Femur for femoral length measurement	31 Spine
11 Finger	32 Sternum
12 Interatrial septum	33 Stomach
13 Interventricular septum	34 Thigh
14 Left atrium	35 Thumb
15 Left kidney	36 Tricuspid valve
16 Left ventricle	37 Ulna
17 Liver	38 Umbilical cord
18 Male external genitalia	39 Umbilical vein
19 Metacarpal shaft	40 Urethra
20 Mitral valve	41 Uterine wall
21 Moderator band	42 Vertebral body

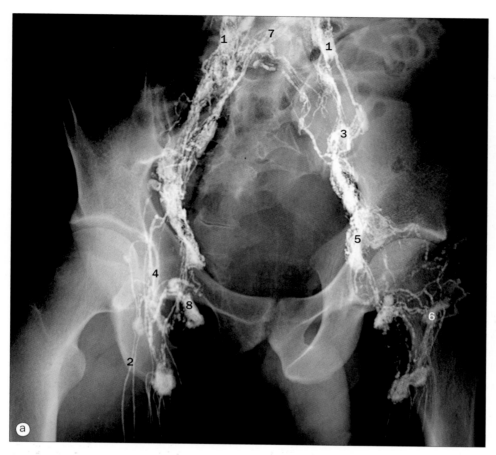

(a) Early filling phase, pelvis.

(b) Late filling phase, pelvis.

1 Ascending lumbar chains
2 Afferent inguinal lymphatics
3 Common iliac nodes
4 Efferent inguinal lymphatics
5 External iliac nodes
6 Superficial inguinal nodes
7 Lumbar crossover
8 Deep inguinal nodes

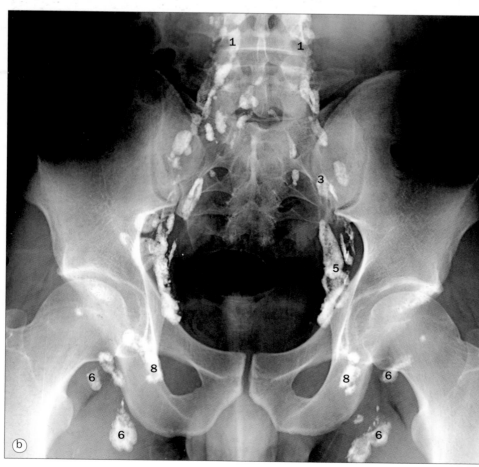

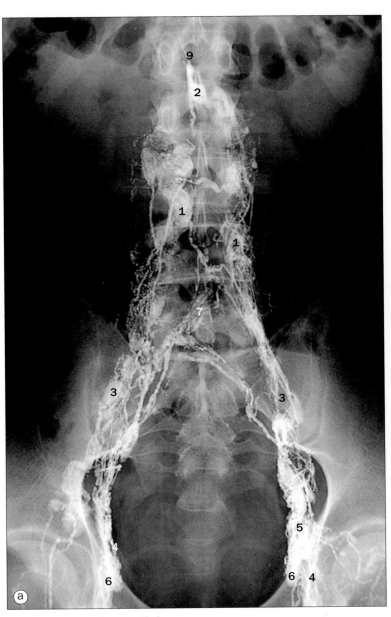

(a) Early filling phase, abdomen.

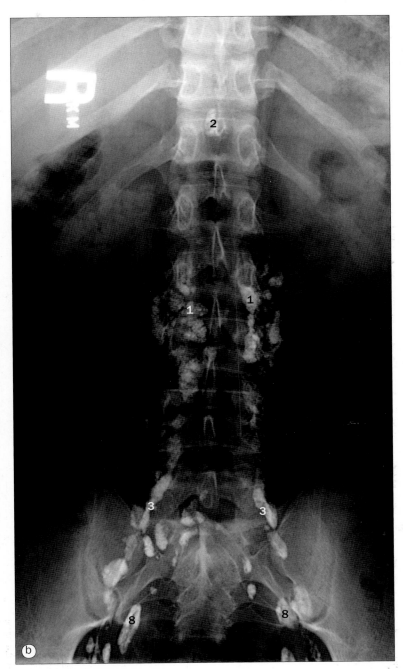

(b) Late filling phase, abdomen.

1 Ascending lumbar chains	6 Inguinal nodes (early filling)
2 Cisterna chyli	7 Lumbar crossover
3 Common iliac nodes	8 Deep inguinal nodes
4 Efferent inguinal lymphatics	9 Thoracic duct
5 External iliac nodes (early filling)	

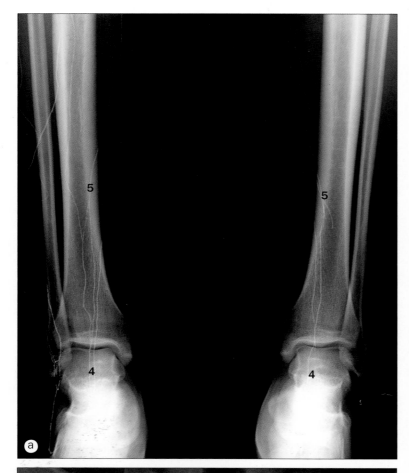

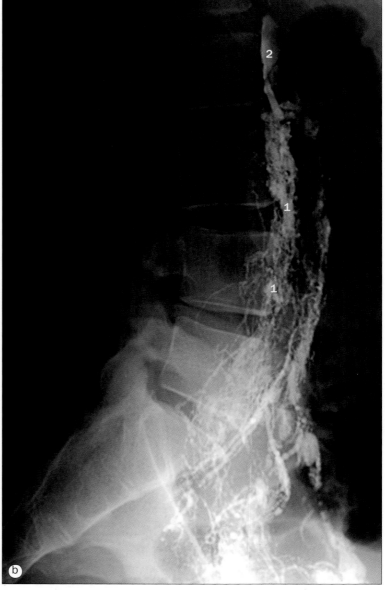

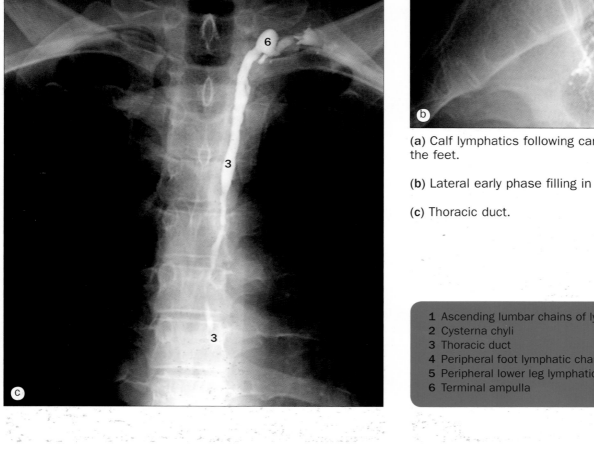

(a) Calf lymphatics following cannulation of lymphatic vessels in the feet.

(b) Lateral early phase filling in abdomen.

(c) Thoracic duct.

1 Ascending lumbar chains of lymph nodes
2 Cysterna chyli
3 Thoracic duct
4 Peripheral foot lymphatic channels
5 Peripheral lower leg lymphatic channels
6 Terminal ampulla

7   Lower limb

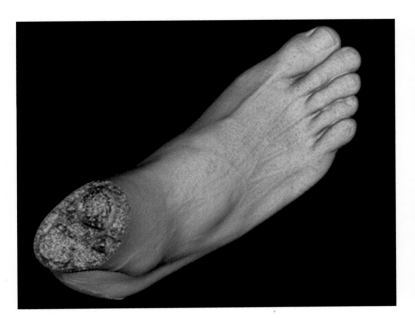

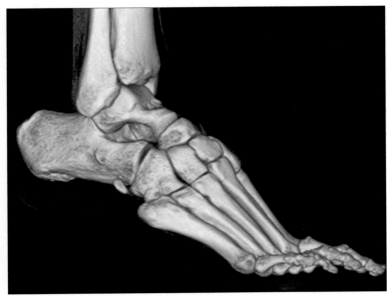

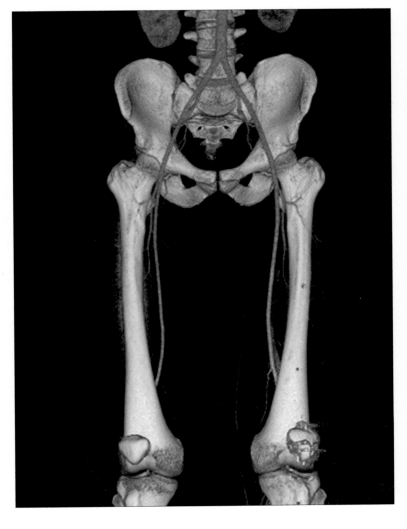

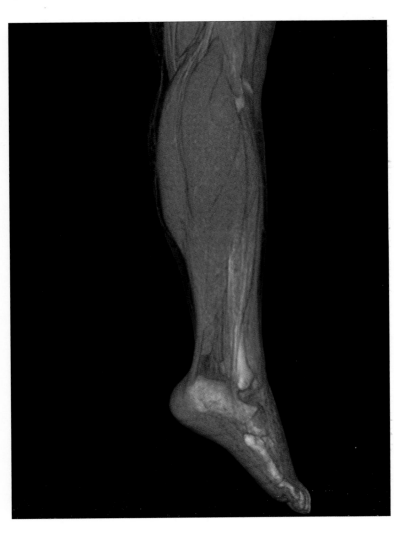

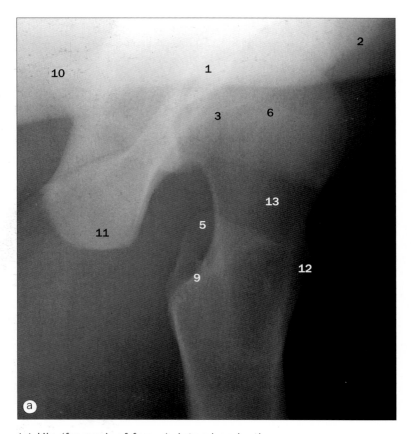

(a) Hip (for neck of femur), lateral projection.

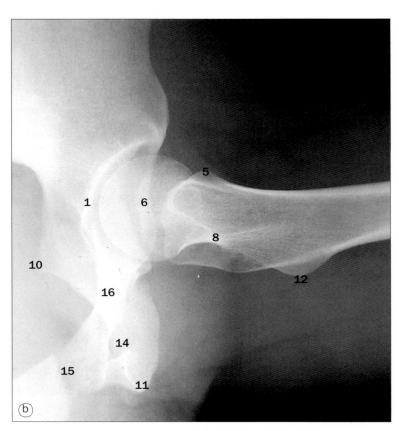

(b) Hip, lateral projection.

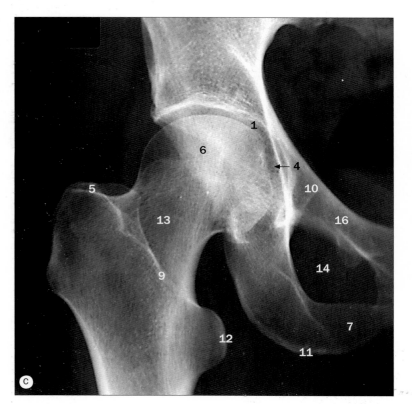

(c) Hip, anteroposterior projection.

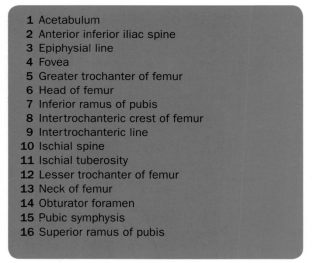

 1 Acetabulum
 2 Anterior inferior iliac spine
 3 Epiphysial line
 4 Fovea
 5 Greater trochanter of femur
 6 Head of femur
 7 Inferior ramus of pubis
 8 Intertrochanteric crest of femur
 9 Intertrochanteric line
10 Ischial spine
11 Ischial tuberosity
12 Lesser trochanter of femur
13 Neck of femur
14 Obturator foramen
15 Pubic symphysis
16 Superior ramus of pubis

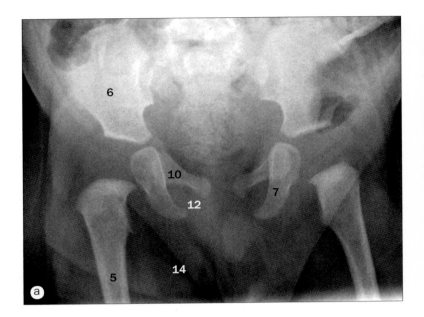

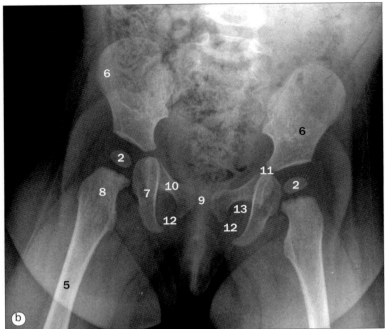

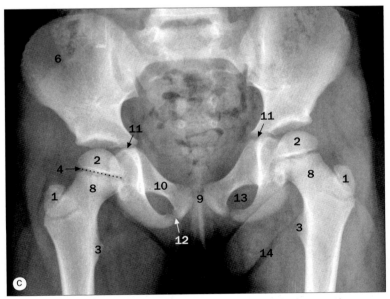

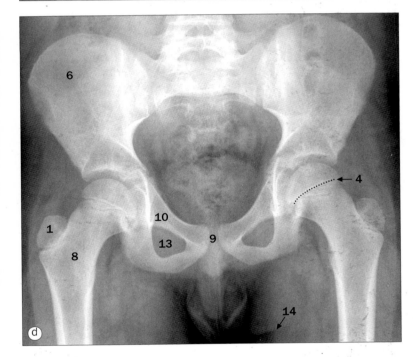

Pelvis, (a) of a 4-month-old girl, (b) of a 9-month-old girl, (c) of a 6-year-old girl, (d) of an 11-year-old girl.

1	Centre for greater trochanter	8	Neck of femur
2	Centre for head of femur (femoral capital epiphysis)	9	Pubic symphysis
3	Centre for lesser trochanter	10	Pubis
4	Epiphysial line	11	Triradiate cartilage
5	Femur	12	Unossified junction between ischium and pubis
6	Ilium	13	Obturator foramen
7	Ischium	14	Fat creases

INNOMINATE (HIP)	Appears	Fused
Ilium	2–3 miu	7–9 yrs
Ischium	4 miu	7–9 yrs
Pubis	4 miu	7–9 yrs
Acetabulum	11–14 yrs	15–25 yrs
Ant. sup. iliac spine	Puberty	15–25 yrs
Iliac crest/sup. spines	Puberty	15–25 yrs
Ischial tuberosity	Puberty +	15–25 yrs

FEMUR (c)		
Shaft	7 wiu	
Head	4–6 mths	14–18 yrs
Greater trochanter	2–4 yrs	14–18 yrs
Lesser trochanter	10–12 yrs	14–18 yrs
Distal end	9 miu	17–19 yrs

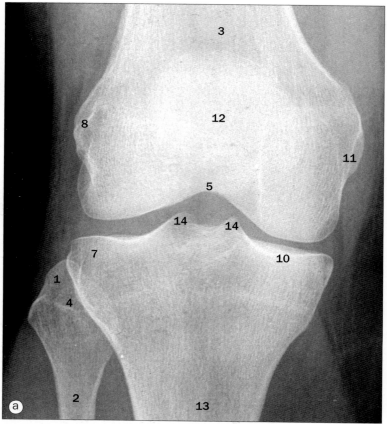

(a) Anteroposterior projection.

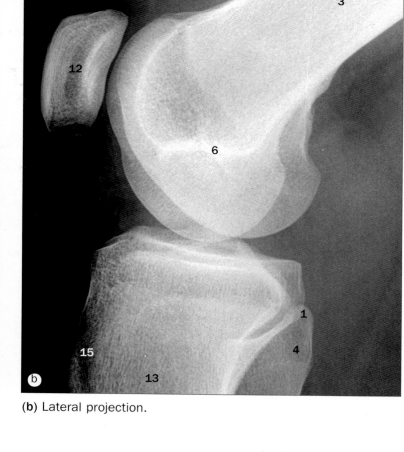

(b) Lateral projection.

1 Apex (styloid process) of fibula
2 Fibula neck
3 Femur
4 Head of fibula
5 Intercondylar fossa
6 Lateral condyle of femur
7 Lateral condyle of tibia
8 Lateral epicondyle of femur
9 Medial condyle of femur
10 Medial condyle of tibia
11 Medial epicondyle of femur
12 Patella
13 Tibia
14 Tubercles of intercondylar eminence
15 Tuberosity of tibia

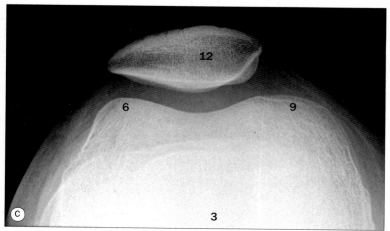

(c) Inferosuperior (skyline) projection.

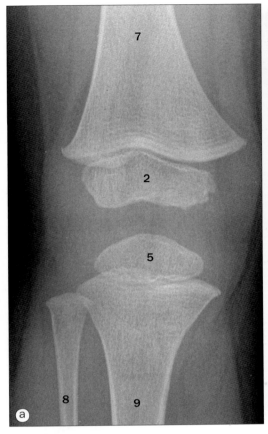

(a) 2-year-old girl.

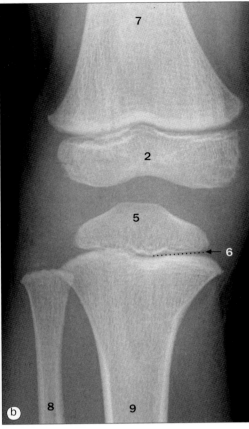

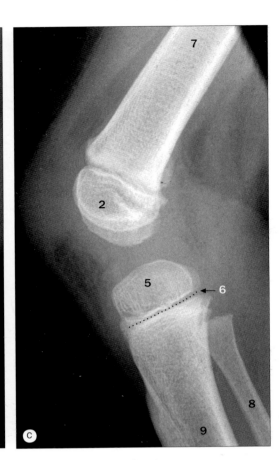

(b) and (c) 5-year-old girl.

1 Antero-inferior extension of proximal
   tibial centre for tuberosity of tibia
2 Centre for distal femur
3 Centre for head of fibula
4 Patella
5 Centre for proximal tibia
6 Epiphysial line
7 Femur
8 Fibula
9 Tibia

PATELLA (c)	Appears	Fused
1–3 centres	3–5 yrs	Puberty
TIBIA (c)		
Shaft	7 wiu	
Proximal/plateau	9 miu	16–18 yrs
Tuberosity	10–12 yrs	12–14 yrs
Distal end	4 mths–1 yr	15–17 yrs
FIBULA (c)		
Shaft	8 wiu	
Proximal end/head	2–4 yrs	17–19 yrs
Distal end	6 mths–1 yr	15–17 yrs

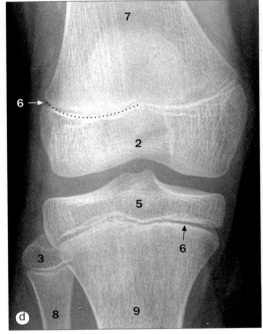

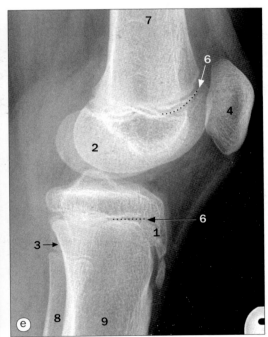

(d) and (e) 12-year-old girl.

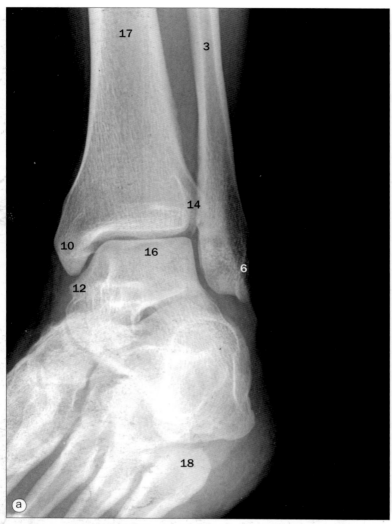

(a) Ankle joint, anteroposterior projection.

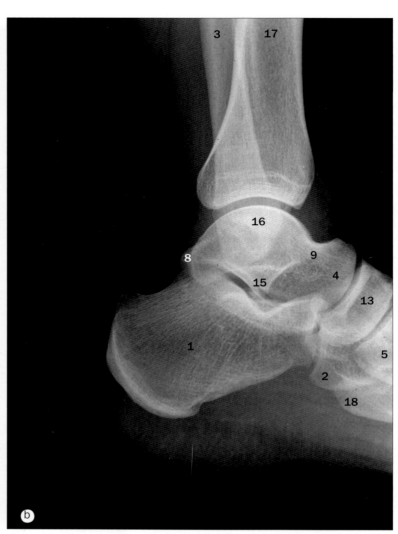

(b) Ankle joint, lateral projection.

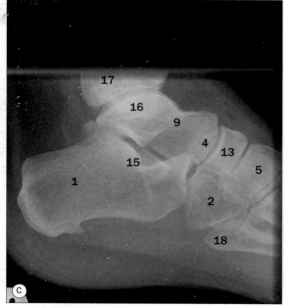

(c) Calcaneus, lateral projection.

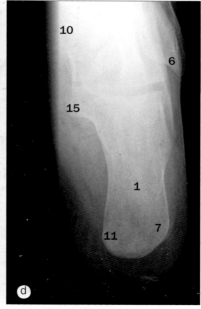

(d) Calcaneus, axial (caudo cranial) projection.

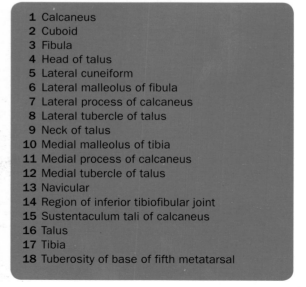

1 Calcaneus
2 Cuboid
3 Fibula
4 Head of talus
5 Lateral cuneiform
6 Lateral malleolus of fibula
7 Lateral process of calcaneus
8 Lateral tubercle of talus
9 Neck of talus
10 Medial malleolus of tibia
11 Medial process of calcaneus
12 Medial tubercle of talus
13 Navicular
14 Region of inferior tibiofibular joint
15 Sustentaculum tali of calcaneus
16 Talus
17 Tibia
18 Tuberosity of base of fifth metatarsal

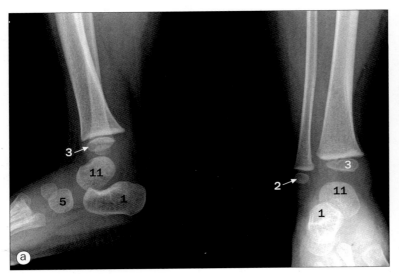

(a) Ankle of a 3-year-old girl.

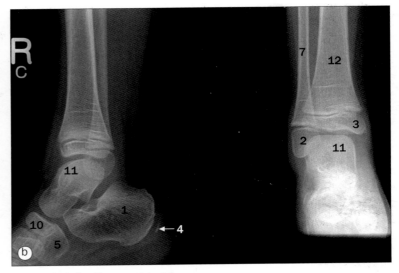

(b) Ankle of a 5-year-old girl.

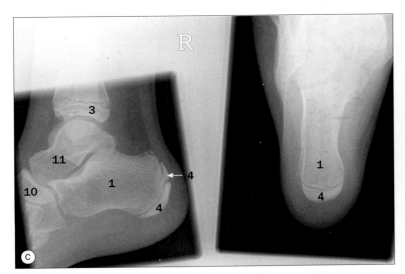

(c) Ankle of a 13-year-old girl.

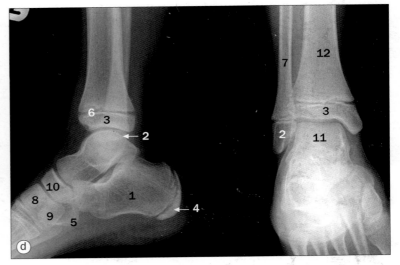

(d) Calcaneus of a 10-year-old girl.

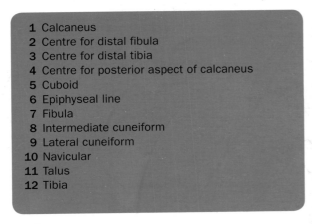

 1 Calcaneus
 2 Centre for distal fibula
 3 Centre for distal tibia
 4 Centre for posterior aspect of calcaneus
 5 Cuboid
 6 Epiphyseal line
 7 Fibula
 8 Intermediate cuneiform
 9 Lateral cuneiform
10 Navicular
11 Talus
12 Tibia

TARSAL BONES (c)	Appears	Fused
Calcaneus	3 miu	14–16 yrs
Talus	6 miu	
Navicular	3 yrs	
Cuneiform lateral	6 mths–1 yr	
Cuneiform intermediate	2–3 yrs	
Cuneiform medial	1–2 yrs	
Cuboid	9 miu	

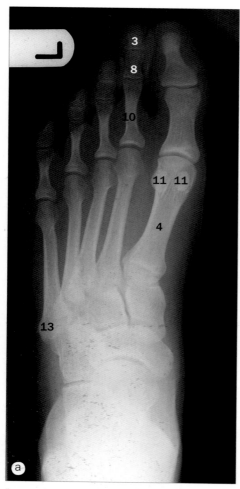

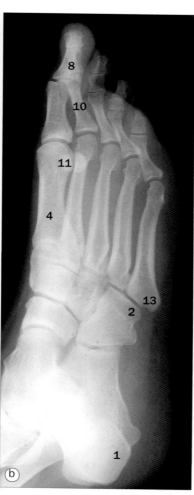

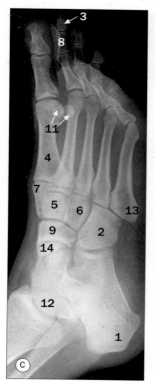

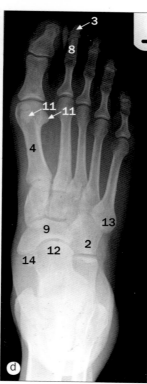

Foot, (a) dorsoplantar projection, (b) dorsoplantar oblique projection, (c) and (d) os naviculare.

1 Calcaneus
2 Cuboid
3 Distal phalanx of second toe
4 First metatarsal
5 Intermediate cuneiform
6 Lateral cuneiform
7 Medial cuneiform
8 Middle phalanx of second toe
9 Navicular
10 Proximal phalanx of second toe
11 Sesamoid bones in flexor hallucis brevis muscle
12 Talus
13 Tuberosity of base of fifth metatarsal
14 Os naviculare

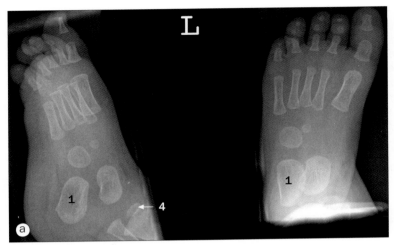

(a) Foot of an 11-month-old girl.

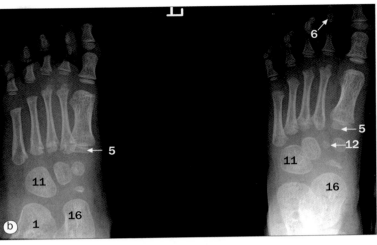

(b) Foot of a 3-year-old girl.

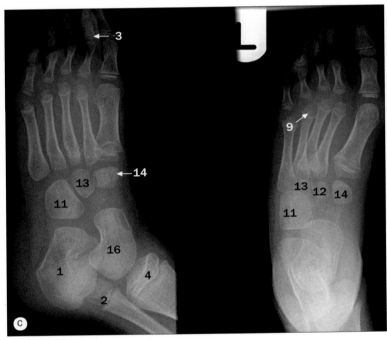

(c) Foot of a 6-year-old girl.

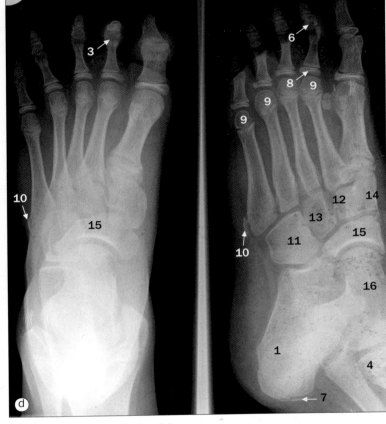

(d) Foot of a 12-year-old girl.

1 Calcaneus
2 Centre for distal fibula
3 Centre for distal phalanx of second toe
4 Centre for distal tibia
5 Centre for first metatarsal
6 Centre for middle phalanx of second toe
7 Centre for posterior aspect of calcaneus
8 Centre for proximal phalanx of second toe
9 Centre for second metatarsal (applies to second to fifth metatarsal)
10 Centre for tuberosity of base of fifth metatarsal
11 Cuboid
12 Intermediate cuneiform
13 Lateral cuneiform
14 Medial cuneiform
15 Navicular
16 Talus

METATARSALS (c)	Appears	Fused
Shafts	9 wiu	
Heads (2–5) or base (1)	3–4 yrs	17–20 yrs
Tuberosity of 5	10–12 yrs	13–15 yrs
PHALANGES (c)		
Shaft	9–12 wiu	
Bases (variable)	1–6 yrs	14–18 yrs

TARSAL BONES (c)	Appears	Fused
Calcaneus	3 miu	14–16 yrs
Talus	6 miu	
Navicular	3 yrs	
Cuneiform lateral	6 mths–1 yr	
Cuneiform intermediate	2–3 yrs	
Cuneiform medial	1–2 yrs	
Cuboid	9 miu	

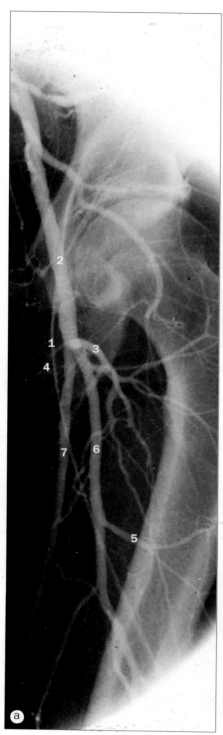

(a) Femoral arteriogram.
The femoropopliteal and tibial arteries are imaged by catheterising the distal abdominal aorta and injecting contrast medium. The column of contrast is then followed as it passes down the legs. If only one leg is to be imaged, an injection into the ipsilateral femoral artery suffices. The external iliac artery continues as the common femoral artery, which originates deep to the inguinal ligament, dividing into the superficial and deep (profunda) femoral arteries. An oblique view is often useful to image the femoral bifurcation and to identify atheroma at the origins of these vessels.

1 Catheter introduced into distal abdominal aorta via left femoral artery
2 Common femoral artery
3 Lateral circumflex femoral artery
4 Medial circumflex femoral artery
5 Perforating artery
6 Profunda femoris artery
7 Superficial femoral artery

(b) Popliteal arteriogram.
The superficial femoral artery becomes the popliteal artery as it passes through the hiatus in the adductor magnus muscle. The popliteal artery terminates at the lower border of the popliteus muscle, dividing into the anterior and posterior tibial arteries.

1 Anterior tibial artery
2 Inferior lateral genicular artery
3 Inferior medial genicular artery
4 Muscular branches of anterior tibial artery
5 Muscular branches of posterior tibial artery
6 Peroneal artery
7 Popliteal artery
8 Posterior tibial artery
9 Superior lateral genicular artery
10 Superior medial genicular artery

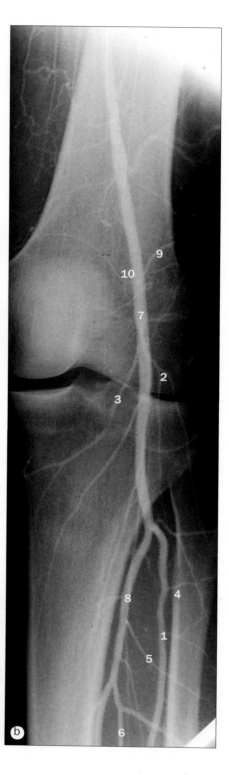

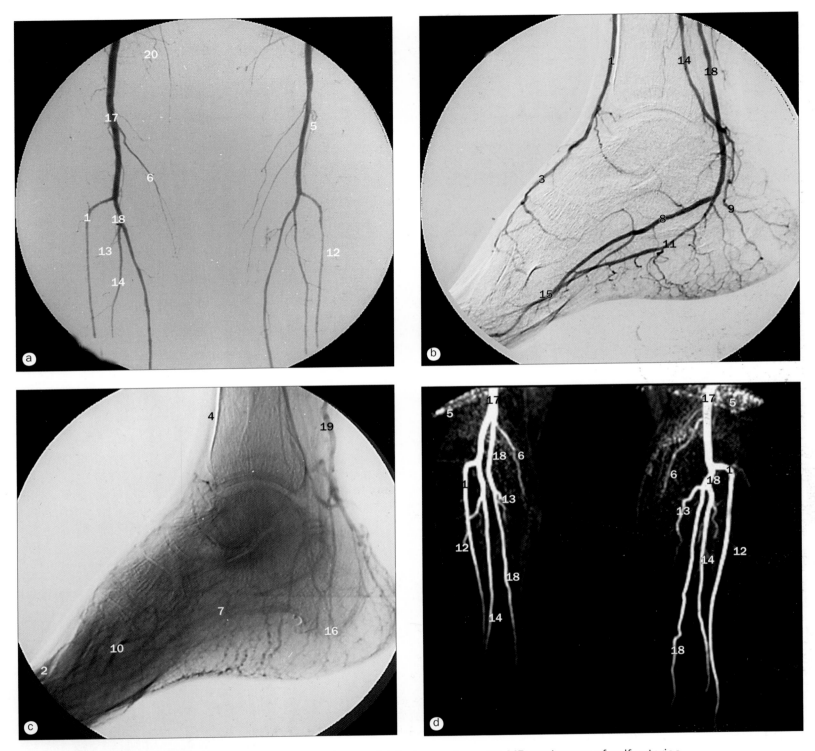

(a) Popliteal arteriogram, (b) foot arteriogram, lateral image, (c) foot venogram, (d) MR angiogram of calf arteries.

1 Anterior tibial artery
2 Dorsal venous arch
3 Dorsalis pedis artery
4 Great saphenous vein
5 Inferior lateral genicular artery
6 Inferior medial genicular artery
7 Lateral marginal vein

8 Lateral plantar artery
9 Medial calcaneal artery
10 Medial marginal vein
11 Medial plantar artery
12 Muscular branches of anterior tibial artery
13 Muscular branches of posterior tibia!
   artery

14 Peroneal artery
15 Plantar arch
16 Plantar cutaneous venous plexus
17 Popliteal artery
18 Posterior tibial artery
19 Small saphenous vein
20 Superior medial genicular artery

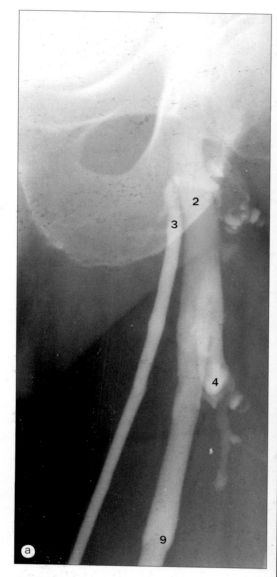

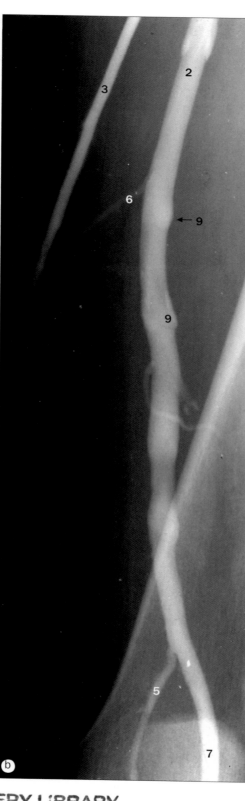

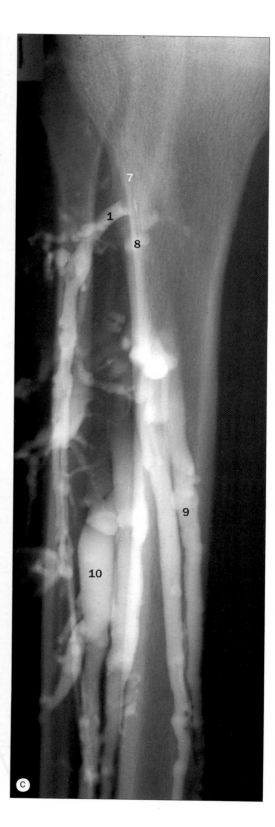

(a)–(c) Lower limb venograms.

1 Anterior tibial vein
2 Femoral vein
3 Great (long) saphenous vein
4 Lateral circumflex vein
5 Muscular tributary of femoral vein
6 Perforating vein
7 Popliteal vein
8 Posterior tibial veins
9 Venous valves
10 Venous calf plexus

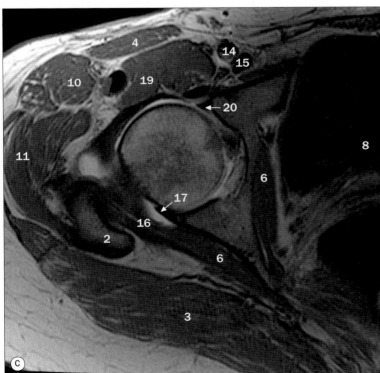

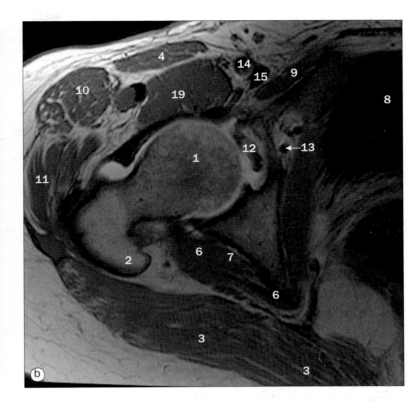

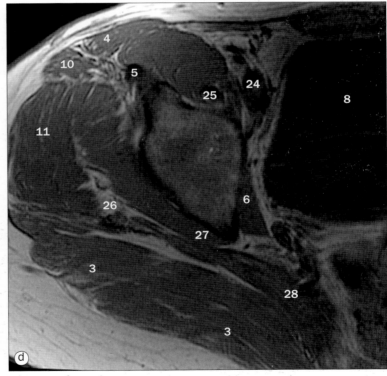

(a)–(d) Hip, axial MR images, from superior to inferior.

1 Femoral head	**8** Bladder	**16** Tendon of obturator internus muscle
2 Greater trochanter	**9** Pectineus muscle	**17** Posterior acetabular labrum
3 Gluteus maximus muscle	**10** Tensor fascia lata muscle	**18** Vastus intermedius muscle
4 Sartorius muscle	**11** Vastus lateralis muscle	**19** Iliopsoas muscle
5 Tendon of rectus femoris muscle	**12** Ligamentum teres	**20** Anterior acetabular labrum
6 Obturator internus muscle	**13** Obturator nerve	**21** Adductor longus muscle
7 Superior gemellus muscle	**14** Femoral artery	
	15 Femoral vein	

22 Adductor brevis muscle	
23 Adductor magnus muscle	
24 Semitendinosus muscle	
25 Profunda femoris artery	
26 External iliac artery	
27 Gluteus minimus muscle	
28 Gluteus medius muscle	

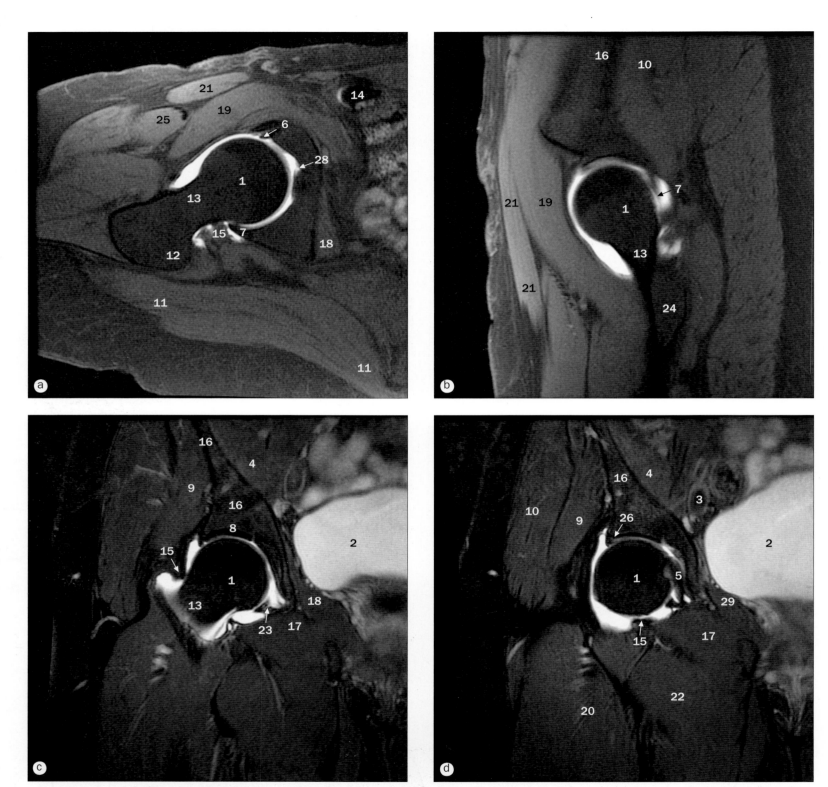

Hip, MR arthrogram images, (a) axial, (b) sagittal, (c) and (d) coronal.

1 Femoral head	11 Gluteus maximus muscle	21 Sartorius muscle
2 Bladder	12 Greater trochanter	22 Adductor longus muscle
3 External iliac artery	13 Femoral neck	23 Transverse acetabular ligament
4 Iliacus muscle	14 Femoral artery	24 Quadratus femoris muscle
5 Ligamentum teres	15 Zona orbicularis (circular fibrous capsule)	25 Rectus femoris muscle
6 Anterior acetabular labrum	16 Iliac bone	26 Superior acetabular labrum
7 Posterior acetabular labrum	17 Obturator externus muscle	27 Gemellus muscle
8 Acetabular roof	18 Obturator internus muscle	28 Acetabular notch (pulvinar)
9 Gluteus minimus muscle	19 Iliopsoas muscle	29 Pectineus muscle
10 Gluteus medius muscle	20 Vastus intermedius	

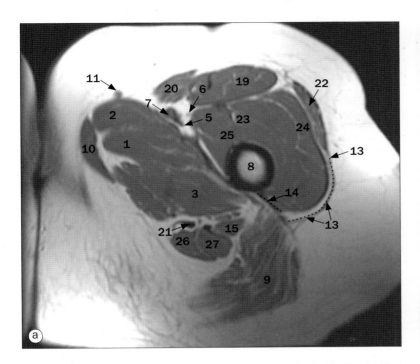

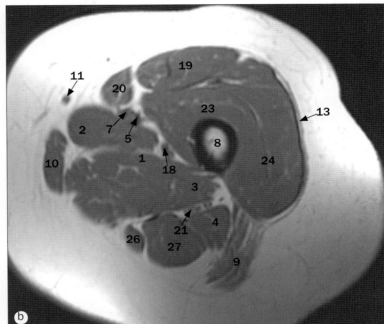

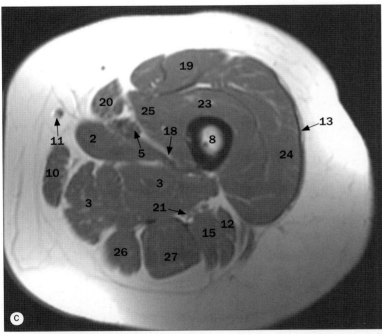

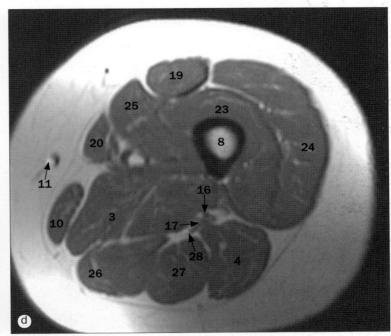

(a)–(d) Axial MR images of the thigh.

1 Adductor brevis muscle	**11** Great (long) saphenous vein	**21** Sciatic nerve
2 Adductor longus muscle	**12** Short head of biceps femoris muscle	**22** Tensor fasciae latae muscle
3 Adductor magnus muscle	**13** Iliotibial tract	**23** Vastus intermedius muscle
4 Biceps femoris muscle	**14** Lateral intermuscular septum	**24** Vastus lateralis muscle
5 Femoral artery	**15** Long head of biceps femoris muscle	**25** Vastus medialis muscle
6 Femoral nerve	**16** Popliteal artery	**26** Semimembranosus muscle
7 Femoral vein	**17** Popliteal vein	**27** Semitendinosus muscle
8 Femur	**18** Profunda femoris artery	**28** Tibial nerve
9 Gluteus maximus muscle	**19** Rectus femoris muscle	
10 Gracilis muscle	**20** Sartorius muscle	

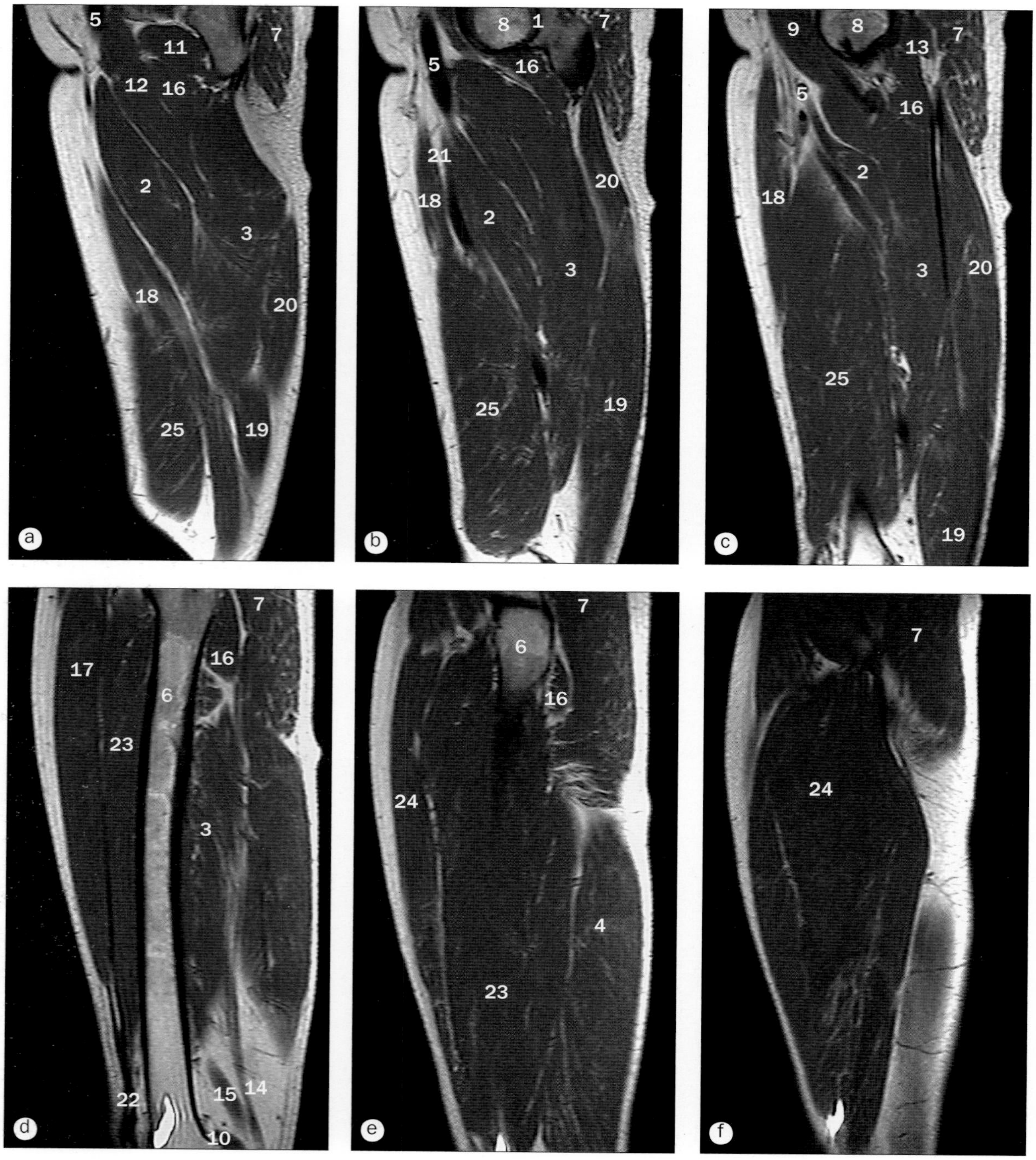

(a)–(f) Thigh, sagittal MR images.

1 Acetabulum
2 Adductor longus muscle
3 Adductor magnus muscle
4 Biceps femoris muscle
5 Femoral artery
6 Femur
7 Gluteus maximus muscle
8 Head of femur
9 Iliopsoas muscle
10 Lateral head of gastrocnemius muscle
11 Obturator externus muscle
12 Pectineus muscle
13 Piriformis muscle
14 Popliteal artery
15 Popliteal vein
16 Quadratus femoris muscle
17 Rectus femoris muscle
18 Sartorius muscle
19 Semimembranosus muscle
20 Semitendinosus muscle
21 Subsartorial canal (Hunter's canal)
22 Tendon of quadriceps muscle
23 Vastus intermedius muscle
24 Vastus lateralis muscle
25 Vastus medialis muscle

(a)–(f) Thigh, coronal MR images.

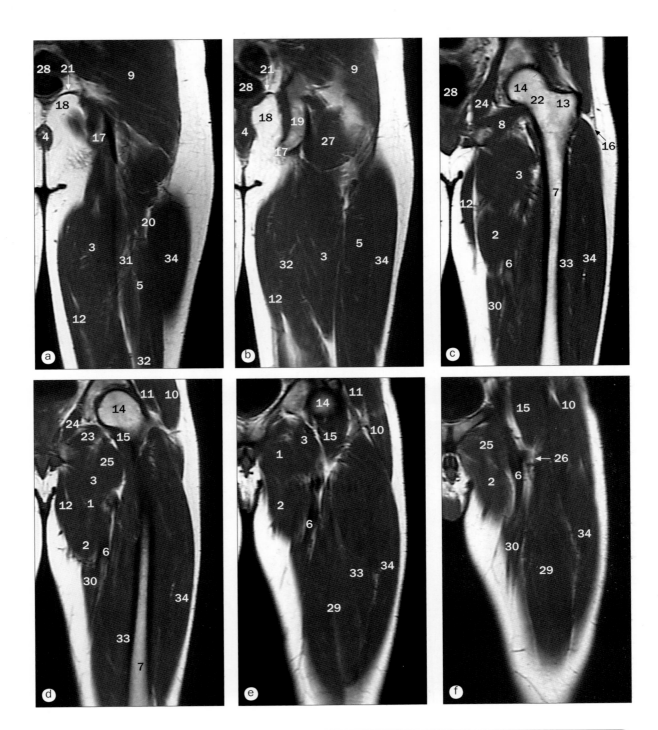

1 Adductor brevis muscle	**13** Greater trochanter of femur	**25** Pectineus muscle
2 Adductor longus muscle	**14** Head of femur	**26** Profunda femoris artery
3 Adductor magnus muscle	**15** Iliopsoas muscle	**27** Quadratus femoris muscle
4 Anal canal	**16** Iliotibial tract	**28** Rectum
5 Biceps femoris muscle	**17** Ischial tuberosity	**29** Rectus femoris muscle
6 Femoral artery	**18** Ischio-anal fossa	**30** Sartorius muscle
7 Femur	**19** Ischium	**31** Semimembranosus muscle
8 Gemellus muscle	**20** Lateral intermuscular septum	**32** Semitendinosus muscle
9 Gluteus maximus muscle	**21** Levator ani muscle	**33** Vastus intermedius muscle
10 Gluteus medius muscle	**22** Neck of femur	**34** Vastus lateralis muscle
11 Gluteus minimus muscle	**23** Obturator externus muscle	
12 Gracilis muscle	**24** Obturator internus muscle	

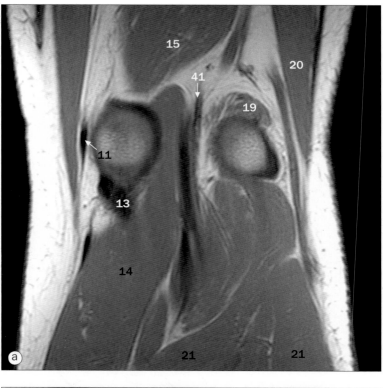

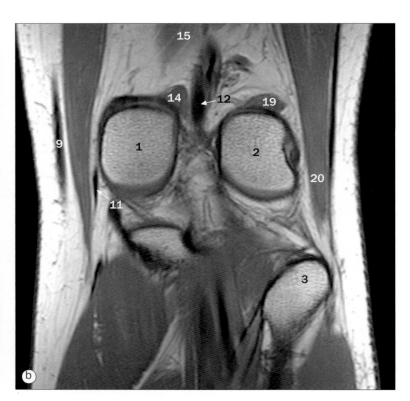

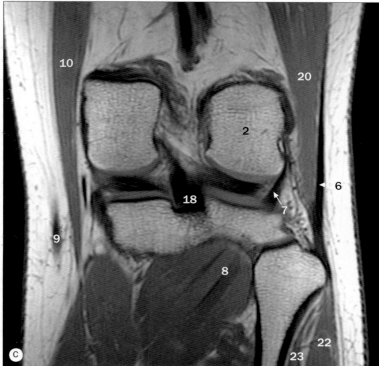

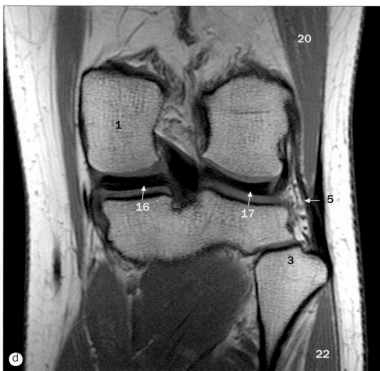

(a)–(h) Knee, coronal MR images, from posterior to anterior.

1 Medial femoral condyle	**9** Great (long) saphenous vein	**17** Posterior horn lateral meniscus
2 Lateral femoral condyle	**10** Sartorius muscle	**18** Posterior cruciate ligament
3 Head of fibula	**11** Tendon of gracilis muscle	**19** Lateral head of gastrocnemius
4 Proximal tibiofibular joint	**12** Popliteal artery	**20** Biceps femoris muscle
5 Lateral collateral ligament	**13** Common peroneal (fibular) nerve	**21** Soleus muscle
6 Iliotibial tract	**14** Medial head of gastrocnemius muscle	**22** Peroneus (fibularis) longus muscle
7 Tendon of popliteus muscle	**15** Semimembranosus muscle	**23** Extensor digitorum longus muscle
8 Popliteus muscle	**16** Posterior horn medial meniscus	**24** Anterior cruciate ligament

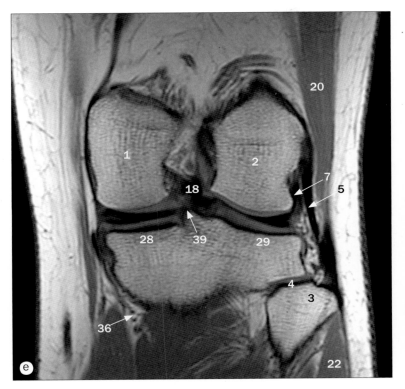

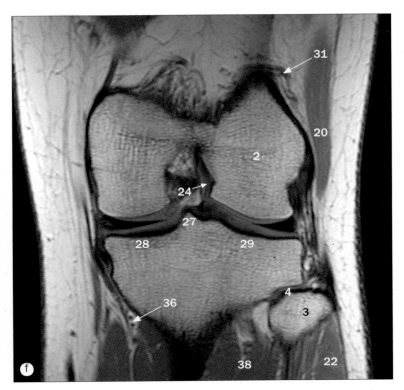

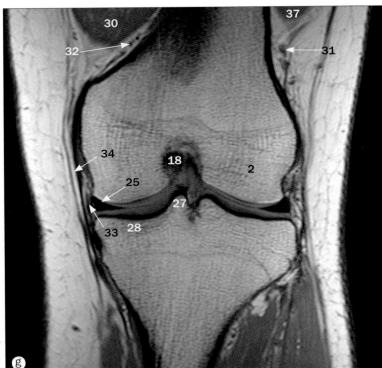

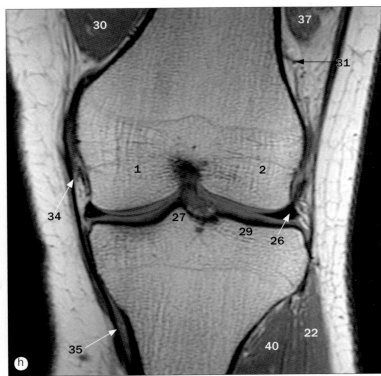

(a)–(h) Knee, coronal MR images, from posterior to anterior.

25 Body of medial meniscus
26 Body of lateral meniscus
27 Tibial spine
28 Medial tibial condyle
29 Lateral tibial condyle
30 Vastus medialis muscle

31 Lateral superior genicular artery
32 Medial superior genicular artery
33 Medial collateral ligament deep portion
34 Medial collateral ligament superficial portion
35 Pes anserinus (muscle attachments)

36 Medial inferior genicular artery
37 Vastus lateralis muscle
38 Tibialis posterior muscle
39 Root of posterior horn, medial meniscus
40 Tibialis anterior muscle
41 Tibial nerve

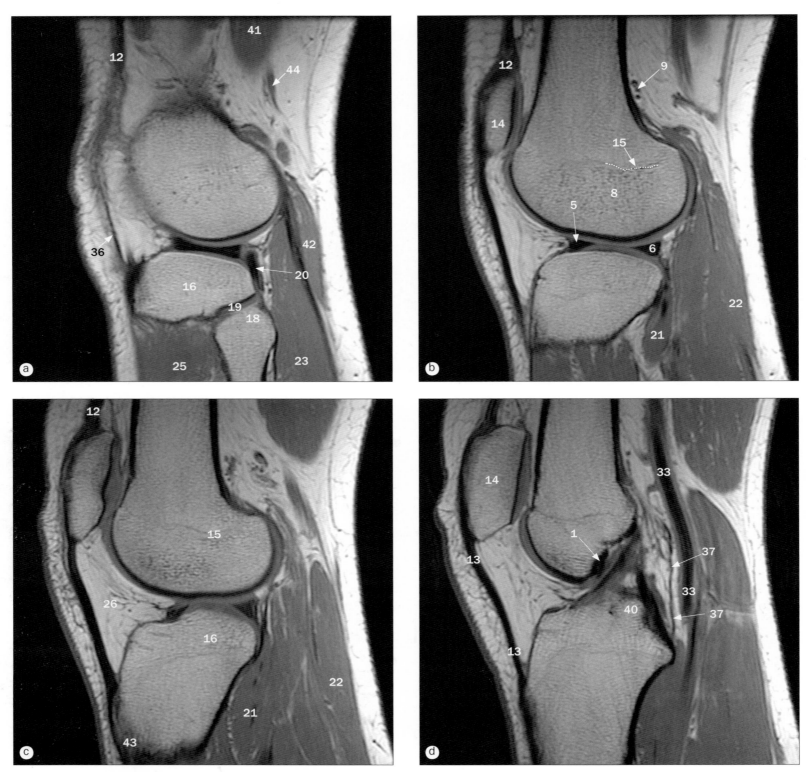

(a)–(h) Knee, sagittal MR images, from lateral to medial.

1 Anterior cruciate ligament	**9** Lateral superior genicular artery and veins	**17** Medial tibial plateau
2 Posterior cruciate ligament	**10** Median intermuscular septum	**18** Fibular head
3 Anterior horn medial meniscus	**11** Medial superior genicular artery	**19** Proximal tibiofibular joint
4 Posterior horn medial meniscus	**12** Quadriceps tendon	**20** Popliteus tendon
5 Anterior horn lateral meniscus	**13** Patellar tendon	**21** Popliteus muscle belly
6 Posterior horn lateral meniscus	**14** Patella	**22** Lateral head of gastrocnemius muscle
7 Medial condyle of femur	**15** Epiphyseal line/scar	**23** Soleus muscle
8 Lateral condyle of femur	**16** Lateral tibial plateau	**24** Vastus medialis muscle

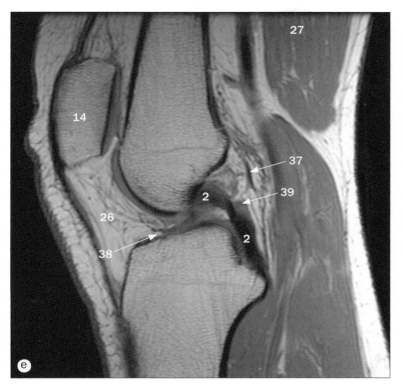

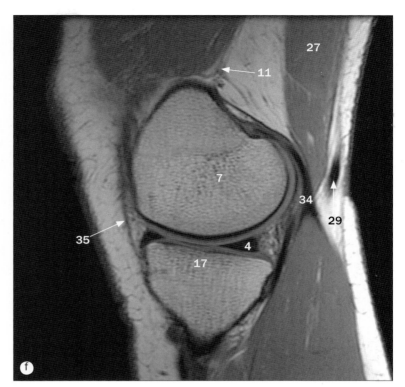

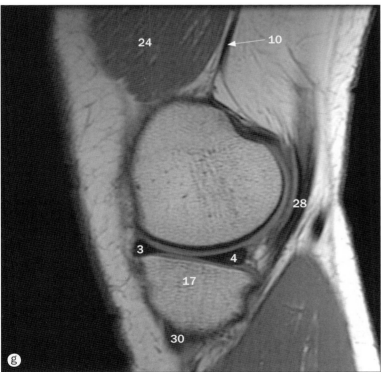

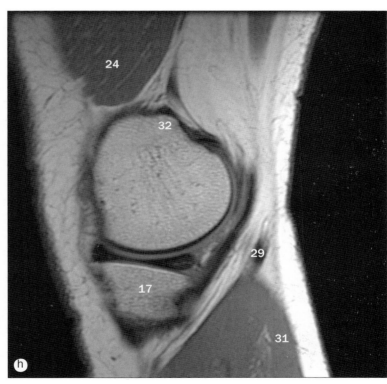

(a)–(h) Knee, sagittal MR images, from lateral to medial.

25 Tibialis anterior muscle	**32** Adductor tubercle	**39** Meniscofemoral ligament (Wrisberg)
26 Infrapatellar fat pad	**33** Popliteal artery	**40** Tibial spine
27 Semimembranosus muscle	**34** Medial head of gastrocnemius tendon	**41** Biceps femoris muscle
28 Semimembranosus tendon	**35** Medial patellar retinaculum	**42** Plantaris muscle
29 Semitendinosus tendon	**36** Lateral patellar retinaculum	**43** Tibial tuberosity
30 Sartorius tendon	**37** Posterior joint capsule	**44** Common peroneal (fibular) nerve
31 Medial head of gastrocnemius muscle	**38** Transverse ligament	

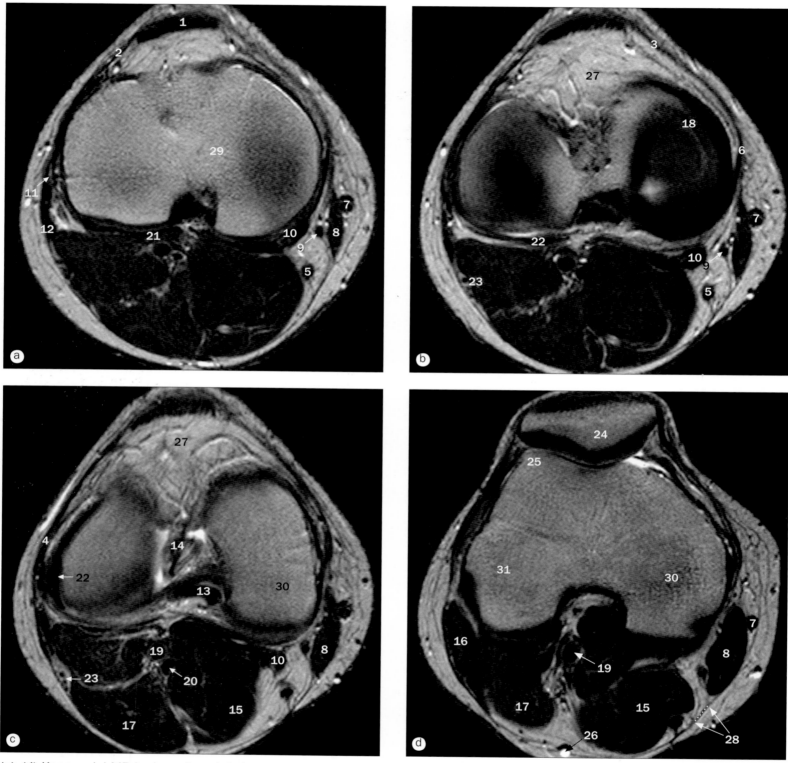

(a)–(d) Knee, axial MR images, from inferior to superior.

1 Patellar tendon
2 Lateral patellar retinaculum
3 Medial patellar retinaculum
4 Iliotibial tract
5 Semitendinosus tendon
6 Medial collateral ligament
7 Long (great) saphenous vein
8 Sartorius muscle
9 Gracilis tendon
10 Semimembranosus tendon
11 Lateral collateral ligament

12 Biceps femoris tendon
13 Posterior cruciate ligament
14 Anterior cruciate ligament
15 Medial head gastrocnemius
   muscle
16 Biceps femoris muscle
17 Lateral head gastrocnemius
   muscle
18 Medial meniscus
19 Popliteal artery
20 Popliteal vein

21 Popliteus muscle
22 Popliteus tendon
23 Common peroneal (fibular) nerve
24 Patella
25 Lateral condylar eminence
26 Short (lesser) saphenous vein
27 Infrapatellar fat pad
28 Deep fascia (fascia lata)
29 Tibial plateau
30 Medial condyle of femur
31 Lateral condyle of femur

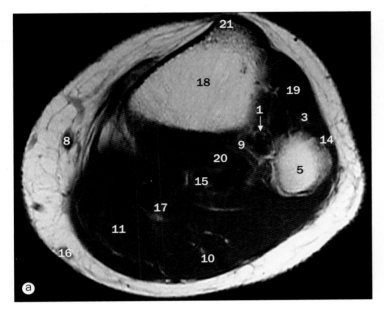

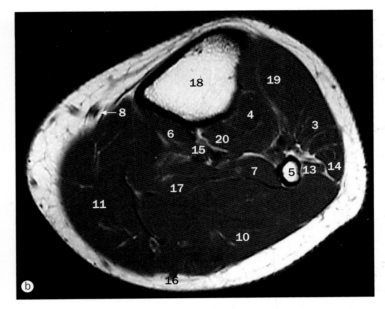

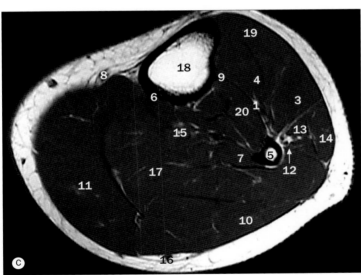

(a)–(e) Calf, axial MR images.

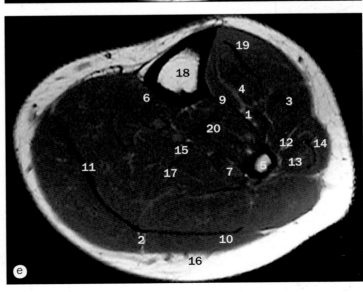

1 Anterior tibial artery
2 Aponeurosis of gastrocnemius muscle
3 Extensor digitorum longus muscle
4 Extensor hallucis longus muscle
5 Fibula
6 Flexor digitorum longus muscle
7 Flexor hallucis longus muscle
8 Great (long) saphenous vein
9 Interosseous membrane
10 Lateral head of gastrocnemius muscle
11 Medial head of gastrocnemius muscle
12 Peroneal artery
13 Peroneus brevis muscle
14 Peroneus longus muscle
15 Posterior tibial artery
16 Small saphenous vein
17 Soleus muscle
18 Tibia
19 Tibialis anterior muscle
20 Tibialis posterior muscle
21 Tuberosity of tibia

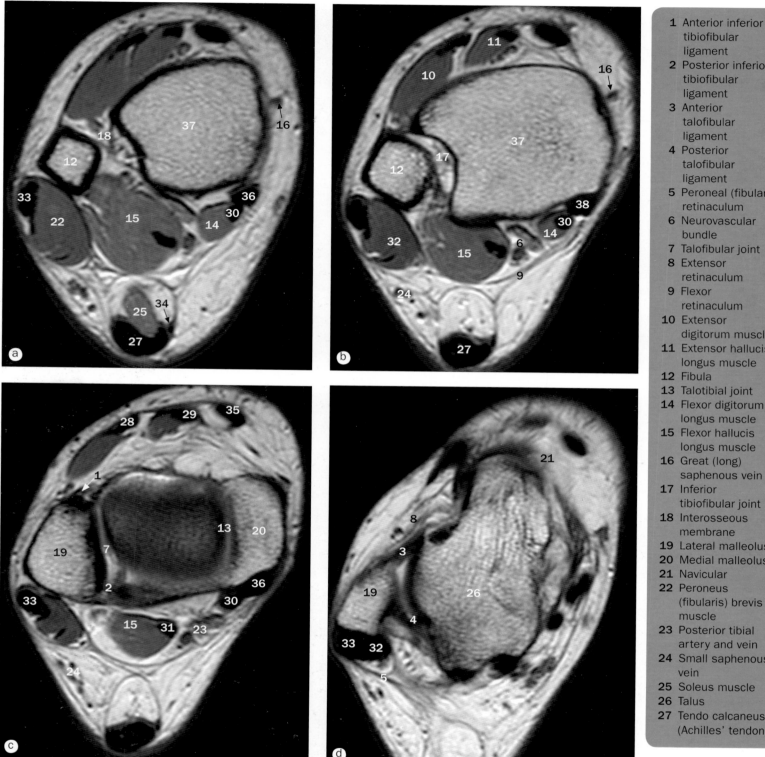

(a)–(h) Axial MR images of the ankle, from superior to inferior.

1 Anterior inferior tibiofibular ligament
2 Posterior inferior tibiofibular ligament
3 Anterior talofibular ligament
4 Posterior talofibular ligament
5 Peroneal (fibular) retinaculum
6 Neurovascular bundle
7 Talofibular joint
8 Extensor retinaculum
9 Flexor retinaculum
10 Extensor digitorum muscle
11 Extensor hallucis longus muscle
12 Fibula
13 Talotibial joint
14 Flexor digitorum longus muscle
15 Flexor hallucis longus muscle
16 Great (long) saphenous vein
17 Inferior tibiofibular joint
18 Interosseous membrane
19 Lateral malleolus
20 Medial malleolus
21 Navicular
22 Peroneus (fibularis) brevis muscle
23 Posterior tibial artery and vein
24 Small saphenous vein
25 Soleus muscle
26 Talus
27 Tendo calcaneus (Achilles' tendon)

28 Tendon of extensor digitorum muscle
29 Tendon of extensor hallucis longus muscle
30 Tendon of flexor digitorum longus muscle
31 Tendon of flexor hallucis longus muscle
32 Tendon of peroneus (fibularis) brevis muscle
33 Tendon of peroneus (fibularis) longus muscle
34 Tendon of plantaris muscle
35 Tendon of tibialis anterior muscle
36 Tendon of tibialis posterior muscle
37 Tibia
38 Tibialis posterior muscle

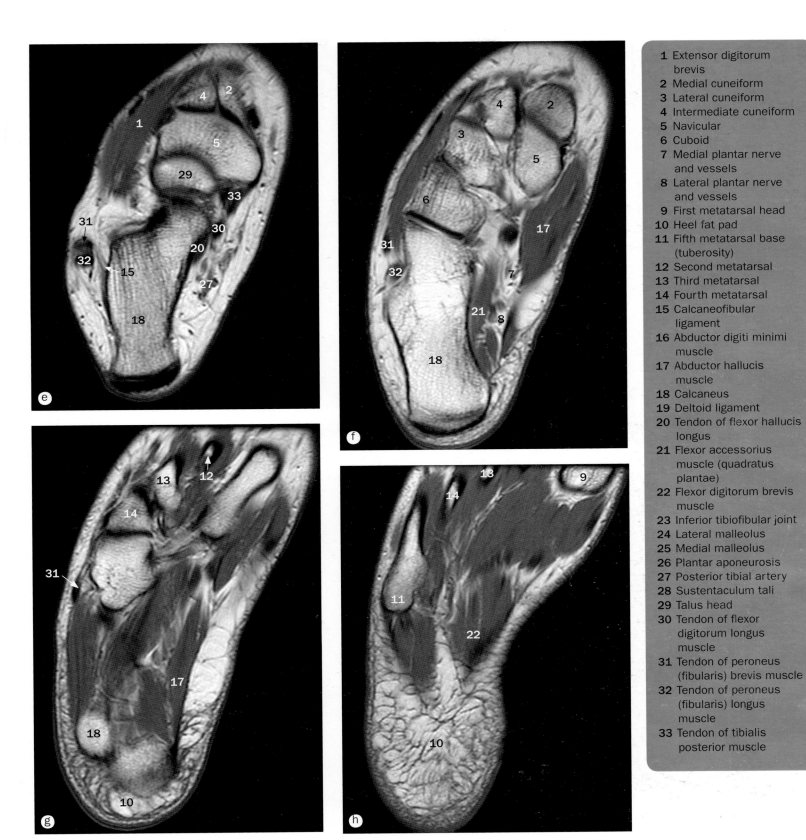

(a)–(h) Axial MR images of the ankle, from superior to inferior.

1 Extensor digitorum brevis
2 Medial cuneiform
3 Lateral cuneiform
4 Intermediate cuneiform
5 Navicular
6 Cuboid
7 Medial plantar nerve and vessels
8 Lateral plantar nerve and vessels
9 First metatarsal head
10 Heel fat pad
11 Fifth metatarsal base (tuberosity)
12 Second metatarsal
13 Third metatarsal
14 Fourth metatarsal
15 Calcaneofibular ligament
16 Abductor digiti minimi muscle
17 Abductor hallucis muscle
18 Calcaneus
19 Deltoid ligament
20 Tendon of flexor hallucis longus
21 Flexor accessorius muscle (quadratus plantae)
22 Flexor digitorum brevis muscle
23 Inferior tibiofibular joint
24 Lateral malleolus
25 Medial malleolus
26 Plantar aponeurosis
27 Posterior tibial artery
28 Sustentaculum tali
29 Talus head
30 Tendon of flexor digitorum longus muscle
31 Tendon of peroneus (fibularis) brevis muscle
32 Tendon of peroneus (fibularis) longus muscle
33 Tendon of tibialis posterior muscle

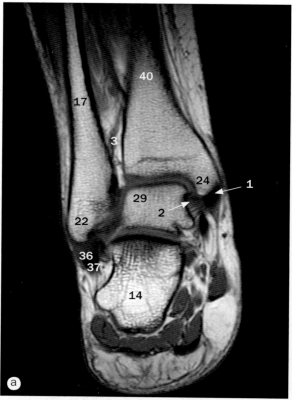

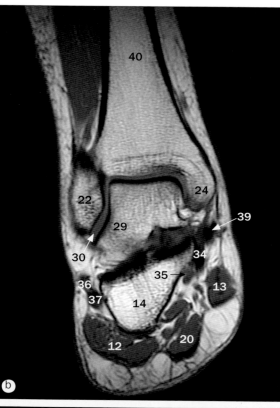

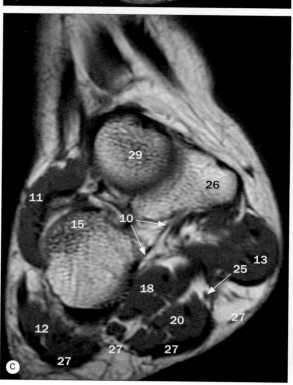

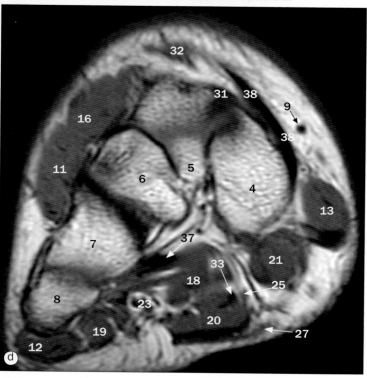

1 Deltoid ligament, superficial portion
2 Deltoid ligament, deep portion
3 Tibiofibular ligament
4 First metatarsal
5 Second metatarsal
6 Third metatarsal
7 Fourth metatarsal
8 Fifth metatarsal
9 Great (long) saphenous vein
10 Plantar calcaneonavicular 'spring' ligament
11 Extensor digitorum brevis
12 Abductor digiti minimi muscle
13 Adductor hallucis muscle
14 Calcaneus
15 Cuboid
16 Extensor digitorum brevis muscle
17 Fibula

(a)–(d) Ankle and foot, coronal MR images.

18 Flexor accessorius muscle
19 Flexor digiti minimi muscle
20 Flexor digitorum brevis muscle
21 Flexor hallucis brevis muscle
22 Lateral malleolus
23 Lateral plantar nerve and vessels
24 Medial malleolus
25 Medial plantar nerve and artery
26 Navicular

27 Plantar aponeurosis
28 Sustentaculum tali
29 Talus
30 Talofibular joint
31 Tendon of extensor digitorum longus muscle
32 Tendon of extensor hallucis longus muscle
33 Tendon of flexor digitorum brevis muscle
34 Tendon of flexor digitorum longus muscle

35 Tendon of flexor hallucis longus muscle
36 Tendon of peroneus (fibularis) brevis muscle
37 Tendon of peroneus (fibularis) longus tendon and muscle
38 Tendon of tibialis anterior muscle
39 Tendon of tibialis posterior muscle
40 Tibia

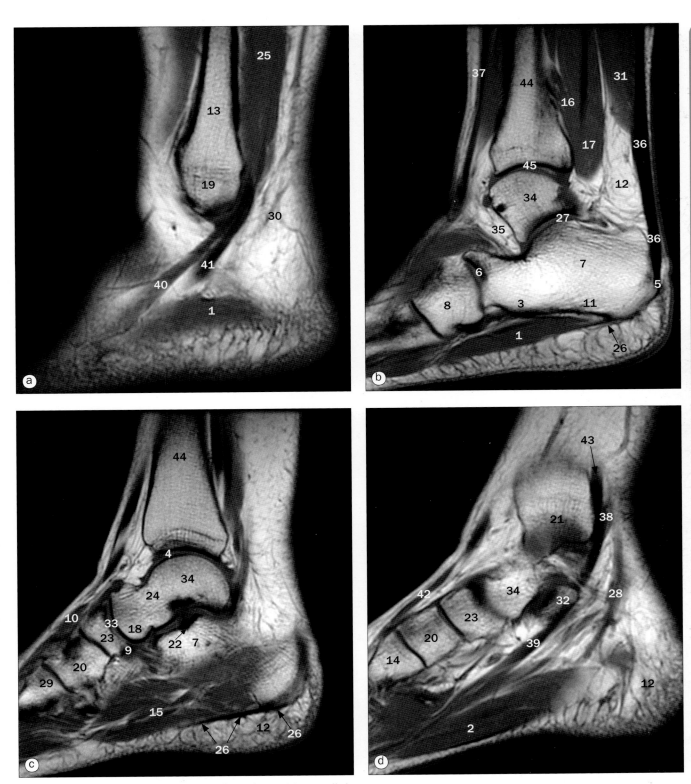

(a)–(d) Ankle, sagittal MR images, from lateral to medial.

1 Abductor digiti minimi muscle
2 Abductor hallucis muscle
3 Anterior tubercle of calcaneus
4 Articular cartilage
5 Insertion of Achilles tendon
6 Calcaneocuboid joint
7 Calcaneus
8 Cuboid
9 Cuneonavicular joint
10 Extensor digitorum brevis muscle
11 Lateral process calcaneus
12 Fat pad
13 Fibula
14 First metatarsal
15 Flexor digitorum brevis muscle
16 Flexor digitorum longus muscle
17 Flexor hallucis longus muscle
18 Head of talus
19 Lateral malleolus
20 Medial cuneiform
21 Medial malleolus
22 Middle facet, subtalar joint
23 Navicular
24 Neck of talus
25 Peroneus brevis muscle
26 Plantar aponeurosis
27 Posterior subtalar joint
28 Posterior tibial artery and vein
29 Metatarsal base
30 Small (short) saphenous vein
31 Soleus muscle
32 Sustentaculum tali

33 Talonavicular joint
34 Talus
35 Tarsal sinus
36 Tendocalcaneus (Achilles' tendon)
37 Tendon of extensor digitorum muscle
38 Tendon of flexor digitorum longus muscle
39 Tendon of flexor hallucis longus muscle
40 Tendon of peroneus brevis muscle
41 Tendon of peroneus longus muscle
42 Tendon of tibialis anterior muscle
43 Tendon of tibialis posterior muscle
44 Tibia
45 Tibiotalar part of ankle joint

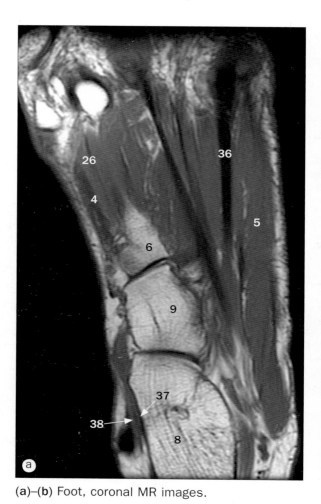

(a)–(b) Foot, coronal MR images.

1	Head of first metatarsal
2	Sesamoid bones in flexor hallucis brevis
3	Flexor digitorum longus
4	Abductor digiti minimi muscle
5	Adductor hallucis muscle and tendon
6	Base of metatarsal
7	Base of proximal phalanx
8	Calcaneus
9	Cuboid
10	Dorsal interossei muscle
11	Extensor digitorum brevis muscle
12	Flexor accessorius muscle (quadratus plantae)
13	Flexor digiti minimi muscle
14	Flexor digitorum brevis muscle
15	Flexor hallucis brevis muscle
16	Head of talus
17	Intermediate cuneiform
18	Interossei muscles
19	Lateral cuneiform
20	Lateral malleolus

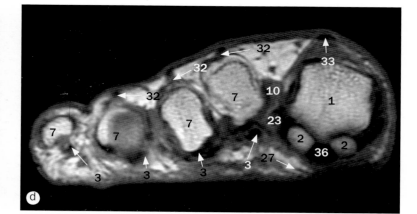

(c)–(d) Foot, axial MR images.

21	Lateral plantar nerve	**27**	Plantar aponeurosis	**33**	Tendon of extensor hallucis longus muscle
22	Medial cuneiform	**28**	Plantar interossei muscle	**34**	Tendon of flexor digitorum brevis muscle
23	Medial plantar nerve and artery	**29**	Shafts of metatarsals 1,2,3,4,5	**35**	Tendon of flexor digitorum longus muscle
24	Navicular	**30**	Talus	**36**	Tendon of flexor hallucis longus muscle
25	Neck of talus	**31**	Tarsal sinus	**37**	Tendon of peroneus brevis muscle
26	Opponens digiti minimi muscle	**32**	Tendon of extensor digitorum longus muscle	**38**	Tendon of peroneus longus muscle

8 Nuclear medicine

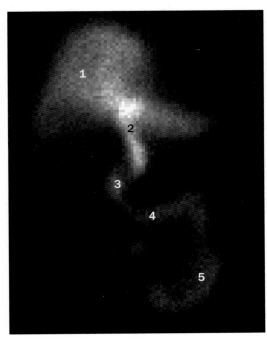

Hepatobiliary scan. The agents injected for this exam are rapidly cleared from the blood. The hepatocytes of the liver extract most of the injected dose and excrete it into the intrahepatic biliary tree. From there, the tracer flows into the hepatic and bile ducts. The agent will often passively fill the gall bladder (not seen in this example for various reasons, e.g. surgically absent, gall bladder is distended or has actively contracted during imaging or patient has had a prolonged fast prior to imaging). The agent then will enter into the duodenum through the ampulla of Vater, and eventually into the small bowel.

1	Liver
2	Bile duct
3	Descending (second) part of duodenum
4	Horizontal (third) part of duodenum
5	Jejunum

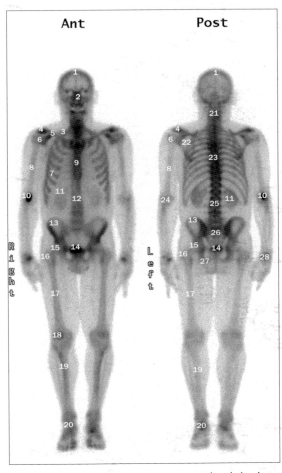

Whole body bone scan. Bone scans use physiologic agents to detect subtle abnormalities in bone metabolism. They are used to define skeletal abnormalities to include infectious, traumatic, congenital, metabolic and malignant conditions. Although the bone takes up the agent, some remains in the blood pool and is eventually excreted by the kidneys.

1	Cranium/skull	14	Urinary bladder
2	Nose and facial bones	15	Femoral head
3	First rib	16	Greater trochanter of femur
4	Acromioclavicular joint	17	Femoral shaft
5	Clavicle	18	Patella
6	Humeral head	19	Tibia
7	Fifth rib	20	Ankle
8	Humeral shaft	21	Cervical spine
9	Sternum	22	Scapula
10	Soft tissue extravasation at injection site in antecubital fossa	23	Thoracic spine
		24	Elbow
11	Right kidney	25	Third lumbar vertebral body
12	Bodies of lumbar spine	26	Sacrum
13	Iliac	27	Ischial tuberosity
		28	Wrist

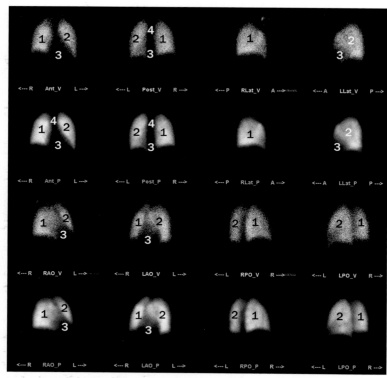

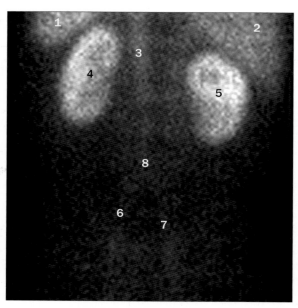

Lung scan. Imaging of the lungs involves both ventilation and perfusion. These two distributions match in the normal state. The order of imaging the ventilation and perfusion depends on the agents being used. Both ventilation and perfusion imaging evaluate the lungs in eight projections (anterior, posterior, right lateral, left lateral, right anterior oblique (RAO), left anterior oblique (LAO), right posterior oblique (RPO) and left posterior oblique (LPO)). The first and third rows are ventilation and the second and fourth rows are the matching perfusion.

1	Right lung	3	Cardiac silhouette
2	Left lung	4	Mediastinum

Renal scan. Renal imaging is performed with the camera placed on the patient's back because the kidneys are closer to the skin surface thus optimising the activity from the kidneys. Depending on the radiopharmaceutical used, relative structure and/or function of the kidneys can be obtained. In general, perfusion and excretion of the agent can be assessed in renal imaging. In the early staging of imaging some of the agent remains in the blood pool allowing visualisation of the surrounding structures.

1	Spleen	5	Right kidney
2	Liver	6	Left common iliac artery
3	Abdominal aorta	7	Right common iliac artery
4	Left kidney	8	Abdominal aortic bifurcation

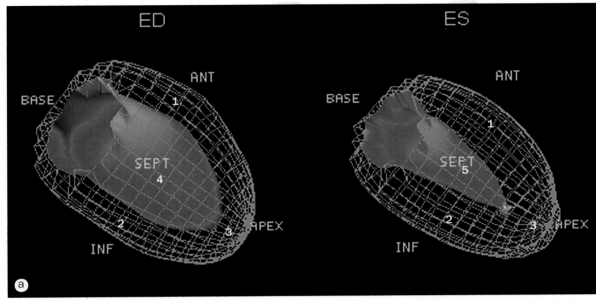

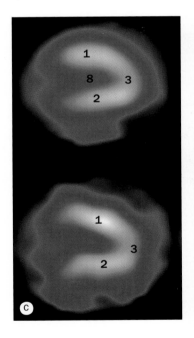

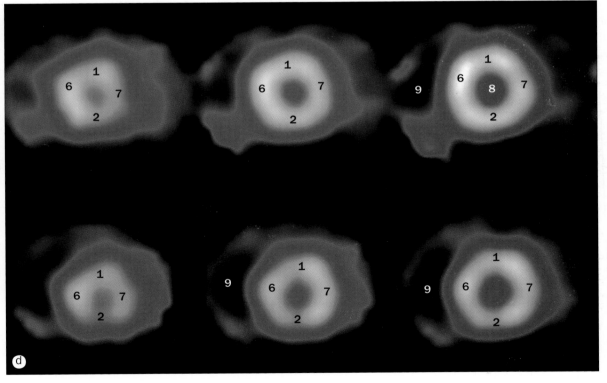

Cardiac scans, (a) 3D reconstructions of the left ventricle at end diastole (ED) and end systole (ES). Subtracting the ventricular volume at end systole from end diastole represents the ejection volume during systole.

Cardiac scans, (b)–(d), images are obtained during stress (exercise or pharmaceutical) represented by the top row of images and during rest represented by the bottom row of images. Comparison of these can determine alterations in cardiac circulation, from acute ischaemia to an old infarction. After imaging, the heart is sliced in different planes to evaluate the specific walls and the circulation that supplies them. The left ventricle appears as a 'horseshoe' shape on the vertical long axis (b) and horizontal long axis (c), and as a 'donut' on the short axis (d) views. The anterior wall, apex and portion of the septum are supplied by the left anterior descending artery (LAD). The right coronary artery (RCA) supplies the inferior wall and part of the septum, and the circumflex artery supplies the lateral wall.

1 Anterior wall of left ventricle
2 Inferior wall of left ventricle
3 Apical portion of left ventricle
4 Blood pool volume within the left ventricle at end diastole
5 Blood pool volume within the left ventricle at end systole
6 Interventricular septum
7 Lateral wall of left ventricle
8 Left ventricle cavity
9 Right ventricle cavity

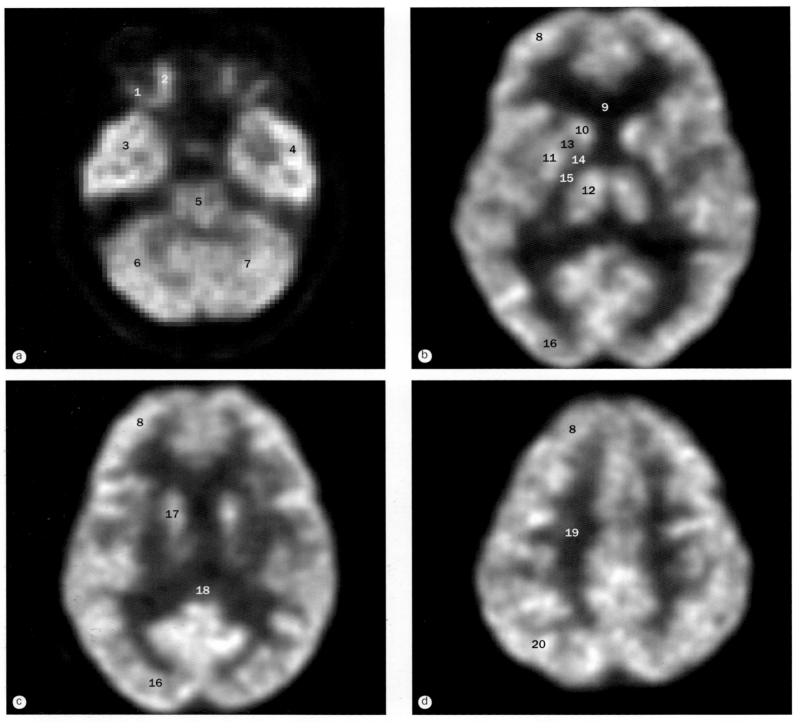

(a)–(d) PET metabolic brain scans. Fluorodeoxyglucose (FDG) is a derivative of glucose. Cells cannot differentiate between glucose and FDG. A major difference is that, once inside the cell, FDG is not metabolised and is trapped. This allows for easy imaging of structures in the body. The brain has high FDG uptake, with grey matter having a higher uptake compared with white matter. The basal ganglia usually have slightly higher uptake than the cortex. It is normal to have areas of increased uptake in the frontal eye fields, visual cortex and Wernicke's region.

1 Lateral rectus muscle	8 Frontal lobe	15 Internal capsule, posterior limb
2 Medial rectus muscle	9 Corpus callosum, genu	16 Occipital lobe
3 Right temporal lobe	10 Caudate nucleus, head	17 Caudate nucleus, body
4 Left temporal lobe	11 Putamen	18 Corpus callosum, splenium
5 Brainstem	12 Thalamus	19 Corona radiata
6 Right cerebellar hemisphere	13 Internal capsule, anterior limb	20 Parietal lobe
7 Left cerebellar hemisphere	14 Internal capsule, genu	

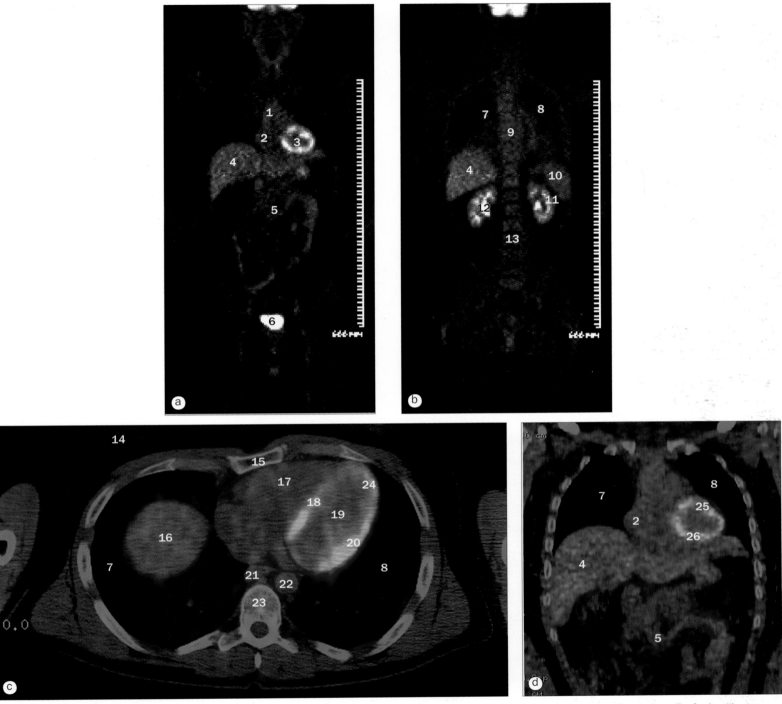

(a)–(d) Whole body PET/CT scans. PET imaging offers physiological function of the tissue and CT offers anatomical information. By fusing these images, precise localisation of areas of interest is made. Figures (a) and (b) are coronal PET images of the body at different depths. Figures (c) and (d) are fused PET/CT images in the axial (c) and coronal (d) projections.

1 Mediastinum
2 Right atrium
3 Left ventricle
4 Liver
5 Small bowel
6 Bladder
7 Right lung
8 Left lung
9 Thoracic spine
10 Spleen
11 Cortex of kidney
12 Kidney, renal pelvis
13 Lumbar spine
14 Right breast tissue
15 Sternum
16 Liver, dome
17 Right ventricle
18 Interventricular septum
19 Left ventricle, cavity
20 Lateral wall of left ventricle
21 Oesophagus
22 Descending thoracic aorta
23 Thoracic vertebral body
24 Apex of left ventricle
25 Anterior wall of left ventricle
26 Inferior wall of left ventricle

Index